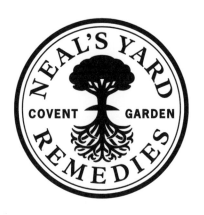

MENTAL
WELLNESS

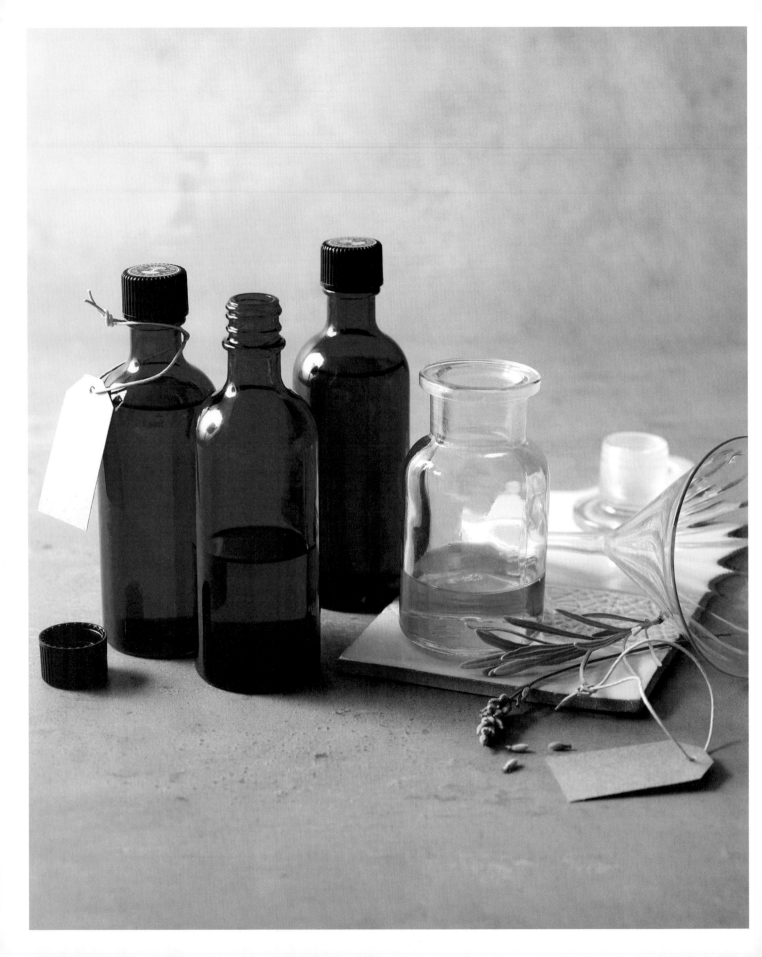

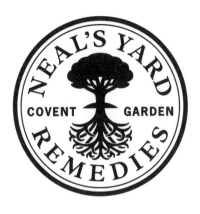

MENTAL
WELLNESS

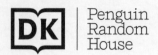

Senior Editor Claire Cross
Senior Art Editors Emma Forge and Tom Forge
Editorial Assistant Kiron Gill
US Editor Karyn Gerhard
US Consultant Jane Wotton
Senior Jacket Designer Nicola Powling
Jacket Coordinator Lucy Philpott
Production Editor Tony Phipps
Senior Producer Luca Bazzoli
Creative Technical Support Sonia Charbonnier
Managing Editor Dawn Henderson
Managing Art Editor Marianne Markham
Art Director Maxine Pedliham
Publishing Director Katie Cowan

Illustrators Ashley Bunten and Mark Scheibmayr
Photographer Tara Fisher
Food Stylist Tamara Vos
Prop Stylist Robert Merrett

First American Edition, 2021
Published in the United States by DK Publishing
1450 Broadway, Suite 801, New York NY 10018

Disclaimer See page 252

A catalog record for this book is available
from the Library of Congress.
ISBN 978-0-7440-3369-4

Printed and bound in China
For the curious
www.dk.com

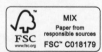

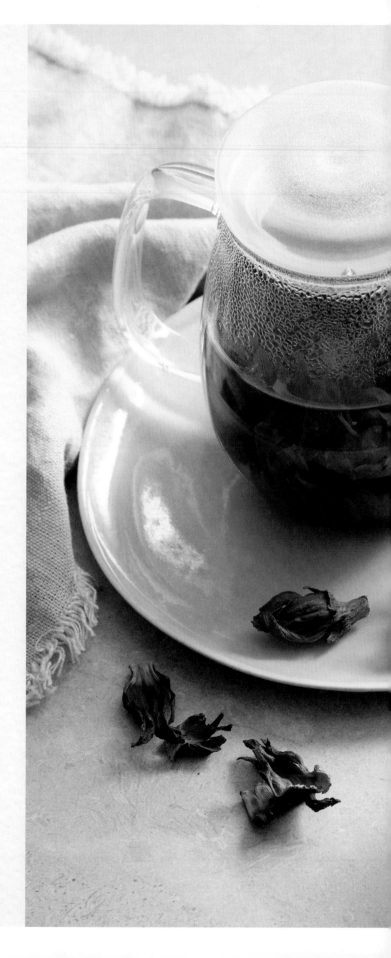

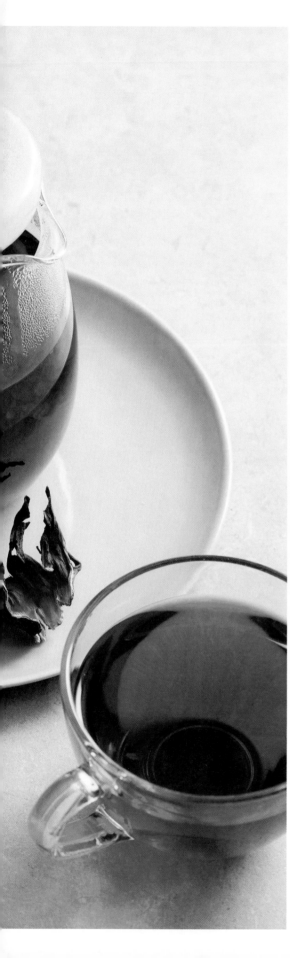

THE AUTHORS

Pat Thomas is the consultant editor for this book. Pat is a qualified psychotherapist and an advocate for natural health, sustainable living, and a clean environment. She is a journalist and is author and editor of the *Natural Health News* website. In addition to her own books, such as the guide to alternative healthcare *What Works, What Doesn't*, she has contributed to several Neal's Yard Remedies' titles, including *Healing Foods, Essential Oils, The Beauty Book*, and *Complete Wellness*.

Inna Duckworth MSc, MNIMH, is a practicing medical herbalist who started her herbal journey more than 15 years ago. She now teaches herbal courses and is collaborating with Neal's Yard Remedies. Inna is a member of Perimenopause HUB, featured on the BBC, and is a founder of *Perimenopause Naturally*, a resource for women in their 40s experiencing various symptoms linked to hormonal changes. She researches herbal application for mental and spiritual health extensively.

Victoria Plum has been an aromatherapy and massage practitioner since 1996 and feels there is still so much to learn. Victoria specializes in the field of mental and emotional health, which developed and refined her hands-on massage work and led her to train as a craniosacral therapist. She is also a reiki practitioner. She taught for the Tisserand Institute from 1999. When the school closed in 2005, she was invited to teach courses for Neal's Yard Remedies. She believes that practice and teaching the practice feel like mutually inspiring and beneficial activities.

Daphne Lambert is a nutritionist, chef, and author who has cooked, studied, taught, and written about food for most of her working life. Daphne is the founding member of Greencuisine Trust, a food education charity, which runs innovative programs, projects, and events cultivating the food knowledge and skills that enable people to take charge of their own health, eat well, and look after the planet.

CONTENTS

FOREWORD

One in four of us will be affected by poor mental health at some point in our lives. The spectrum of experiences and symptoms ranges from the transient ebb and flow of mood, energy, sleep, and social interactions to life changes such as upheaval, separation, and grief, to serious issues such as chronic depression and anxiety, anger, self-harm, despair, and social withdrawal.

Health authorities such as the World Health Organization argue that there is no health without mental health. As well as a human and social cost, mental illness has an economic cost, as overburdened health services struggle to cope with rising rates of depression, anxiety disorders, aggression, eating disorders, and addictive behaviors. This recognition has led to increasing efforts to encourage more of us to feel comfortable talking about mental well-being and to end the stigma around mental ill health.

Raising awareness and talking about mental health are important, positive steps. But we also need to look to a wide range of resources to help people cope, wherever they find themselves on the mental wellness spectrum.

Neal's Yard Remedies has a long history of encouraging and supporting self-care, through nutritious food, natural remedies, and complementary therapies that focus on the whole health of the person, rather than reducing an individual to a collection of symptoms.

A whole-health approach to wellness recognizes that body and mind are connected and constantly influencing each other. Many people who experience mental or emotional ill health, for instance, also experience a range of physical symptoms, such as digestive problems, skin rashes and irritations, headaches, respiratory distress, and chronic infections.

Ongoing scientific research means that our understanding of the two-way communication between body and mind is becoming much clearer. Key systems in the body—the hypothalamic-pituitary-adrenal (HPA) axis, which regulates a range of hormones and nervous system activity, and the gut–brain axis—control interactions between the mind and the physical body and different

> *" An holistic approach to mental wellness recognizes that our bodies and minds constantly influence each other."*

emotional states have been shown to affect, and be affected by our hormonal, immune, and digestive systems.

We also know now that certain foods, especially those that feed "good" bacteria in our guts, can significantly impact mental wellness. All of this underscores the importance of viewing health challenges in an holistic way.

This book recognizes that self-care—whether by eating well, exercising, getting enough sleep, or using complementary and alternative approaches—can help to manage many mental health symptoms, and may prevent some from worsening.

Written by experts with years of experience in natural health, nutrition, herbal medicine, and aromatherapy, the following pages provide sound guidance to help you understand the fundamentals of mental wellness and to make sense of any symptoms you are experiencing.

Suggestions are given for managing symptoms with herbs, essential oils, foods, exercise, and therapies. Step-by-step techniques show you how to make herbal remedies and essential oil blends, and ideas are given for simple nutrient-dense recipes that help energize and balance moods.

The remedies, recipes, and therapies can be used alone to manage mild or transient symptoms, or alongside conventional approaches to support you on the journey to mental wellness. Wherever you are on that journey, we wish you the best of health.

PAT THOMAS

UNDERSTANDING MENTAL WELLNESS

INTRODUCTION

WHAT IS MENTAL WELLNESS?

There are many facets to our mental wellness. It is very clear that being mentally healthy is more than just the absence of feelings such as sadness, worry, or insecurity, and it is also about more than just being happy. Mental wellness is about our ability to cope with both good and bad times, to realize our own potential, to engage with and feel connected to others, and to make our own unique contribution to the world.

DEVELOPING STRATEGIES

The topic of mental health has, in recent years, become more prominent in the global health agenda, and much of the stigma and embarrassment that people once felt talking about difficult feelings and experiences has begun to disappear. We recognize that, for each of us, there will be times when we feel overwhelmed; times when we need to make self-care a priority; and moments when we need to seek out a little extra help. Good mental health is largely expressed through our behavior, resilience, and how we respond to life's challenges.

Our ability to make healthy choices, not just about everyday things such as food and exercise, but also about our relationships and work, how we spend our leisure time, and how we manage stress, displays mental wellness. Healthy choices can also mean sometimes saying "no" to people or things that have a negative impact on our lives.

Setting realistic goals and boundaries that help us feel fulfilled gives a sense of purpose and lets us reach our potential. This includes being fair to ourselves; judging our appearance and lives by normal standards rather than distorted media ones; being realistic about expectations; and not punishing ourselves when a goal is not reached.

How we cope with change reflects our mental health. Change is a part of life; some changes we plan for and navigate with ease, others take us by surprise. In today's rapidly changing world, our perceptions of ourselves and each other and of what we hope for in the future are subject to constant review. Mental wellness helps us to work through challenges and maintain a sense of stability alongside the ups and downs that come with change.

Our self-confidence and self-esteem can be a measure of mental wellness. In difficult times, the ability to care for ourselves and believe we are worthy of care is

> *"Being realistic about our goals and boundaries can give us a sense of purpose and help us to reach our potential and feel fulfilled."*

demonstrated in small actions such as eating nourishing food, getting enough sleep, and finding joy in day-to-day routines. Self-care nurtures our self-esteem and the feeling that we have a right to be a part of things that help us to forge a successful path in life.

How well we make use of our resources is important for mental wellness. Being mentally well means being resilient and cultivating external and internal resources to draw on when needed. Both conventional and complementary medicines have a great deal to offer in supporting mental wellness. For most people with mild, moderate, or occasional symptoms of poor mental health, a self-help regimen or consulting a complementary practitioner for support may be sufficient to regain equilibrium. Recognizing when we need additional professional medical help with, for example, depression, anxiety, phobias,

or compulsions, and learning to ask for that help is also a key aspect of mental wellness.

THE BIGGER PICTURE

Mental health cannot be separated from physical and spiritual health. These three aspects of our lives are dynamic and constantly interacting. On days when we feel spiritually low, physical exercise may provide a lift. On days when we feel mentally low, spiritual practice, whether through mindfulness, spending time in nature, or engaging in prayer can be uplifting. Viewing our mental wellness in this holistic way can help us to find the resources to cope with changes and challenges.

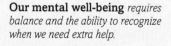

Our mental well-being *requires balance and the ability to recognize when we need extra help.*

OUR MENTAL LANDSCAPE

Mental well-being is sometimes seen as a choice. It is true that many choices we make about things we can control, such as relationships and diet, influence mental health. However, factors that we cannot control, such as our childhoods or changes of season, also affect us. Mental and emotional balance is about recognizing what we can change and accepting or finding coping strategies for what is beyond our control.

OUR EXPERIENCES

Changes in mental wellness, when they happen, can sometimes feel as if they come out of the blue. Aspects of our lives that we have little or no control over shape our mental and emotional well-being. Fortunately, our understanding of how we can better equip ourselves to cope is growing.

Childhood experiences can influence mental health throughout our lives. Being nurtured and cared for sets us up with a strong foundation for robust mental health and resilience when we are older. However, neglect, abuse, or trauma in childhood, without support and healing, can affect us as adults. In addition, there is some evidence that if a parent had mental health issues, this can increase the chance that their children may experience similar problems, so being aware of the warning signs and acting on these is important.

Life stages impact our mental health landscape. Every significant life stage or event, including puberty, moving out of our childhood home, committing to a relationship, buying a home of our own, separation, job loss, childbirth, and bereavement, all present significant emotional challenges. For women, certain life phases such as the onset of menstruation, pregnancy, and menopause bring significant hormonal fluctuations that can influence mood and our ability to cope with life's ups and downs.

Changes in our natural environment, such as lower levels of sunlight in the fall and winter, can trigger a form of depression known as seasonal affective disorder (SAD) in some susceptible individuals.

Our physical environment is thought to influence mental well-being. Studies show that city dwellers without access to green spaces may be more prone to depression and anxiety, while rural residents can face challenges such as

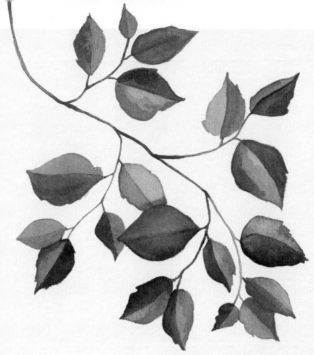

The seasons *and being in nature can directly affect our mood.*

isolation. Where possible, making sure we spend time in natural environments and ensuring we stay connected with others will help to support our mental well-being.

Adult trauma can be a major challenge to mental health. Being a victim of crime or in a situation where we fear for our safety, such as combat, can be emotionally scarring.

Physical health is intertwined with mental well-being. There are obvious physical causes of mental and emotional issues, such as head injury or epilepsy. Those who suffer from chronic pain, for example, with back problems or fibromyalgia, are more vulnerable to depression. Other factors are also influential. For example, the nutrients we eat daily support or hamper our mental and physical health (see pp.20–21).

Our relationships can play an important role in mental well-being. A mutually supportive and loving relationship can help us cope with challenges. But unhappy, dysfunctional, or abusive relationships erode well-being. Social isolation or loneliness also significantly impact mental wellness; and bereavement can profoundly affect us. Similarly, long-term carers can be more vulnerable to mental health problems.

Financial stress affects mental health. Whether it's not having enough money to meet basic needs, for example, or the loss of a job or business, financial instability can cause emotional and mental distress.

HOW WE COPE

These factors can work individually, or at the same time, through our lives. The more challenges we face, the harder it can be to maintain balance. Poor lifestyle choices and turning to props such as alcohol or drugs to escape pain, disrupt our ability to develop healthy coping skills. Instead we need to find positive ways to cope (see pp.20–21).

" Every significant life stage or event presents emotional challenges."

LOOKING AT LIFESTYLE

Most people facing mental health issues can benefit from the support of some form of therapy, and creating a safe space to discuss problems and work through issues with another trusted person can be vital. As well as knowing when to seek help, lifestyle changes that we can make on our own can be powerfully therapeutic for our mental and emotional well-being.

OPTIMIZING MENTAL WELLNESS

Making lifestyle changes, and sticking to them, brings physical and emotional benefits and a sense of control and accomplishment. A lot of small actions, taken together, can significantly improve symptoms of anxiety, depression, self-worth, and self-confidence. Many of these lifestyle activities are also effective ways of managing stress.

Exercise has measurable effects on well-being. Regular exercise can have a profoundly positive impact on stress, depression, anxiety, and conditions such as post-traumatic stress disorder (PTSD) and attention deficit hyperactivity disorder (ADHD). If something supports heart health, it is generally good for mental wellness, as it strengthens blood vessels, improving circulation and oxygenation to the brain and central nervous system. Those who exercise regularly report a tremendous sense of well-being, more energy, improved sleep and memory, and a more positive outlook.

Eating whole foods maximizes brain health. Leafy green vegetables, fruit, legumes, whole grains, lean meats, and seafood provide key nutrients such as folate, zinc, magnesium, and essential fatty acids and antioxidants, all necessary for optimal brain function. As well as choosing the right foods, a healthy diet is also about balance. The occasional cup of coffee can give us an energy boost, and drinking alcohol in controlled moderation can relax us and help us socialize. In excess, though, these can be harmful.

Sleep is as key to mental and emotional health as regular activity. It allows the body to rest, digest food, and repair itself. Good sleep habits—adjusting light and temperature in bedrooms, having a regular bedtime, and reducing screen time before bed, give the body and mind recovery time.

Getting out of artificial environments and spending time in a green space such as a local park, the countryside, or by the ocean de-stresses and connects us with the real world.

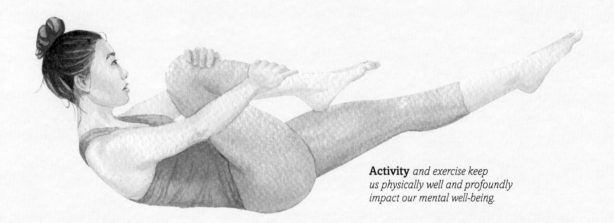

Activity *and exercise keep us physically well and profoundly impact our mental well-being.*

It exposes our senses to new sights and sounds and our bodies to beneficial sunshine; sunlight synthesizes vitamin D in the body, which helps regulate sleep–wake cycles.

Cultivating healthy relationships boosts well-being. Positive relationships provide strength and support. Those who are socially connected to family, friends, or their community tend to be happier, healthier, and live longer. They also tend to experience fewer mental health problems than those who are less well-connected. It is not just about how many people you know; the quality and depth of relationships matter, too.

Regular hobbies and activities benefit mental health. Whether interests are athletic, creative, or intellectual, spending time doing something we enjoy improves well-being. Those with hobbies are less likely to experience stress, low mood, and depression. Group activities such as team sports also improve social skills and confidence.

Cultivating spirituality, in whatever form is meaningful to us, can give insight, hope, and peace of mind. It can also help us cope with stress, to accept and live with ongoing problems, and find strength to make changes. Exploring spirituality can also encourage altruism and a sense of service to the wider community, which has been shown to encourage a greater sense of self-worth.

WHAT TO AVOID

Unhealthy lifestyle choices can be hugely detrimental to mental wellness and physical health. Part of embracing a healthy lifestyle is knowing what to avoid. A sedentary lifestyle that doesn't stimulate circulation and stiffens our bodies and insufficient sleep make us sluggish and below par mentally and physically. In addition, refined, processed foods high in salt and sugar (see p.106); drinking more than advised levels of alcohol; smoking; and using recreational drugs impact our emotional balance and brain function.

"A series of small lifestyle changes can significantly improve well-being."

OUR RESPONSE TO STRESS

Though most of us are unaware of it, our bodies actually have two "brains." The brain in our head is connected to our central nervous system. We also have a "second brain" in our gut, known as the enteric nervous system, which controls digestion and local circulation. These two brains are in constant communication with each other, and how our bodies deal with stress affects both systems.

THE GUT–BRAIN AXIS

Our two nervous systems, in the brain and the gut, are linked by the vagus nerve, the longest of all the cranial nerves. The vagus nerve stretches from the brainstem through the neck and ends in the abdomen, providing a continuous two-way line of communication between the gut and the brain. Within this system, the hypothalamic–pituitary–adrenal axis (HPA axis) also aids communication between the gut and the brain. This system of connections and communication between the gastrointestinal tract and the brain is referred to as the "gut–brain axis."

There is ample evidence that these systems mirror each other. During sleep, the head's brain produces 90-minute cycles of slow-wave sleep, punctuated by periods of rapid eye movement (REM) sleep, in which dreams occur. During the night, the gut's brain produces 90-minute cycles of slow-wave muscle contractions punctuated by short bursts of rapid muscle movements.

In addition, what affects one system can affect the other. For example, those with bowel problems have also been shown to have abnormal REM sleep—a finding that helps explain the observed link between indigestion and nightmares. And those suffering from Alzheimer's and Parkinson's diseases often suffer from constipation.

Drugs designed to work on the brain are likely to have an effect on the gut. For instance, antidepressants that alter serotonin levels can also cause gastrointestinal problems such as nausea, diarrhea, and constipation.

AN INSIGHT INTO MENTAL HEALTH

This direct link between our brains and our digestive tracts has changed our thinking about mental wellness. Doctors and scientists who have studied the gut–brain axis now suspect that it has a role to play in bipolar disorder, schizophrenia, and other psychological or neurological problems. Specifically, it is thought that

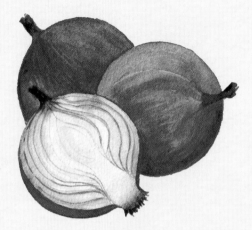

Prebiotic foods *such as onions feed the healthy bacteria already in our guts.*

disruptions or imbalances in the microbiome—the diverse population of microbes, or bacteria, that live in our gastrointestinal (GI) tracts—may be influential.

Recent studies suggest that a healthy gut in infancy can, in addition to helping maintain immunity, have a profound effect on our minds and emotional health during our adult lives. Other data suggests the communication between bacteria in our guts and our brains plays an important role in the development not just of psychiatric illnesses but also of intestinal diseases and probably other health problems, including obesity.

THE EFFECT OF STRESS HORMONES

The response of the gut–brain axis to stress is also thought to have a profound effect on our moods. The organs in the HPA axis, particularly the adrenal glands, release a cascade of stress hormones, including cortisol, epinephrine (adrenaline), and norepinephrine (noradrenaline) into our bodies to help us cope in times of stress. These hormones have a stimulant effect, and their release is an ancient physiological reaction in the human body that gives us the strength to fight or take flight in times of danger or attack. However, a continued release of these hormones can have a rebound effect—adrenal fatigue and a drop in adrenal efficiency, which can lead to profound exhaustion with accompanying mood swings and sleep disruption.

Taking care of our two brains requires a range of measures. Eating healthy whole foods is key, including prebiotics to feed good gut bacteria, found in foods such as onions and other plant foods, and probiotics that provide healthy bacteria, found in live yogurt and fermented foods. Lifestyle actions such as reducing stress and improving sleep quality are also key. Taking these steps encourages the growth and survival of our microbiomes and reduces levels of stress hormones in the body, in turn improving overall mental and emotional well-being.

"The gut–brain axis, the direct link between our brains and digestive tracts, plays a key role in mental well-being."

AN HOLISTIC APPROACH

To view mental health as simply concerning the mind underestimates its impact and also unnecessarily limits the resources we can choose from to maintain mental equilibrium or find a path back to wellness. Multiple studies show that physical symptoms often accompany mental and emotional ones, and vice versa. Therapies that treat body, mind, and spirit as one allow for truly holistic mental health and healing.

HOLISTIC THERAPIES

As well as the connection between our mental, emotional, and physical health, mental wellness can also affect and be affected by things going on in our environment. Where we live, who we live with, where we work, and what is happening in our countries and the wider world.

An holistic, or whole person, approach to mental health takes account of these factors and uses safe, effective natural remedies and therapies that complement each other and work with more conventional approaches, to treat mind, body, and spirit.

Herbal remedies have been used for thousands of years to heal and to maintain wellness. Many of the conventional pharmaceuticals that we use today are synthesized versions of traditional herbal remedies. For mild to moderate symptoms, herbal remedies can nudge us back to wellness without the debilitating side effects that can

sometimes accompany conventional medications. Pages 38 to 71 look at key herbs for mental wellness, what their benefits are, and offer suggestions for simple remedies to use in infusions, decoctions, tinctures, and capsules.

Aromatherapy is the therapeutic use of essential oils. Multiple studies have shown that different aromas provoke emotional states, whether to lift mood, calm, or ground us in the here and now. Many healthcare environments now make use of calming or uplifting essential oils such as lavender or citrus to help comfort patients. Pages 72 to 101 explore the key essential oils for mental wellness, how these can be blended to enhance their effects, and how aromatherapy can be used in massage oils, facial spritzes, diffusers, and rollerballs.

Foods and supplements have a direct effect on the body and mind. Foods supply us with essential nutrients and many of these, in turn, are involved in the regulation of

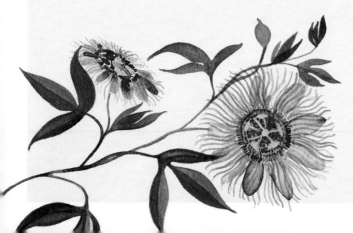

Calming passionflower *eases anxiety and its sedative properties are helpful for insomnia.*

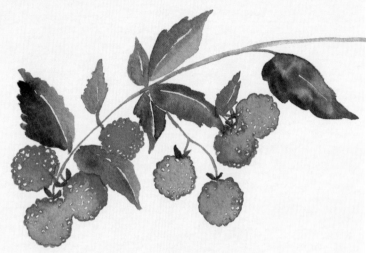

Summer berries *are high in vitamin C, needed to synthesize mood-regulating serotonin.*

mood and mental clarity. Pages 102 to 175 provide information on the importance of whole foods and a diet that provides seasonal variety, and explores how ingredients directly impact mood. Where nutrients may be lacking, key supplements for long-term mental wellness are advised.

Movement and exercise can come in many forms. Our bodies are meant to move, to bend and stretch and breathe hard. Studies show that a sedentary lifestyle and mental health symptoms such as lethargy, low mood, and lack of motivation go hand in hand. Pages 176 to 201 provide information on the different types of exercise and movement to suit all ages and levels of fitness.

Therapeutic practices offer a path to mental wellness. There are a range of helpful therapies and practices that work with mind, body, and spirit and which can be part of a day-to-day self-care routine, or an individual or group

therapy. Pages 202 to 241 look at therapies that involve touch, breath, sound, and mindfulness. Some also work on our energy flow, to bring the mind and emotions back into balance. Information is given on how each therapy works and what its specific benefits for mental wellness are, to make it simple to choose what is right for you.

SYMPTOM CHECKER

For all but the most serious mental health issues it is good to start with a wellness check, looking at whether, for example, you are feeling fatigued, depressed, anxious, withdrawn, or are lacking focus or motivation. These are states we all experience to varying degrees at times. They may be chronic and a sign that you need help; transient and linked to life stages; stress-related; or from a loss of work–life balance. Pages 26 to 37 explore how you are feeling now, offer an insight into cause, and point to the natural approaches in the book that may work best.

HOW DO I FEEL NOW?

INTRODUCTION

TUNING IN

"How do I feel now?" is not a question we often ask ourselves, and if we do, we tend to focus on our bodies rather than our mind and emotions. Most of us "check in" with our physical well-being. We assess the condition of our skin and hair, weigh ourselves, check under-eye bags, and respond to joint or muscle pain by adjusting our activities. Since our mental health is integral to our overall health, checking in on this is just as vital.

THE IMPACT OF MENTAL HEALTH

We live in a society where, for the most part, we are expected to put our feelings aside and get on with our daily lives. However, when mental health challenges arise they can make getting on with things difficult. This is because the state of our mental health determines how we think, feel, and act.

ASSESSING HOW WE FEEL

As with physical health, prevention is better than cure, which is why it is important to check in with how you feel from time to time. Signs of mental unwellness can range from the mild and transient to acute and deep-seated problems. Regularly making time to check your feelings and needs can help you fine tune your responses and even out the often exhausting cycle of highs and lows. However, few of us have developed the habit of regularly checking our emotional and mental well-being. Are we feeling low, worried, angry, or withdrawn? Is it hard to focus? Do we struggle to stop crying? Or are we acting out in ways that suggest hidden emotional conflicts?

Given that we all feel overwhelmed from time to time, how can you tell if the feelings you are experiencing are something to worry about or not?

Your vulnerability to major mental health issues can depend on multiple social, psychological, and biological factors. Issues in the early years, such as whether you felt safe, loved, and secure as a child, are a major factor. Poor mental health is also associated with rapid social change, stressful work conditions, gender discrimination, social exclusion, and abuse. Unhealthy lifestyle and physical ill health also influence long-term mental well-being.

Rather than being happy all the time, mental health is a dynamic state where different components of well-being, such as the physical and social, are very much interconnected. This means that sometimes symptoms

"As with your physical health, prevention is better than cure for mental well-being, so it is important to check in with how you feel."

of a mental health disorder appear as physical problems, such as stomach pain, back pain, headaches, or other unexplained aches and pains.

Once acknowledged, mild to moderate mental health symptoms can be managed and mitigated through behavioral change and self-care choices to prevent things from getting out of hand. The key is knowing when self-care is appropriate and when you need extra help.

The Symptom Checker pages that follow explore some of the common early warning signs of mental health concerns and their causes. If what you are experiencing is seasonal, such as seasonal affective disorder (SAD), or situational, for instance, related to life changes, exams, or work stresses, the simple self-help suggestions in this chapter and throughout this book can help you care for yourself. If what you are going through is acute and part of a long-standing pattern of mental distress, then while self-care is crucial, more important still is to always seek professional help.

QUESTIONS TO ASK YOURSELF

What are the major stressors in my life—are they constant or temporary?

How well do I feel I am coping with stress?

Are there important feelings I am hiding from myself and others?

Do I have physical symptoms that I am ignoring?

Is my impulse right now toward self-care or self-harm?

What would make things better for my emotional and mental well-being?

Do I have a support system in place and am I making good use of it?

SYMPTOM CHECKER

Being aware of signs and symptoms of changes in mental equilibrium can help us notice when our mental well-being is below par and take preventative measures. This chapter explores some key "red flags" and provides pointers to the natural remedies, foods, exercises, and therapeutic practices discussed throughout that can work together to help restore balance and harmony.

LOW MOOD

Mild, low-grade depression is often dismissed as part of life. No one is constantly happy, but chronic sadness can affect day-to-day function. When life is stressful, it can intensify, leading to emotional vulnerability and mood swings. Low mood can also be linked to conditions such as diabetes or poor circulation.

HERBAL REMEDIES

Adaptogenic herbs (p.40) such as rhodiola (p.64) and schisandra (p.65) alleviate stress symptoms such as fatigue, irritability, anxiety, low mood, and a feeling of losing control.

Antioxidants (p.41) include rosemary (p.64) and turmeric (p.49), whose active ingredient, curcumin, helps balance neurotransmitters, easing symptoms such as sadness, fatigue, an inability to focus, and anxiety.

AROMATHERAPY

Pungent, focusing essential oils (p.76) clear the mind. Rosemary (p.99) invigorates to motivate and lift a low mood, while stimulating juniper (p.91) helps those suffering with depression.

Uplifting oils (p.75) such as may chang (p.95) and citrus oils such as sweet orange (p.88) have a joyous, optimistic effect, promoting vitality, helpful when a low mood makes you feel "stuck."

FOODS & SUPPLEMENTS

Fatty fish (p.154) provide omega-3 fatty acids and vitamins B12 and D, all of which support the nervous system.

Mineral-rich cacao (p.169) stimulates the brain to release neurotransmitters that trigger positive emotions.

Foods that promote a healthy gut (p.105) such as sauerkraut (p.112) or whole fermented soybean products (p.147) support brain health via the gut–brain axis.

B complex supplements (p.174) can raise low folic acid levels, linked to depression; magnesium (p.175) helps restore a sense of balance and calm.

EXERCISE & MOVEMENT

Aerobic exercise (p.180), yoga (p.184), and Pilates (p.190) stimulate the brain.

THERAPEUTIC PRACTICES

Homeopathy (p.216) has a long history in treating low mood and depression.

REMEDY

Juniper oil

Combine a few drops each of juniper and rosemary essential oils in a diffuser to stimulate the mind and improve concentration.

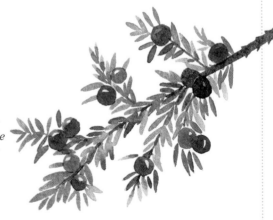

"Zingy, uplifting citrus essential oils such as lemon can help to lift 'brain fog' and re-energize."

POOR FOCUS

Difficulty concentrating can result from stress, insomnia, poor diet, normal hormonal changes, illness, and medication. Confusion, uncertainty, indecisiveness, and an inability to be organized can provoke feelings of helplessness or failure, particularly if these states are new.

HERBAL REMEDIES

Anxiolytic herbs (p.41) such as lemon balm (p.58) sharpen acuity and calm the autonomic nervous system.

Tonic herbs (p.42) such as Korean ginseng (p.63) aid focus by reducing corticosteroid stress hormones. Ginkgo (p.54) aids cerebral blood flow, and licorice (p.54) supports the adrenals.

AROMATHERAPY

Grounding oils (p.75) such as cedarwood Atlas (p.82) still the mind; a clearing oil such as cardamom (p.90) helps when overwhelmed by work.

Focusing oils (p.76) such as rosemary (p.99) and juniper (p.91) clear the mind (see remedy, opposite). Lemon (p.86) helps lift "brain fog," and grapefruit (p.86) energizes.

FOODS & SUPPLEMENTS

Brassicas (p.112) such as cauliflower and broccoli contain sulforaphane, which prevents the buildup of plaque linked to Alzheimer's disease.

Cacao (p.169) has antioxidant flavanols, which help improve circulation to the brain, supporting brain function.

Vitamin D-rich foods such as eggs (p.157) support the synthesis of GABA, a neurotransmitter that aids learning, memory, attention, and focus.

For low iron levels, a supplement (p.175) helps transport oxygen to the brain and synthesize serotonin, both aiding focus, attention, and memory.

EXERCISE & MOVEMENT

Yoga (p.184) and t'ai chi movements (p.196) aid focus and concentration.

THERAPEUTIC PRACTICES

Meditation (p.206) is relaxing and helps improve attention span.

Mind exercises (p.210) can keep your mind active and stimulated.

FATIGUE

This can be caused by life changes, chronic stress, hormonal fluctuations, illness, medication, or insomnia. It is also common with depression. When depressed, it can be hard to fall or stay asleep, and we may wake too early. Depression is linked to changes in neurotransmitters such as dopamine, norepinephrine, and serotonin, which help regulate energy levels, sleep, appetite, motivation, and pleasure. Setting limits on work and devices can avoid feeling overloaded.

HERBAL REMEDIES

Adaptogenic herbs (p.40) lower stress hormones to help the body respond to stress. Try Korean ginseng (p.63), Siberian ginseng (p.50), reishi (p.51), schisandra (p.65), and rhodiola (p.64). Ashwagandha (p.71) helps lower stress hormones to ease adrenal fatigue.

Sedative herbs (p.42) such as valerian (p.70), passionflower (p.63), and chamomile (p.57) induce restful sleep.

Enjoy balancing infusions in place of caffeine. Try peppermint (p.59), hibiscus (p.55), or lemon balm (p.58).

AROMATHERAPY

Oils to energize (p.75) include sweet orange (p.88), rosemary (p.99), and lemon (p.86). Frankincense (p.78) helps balance the nervous system. Lavender (p.94) is a proven aid for restful sleep.

FOODS & SUPPLEMENTS

Slow energy-release foods such as legumes (p.144) and grains (p.148) ensure a steady supply of energy.

Supplement, where needed. B12 (p.174) aids energy release; vitamin D (p.174) lifts fatigue; and iron (p.175) helps transport oxygen in the blood.

Dehydration can cause blood pressure to drop, decreasing blood flow to the brain, leading to tiredness. Hydrating foods such as celery (p.123) can help.

EXERCISE & MOVEMENT

Regular aerobic (p.180), stretching, and strength-bearing activity energizes. Alexander technique (p.200) corrects posture that may be affected by stress.

THERAPEUTIC PRACTICES

Massage (p.222) and time outside (p.212) stimulate and energize the body and mind.

ANXIETY

Feelings of anxiety cover a broad spectrum from mild apprehension to dread and panic. When anxious, the mind is highly alert and restless. While it is normal to feel some anxiety, for instance in response to stressful situations or life changes, the longer it goes on the more likely we will experience physical symptoms such as headaches, heart palpitations, sweating, tight chest, and upset stomach. Anxiety, like any emotion, can become a habitual response that makes day-to-day functioning hard.

HERBAL REMEDIES

Try antispasmodic herbs (p.41) such as California poppy (p.50); anxiolytic (p.41) and adaptogenic (p.40) herbs, such as antidepressant saffron (p.48), which eases anxiety, helping reduce stress hormones; and balancing motherwort (p.57). Rhodiola (p.64) eases fatigue, irritability, and anxiety. Ginseng (Siberian and Korean) (p.50 and p.63) calms a rapid heartbeat.

Nervines (p.42) calm the nervous system. Try sage (p.65) or skullcap (p.68) to balance neurotransmitters such as serotonin. Sedative lime flower (p.69) aids restlessness, and passionflower (p.63) calms the mind when there is a tendency to overthink.

AROMATHERAPY

Unwinding essential oils (p.74) such as palmarosa (p.89) ease tension, while frankincense's meditative quality (p.78) is a powerful remedy for panic and anxiety. Choose ylang ylang (p.79) when past trauma causes you to "freeze."

Think oranges. Most citrus oils—bergamot, mandarin, neroli, sweet orange, and petitgrain (pp.84–8) are profoundly uplifting and balancing.

FOODS & SUPPLEMENTS

Prebiotic foods (p.105) such as Jerusalem artichoke (p.120) feed good bacteria in the gut, which play a key role in regulating brain functions, including our stress response.

Vitamin C (p.174) is a vital antioxidant molecule in the brain and a cofactor in the synthesis of neurotransmitters that regulate anxiety and happiness and balance mood.

EXERCISE & MOVEMENT

Aerobic and everyday exercise (p.180 and p.182) promote relaxation to help ease general anxiety. Practices such as yoga (p.184) and t'ai chi (p.196) that have a meditative element are excellent for releasing anxiety.

THERAPEUTIC PRACTICES

Cognitive behavioral therapy (CBT) (p.236) can help adjust our response to anxiety-provoking situations.

Mindful meditation (p.206) and breathwork (p.208) help us to manage stress, control anxiety, focus, and balance and manage emotions.

Osteopathy and chiropractic (p.234) ease tension that we can hold in our muscles when anxious and stressed.

Mind exercises (p.210) help to shift focus away from immediate problems and reduce levels of stress and anxiety.

Time in nature (p.212) is restorative and has been shown to reduce feelings of anxiety significantly.

FEELING OVERWHELMED

Intense emotions that are difficult to manage can lead to a feeling of being overwhelmed, making it hard to focus on anything except your feelings and problems. Stress, traumatic life events, such as bereavement, financial insecurity, and relationship issues can lead to this feeling. Being physically ill or suffering with anxiety or depression makes us more prone to feeling this way. If the feeling lasts for an extended time, seeking professional help is advisable.

HERBAL REMEDIES

Gentle sedatives (p.42) such as chamomile (p.57) or lemon balm (p.58) promote sleep. Milky oats (p.44) can be used as a tonic for recovery after uncomfortable emotional events.

For nerves and stress-related stomach upsets, wood betony (p.68) is calming.

AROMATHERAPY

Hormone-balancing essential oils (p.74) such as palmarosa (p.89) help with anxiety and being overwhelmed in pregnancy; juniper (p.91) eases a feeling of being alone, or "lost," or of feeling overwhelmed by stress-related menopause symptoms.

Try clearing, grounding oils (pp.75–6). Cardamom clears the head (p.90); rosemary (p.99) and lemon (p.86) ease

" Juniper is supportive when feeling overwhelmed by stress-related menopausal symptoms."

"brain fog." Rose (p.98) grounds when erratic thoughts overwhelm.

FOODS & SUPPLEMENTS

Magnesium-rich foods such as broccoli (p.113), watercress, arugula (p.114), sunflower seeds (p.167), and cacao (p.169) calm nervous anxiety.

Butternut squash (p.127) is an excellent source of vitamin B6 as well as B2, B3, folate, and pantothenic acid, which reduce fatigue and calm.

Shiitake mushrooms (p.130) contain selenium, adequate levels of which help prevent anxiety.

Vitamin C (p.174) helps protect your immune system in times of stress.

EXERCISE & MOVEMENT

T'ai chi's (p.196) meditative movement focuses the mind and slows breathing.

THERAPEUTIC PRACTICES

Bach flower remedies (p.218) can help with feeling overwhelmed by life transitions or exams.

Counseling (p.236) and music therapy (p.238) can help us learn how to cultivate coping skills.

SOCIAL WITHDRAWAL

Time to ourselves is self-care, but we also need to connect with others. Being introvert or extrovert, shy, or having low self-esteem can be influential, but chronic withdrawal can signal underlying anxiety. Those with anxiety often have a strong desire to retreat socially, which can become habitual. When extreme, this is called social anxiety withdrawal and can cause nausea, shaking, or faintness when around others.

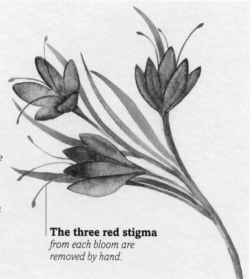

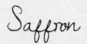

FOCUS ON

Saffron

PROFILE
Native to Iran and the Mediterranean, this golden culinary and medicinal spice has a rich, exotic aroma.

PROPERTIES
Strongly antioxidant, saffron helps protect the body from inflammation, promoting healthy brain function.

The three red stigma *from each bloom are removed by hand.*

HERBAL REMEDIES

Anxiolytic herbs (p.41) help treat anxiety. Try lemon balm (p.58) for heart palpitations, nervousness, and constant worrying. Skullcap (p.68) dispels giddiness and confusion, especially related to stressful events.

Adaptogenic herbs (p.40) bring balance. Siberian ginseng (p.50) calms the heart and reduces anxiety. Rhodiola (p.64) eases symptoms of irritability and a feeling of losing control. Bacopa (p.45) helps restore control and the ability to function every day.

AROMATHERAPY

Use calming oils (p.74) to soothe heart and lungs. Try Roman chamomile (p.78) to ease panic attacks where breathing is fast; may chang (p.95) for stress-related palpitations or asthma; or marjoram (p.96) for over-reactive states that lead to palpitations and shallow breathing.

Try cheerful citrus oils such as mandarin (p.87) to boost confidence. This brings optimism and dispels gloom and fretfulness.

FOODS & SUPPLEMENTS

Eat easy-to-digest foods. Too much serotonin is linked to social withdrawal. Easily digested, low-fiber foods, such as eggs (p.157), bananas (p.138), sweet potatoes (p.119), avocado (p.129), oily fish (p.154), and oatmeal lower levels.

Antioxidant-rich foods (p.104) can reduce anxiety. Include watermelon, fruits, and berries (pp.132–43) in your diet. Steamed or fermented vegetables retain nutrients and digest easily.

A B12 supplement (p.174), if levels are low, boosts your response to stress. Vitamin D tends to be low with anxiety.

EXERCISE & MOVEMENT

T'ai chi (p.196) calms. Being non-competitive, it offers a group activity but with a sense of space.

THERAPEUTIC PRACTICES

Counseling and CBT (p.236) can help if social withdrawal has become a habit we find hard to break.

Bach flower remedies (p.218) work at an emotional level.

CHANGES IN APPETITE

Hunger can change in response to your daily life, your mood, and, in particular, your levels of physical exercise. An increase or decrease in appetite can also be your body's response to what else is going on in your life: your stress levels, normal hormonal changes, illness or infection, and medication use. Habitually eating more or less than is healthy, however, can deplete the body of essential nutrients, increasing mood swings, lethargy, and low self-esteem.

HERBAL REMEDIES

The antioxidant herb (p.41) hibiscus (p.55) can help reduce cravings.

Tonic antidepressant herbs (p.42) such as St. John's wort (p.56) help balance serotonin levels, reducing the desire to indulge cravings or to binge.

AROMATHERAPY

Appetite stimulants such as cinnamon (p.82) can stimulate low appetite due to ongoing anxiety, grief, and despair. Try coriander (p.89) or cardamom (p.90) when appetite loss is due to stress, anxiety, or depression.

Uplifting oils (p.75) such as sweet orange (p.88) help when painful emotions lead either to a loss of appetite entirely, or to comfort eating.

FOODS & SUPPLEMENTS

Aim for balance. Cravings can be a sign that your body needs a particular nutrient. A varied diet of fresh whole foods can help calm the urge to snack.

Keep hydrated. Many people mistake thirst for hunger. Before having a snack, drink a glass of water. Eat hydrating foods such as celery (p.123).

Graze by eating several smaller meals throughout the day to provide sufficient nourishment when the appetite is small.

Low GI foods such as sweet potatoes (p.119) and oats (p.148) release energy slowly, helping to regulate appetite.

Zinc deficiency can cause taste and appetite changes. Eat zinc-rich foods such as lentils (p.144) and dulse (p.131).

Thiamine (B1) deficiency can cause a loss of appetite, and is an early sign of anorexia. Peas (p.145) and chicken (p.156) are good sources.

Healthy fats (p.106) such as coconut oil (p.160) and omega-3s help even out appetite highs and lows. Eat foods such as oily fish (p.154) and hemp (p.166).

EXERCISE & MOVEMENT

Regular exercise (pp.180–83) helps to regulate low and excessive appetite.

THERAPEUTIC PRACTICES

Counseling and CBT (p.236) can help if bulimia or anorexia are the cause of unbalanced appetite.

Aromatherapy massage (p.222) and reflexology (p.230) can help us to feel back in touch with our bodies.

ANGER AND IRRITABILITY

Anger, irritability, frustration, and impatience are a fact of life. Life stressors, a lack of sleep, low blood sugar levels, and cyclical hormonal changes can make us more irritable than usual. Illnesses such as an infection can also be a cause. Taking a break or changing your routine can usually restore balance. If feelings of extreme irritability last for an extended period, there could be underlying depression or anxiety. Increased irritability or anger can also often go hand in hand with risk-taking and substance abuse.

HERBAL REMEDIES

Herbs such as vervain (p.71) and turmeric (p.49) support the liver and help treat anxiety. In traditional Chinese medicine, anger is linked with liver function.

Sedative herbs (p.42) are helpful if irritation is caused by lack of sleep. Herbs such as valerian (p.70) and California poppy (p.50) have a calming effect and can help you sleep.

RECIPE

Berry oats

Add a handful of blackberries and other summer berries and a scattering of sunflower seeds to a calming bowl of porridge oats.

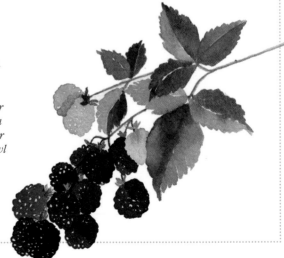

AROMATHERAPY

Cooling and calming essential oils (p.74) such as lavender (p.94) or palmarosa (p.89) help calm feelings of irritability. Roman chamomile (p.78) is a go-to remedy for soothing agitated feelings. Citrus oils (pp.84–8), particularly grapefruit, can have an uplifting effect, while petitgrain (p.85) is also gently sedating and can help dispel feelings of bubbling irritability.

FOODS & SUPPLEMENTS

Berries (p.132) are rich in antioxidants (p.104). Anger stresses the body, increasing its need for nutrients. Fresh or frozen blueberries, blackberries, strawberries, and cranberries help reduce inflammation and support brain health. See recipe, opposite.

Eat energizing foods (p.104). Slow-release carbs such as whole grains (p.148), legumes (p.144), and veggies (pp.108–29) give sustained energy as well as feed good bacteria in the gut.

If low, try increasing your intake of vitamin C and B vitamins (p.174); B5, B6, and B12 are very helpful.

EXERCISE & MOVEMENT

Exercise (pp.180–183) releases feel-good endorphins. If feeling irritated, try going for a walk or jog.

Join a yoga class (p.184) to unwind.

THERAPEUTIC PRACTICES

Acupuncture (p.220) helps to calm the mind and to restore balance in the body and mind.

Try mindful meditation (p.206) to help ground emotions and focus the mind inward, away from external stressors. This helps to let go of irritations and reevaluate.

Break the habit. If anger has become a habitual response to minor stressors, CBT and counseling (p.236) can help to understand and change negative behavior patterns.

Aromatherapy massage (p.222) and reflexology (p.230) can help bring you back in touch with your body.

GUILT

Guilt sits in a spectrum of emotions that includes remorse, regret, shame, and grief. Similar to sadness, it is often more inwardly focused on something we have done wrong or feel we have done wrong that we find hard to forgive ourselves for. Guilt can be a useful red flag, telling us where to make amends. However, it can also be a learned response and a way to chastise ourselves for imagined wrongs or feeling we do not measure up to others' expectations. If guilt interferes with life and relationships it is advisable to seek help.

HERBAL REMEDIES

Hyssop (p.56) is calming and cleansing, creating space for emotional healing.

Adaptogenic herbs (p.40) can help. Holy basil (p.62) brings balance, is antidepressant, and fosters clear thinking. Rhodiola (p.64) can ease the exhaustion of overthinking things.

BEST LEGUMES

Opt for dried lentils and legumes over canned, as these preserve more beneficial nutrients and contain less salt.

AROMATHERAPY

Grounding essential oils (p.75) are helpful. Cedarwood Atlas (p.82) is strengthening and aids meditation and thought. Patchouli (p.97) can take you out of your head back into the reality of your body. Rose (p.98) is comforting and supportive.

Oils to clear your head (p.76) are helpful. Juniper (p.91) aids focus and offers a sense of purpose. Rosemary (p.99) can shift focus away from over-introspection. Cardamom (p.90) promotes clearer thinking.

THERAPEUTIC PRACTICES

Counseling and CBT (p.236) can help us to understand the reasons for guilt and change negative behaviors.

Hypnotherapy and biofeedback (p.240) provide a way to unlearn destructive patterns.

Bach flower remedies (p.218) can help us take responsibility when we need to and to let go when we do not.

Prayer and spirituality (p.214) can bring clarity and a sense of connection.

Massage (p.222) can help us to let go of tension and unhelpful thoughts and ground us more in the physical world.

"Cooling essential oils such as Roman chamomile help to ease irritability."

TEARFULNESS

There are no real guidelines for how much crying is too much. Some people cry easily at books and films. Others are moved to tears less often. There is some evidence that women cry more easily and more often than men, but this is most likely due to social conditioning. While crying can at times bring relief, studies show this is not always the case. Of course, experiences such as bereavement make us sadder and more likely to cry, but otherwise, if you are sadder than usual and have started crying more regularly and cannot seem to stop, this can be despair, depression, or another mood disorder. Seeking professional help is important.

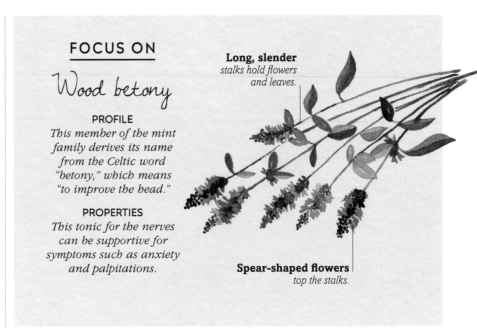

FOCUS ON

Wood betony

PROFILE
This member of the mint family derives its name from the Celtic word "betony," which means "to improve the head."

PROPERTIES
This tonic for the nerves can be supportive for symptoms such as anxiety and palpitations.

Long, slender *stalks hold flowers and leaves.*

Spear-shaped flowers *top the stalks.*

> " *Grounding frankincense oil can be supportive when depleted of energy.* "

HERBAL REMEDIES

Wood betony (p.68) is supportive for emotional shock and grief. Hawthorn (p.48) is physically and emotionally strengthening for the heart, while lime flower (p.69) soothes and nourishes if there is nervous exhaustion and fatigue.

Antioxidant-rich herbs (p.41) support nervous system function. Try ginkgo (p.54) to address symptoms of anxiety and depression. Vervain (p.71) calms, grounds, and lifts the spirits.

AROMATHERAPY

Strengthening and grounding oils (p.75) such as frankincense (p.78) are useful where there is fatigue and a feeling of depletion and hopelessness. Vetiver (p.101) supports a sense of identity. Sandalwood (p.100) and rose (p.98) comfort, restore, and ground.

Uplifting oils (p.75) such as thyme linalool (p.101) enliven the nervous system. Lime (p.83), grapefruit (p.86), and cardamom (p.90) energize.

FOODS & SUPPLEMENTS

Prebiotic foods (p.105) maintain gut health and support the functioning of the hypothalamic-pituitary-adrenal axis, which regulates mood and our response to stress. Try eating more whole grains (p.148), cabbage (p.112), fennel and celery (p.123), plus legumes (p.144), nuts (p.164), linseed (p.168), and sunflower seeds (p.167).

Foods rich in beta-carotene such as mangoes (p.139), sweet potatoes (p.119), apricots (p.143), grass-fed beef (p.152) and hemp oil (p.161) can improve symptoms of depression.

For supplements, an adequate daily intake of anti-inflammatory omega-3 fatty acids (p.175) has been shown to lessen symptoms of depression. Vitamin D (p.174), the sunshine vitamin, helps even out moods and is especially helpful when tearfulness is linked to seasonal affective disorder (SAD).

EXERCISE & MOVEMENT

Aerobic exercise (p.180), preferably outdoors, uplifts and releases feel-good hormones, helping you feel in control and easing anxiety and depression.

THERAPEUTIC PRACTICES

Spiritual practice (p.214) can support and ground us in times of crisis, trauma, and grief.

Homeopathy (p.216) can help to restore emotional balance.

Counseling (p.236) encourages you to understand the roots of sadness and to change your response.

LOW LIBIDO

A loss of interest in sex can be accompanied by apathy, listlessness, and boredom. Libido can be affected by stress, loss of self-confidence, and normal hormonal fluctuations. It can also be a sign of unhappiness in a relationship. If chronic, it can indicate an underlying concern such as high blood pressure or cholesterol, diabetes, and kidney or liver issues.

HERBAL REMEDIES

Tonic herbs (p.42) such as damiana (p.70) energize and adaptogenic herbs (p.40) such as ashwagandha (p.71) restore.

For men, Korean ginseng (p.63) stimulates nerve function and blood supply. For women, shatavari (p.44) nourishes reproductive organs.

AROMATHERAPY

Stress releasers (p.74) such as clary sage (p.99) help when stress affects performance. Patchouli (p.97) aids nervous exhaustion and anxiety, while ylang ylang (p.79) releases inhibitions.

Balancing oils (p.74) such as palmarosa (p.89) help where negative emotions interfere with fulfilment. Jasmine (p.90) promotes well-being and optimism.

For men, cardamom (p.90) relieves stress when overtired. For women, rose (p.98) comforts, uplifts, and supports reproductive and sexual health.

FOODS & SUPPLEMENTS

Lentils (p.144), chickpeas (p.146), oats (p.148), and red meat (p.152) are good sources of zinc, which can boost drive and performance where declining testosterone levels are a problem.

Nuts and seeds, including walnuts, hazelnuts, pumpkin seeds, linseeds, and hemp seeds (pp.164–9), are a useful source of healthy fats, vitamin E, and minerals such as magnesium, to defend against the effects of stress.

Antioxidant vitamin E supports healthy blood flow. Eat foods such as avocado (p.129) and nuts (p.164).

Iron deficiency can lead to listlessness and exhaustion. Consider a supplement (p.175) if levels are low.

EXERCISE & MOVEMENT

Aerobic and other exercise (pp.180–83) boosts mood-lifting hormones.

THERAPEUTIC PRACTICES

Massage (p.224) and reflexology (p.230) relax us and release blocked emotions.

Counseling and hypnotherapy (p.236 and p.240) can help reveal the deeper causes of low libido.

RISKY BEHAVIOR

Some take risks following trauma, to escape feelings. Others may act out hard-to-express emotions. Or risky behavior can be a defense to avoid being hurt. While some risks can be good, chronic risk-taking, such as substance abuse, self-harm, promiscuity, and putting yourself or others in danger can be a cry for help.

HERBAL REMEDIES

Brain-balancing tonics (p.42) such as peppermint (p.59) lower stress hormones and aid serotonin metabolism. Valerian (p.70) fosters inner peace and supports the parasympathetic nervous system. Passionflower (p.63) induces mild euphoria and quiets mental chatter.

Sedating chamomile (p.57) eases anxiety and aids sleep; skullcap (p.68) aids restorative sleep; and lemon balm (p.58) regulates fight-or-flight responses.

AROMATHERAPY

Geranium (p.96) helps those who struggle to express feelings. Frankincense (p.78) connects to inner truths and spirituality.

For self-control, palmarosa (p.89) helps where tension leads to an urge to lash out. Jasmine (p.90) supports where there is a tendency to self-harm or use alcohol or drugs to release or numb painful, intense emotions.

FOODS & SUPPLEMENTS

Balance blood sugar levels. Risk taking can be linked to energy highs and lows. Eat slow-energy-release whole foods such as oats (p.148).

EXERCISE & MOVEMENT

Aerobic exercise (p.180) and Pilates (p.190) can be a healthy way to challenge physical limits.

THERAPEUTIC PRACTICES

Counseling and CBT (p.236) can help to address long-standing patterns.

Meditation (p.206) encourages reflection.

Reiki (p.228) and homeopathy (p.216) help unblock emotions.

WHOLE GOODNESS

Purchase whole, raw seeds as these stay fresh the longest, and store them in an airtight container for freshness.

HERBAL REMEDIES

INTRODUCTION

THE ROLE OF HERBS

Plants and mushrooms have been used traditionally in many cultures for their healing qualities. Herbalists have been learning about their unique qualities for millennia, using the slow art of herbal lore, involving thorough observation of plants and people, to form a robust knowledge of herbs. Today, scientific research, scrutiny, and clinical trials have uncovered increasing evidence to verify this ancient knowledge.

HOW DO HERBS WORK?

Plants contain various chemicals, or compounds, with a range of medicinal properties. These can be similar across different plants, but tend to be in a certain composition within a species. For example, many aromatic plants, such as lemon balm, have the component geraniol, giving them a sweet, citrus smell and calming properties. However, in each plant, geraniol is part of a unique blend of components, like a single note in a perfume, giving it an individual character in that species. This is why herbalists work with the whole plant rather than singling out an ingredient, harnessing the naturally occurring synergy of components, then carefully blending plants into more complex remedies.

HERBS FOR MENTAL WELLNESS

Herbalists take an holistic approach to remedies. Herbal blends are chosen that have been found to work on systems in synergy, using a range of actions to finely balance body, mind, emotions, and spirit. Each herb also has more than one action, making it useful for a range of conditions. The following actions, found in the herbs listed on pages 44 to 71, are all beneficial for mental wellness.

Adaptogenic herbs, such as Siberian and Korean ginseng, ashwagandha, rhodiola, reishi, schisandra, and holy basil help the body adapt to external or internal stressors. They restore vitality by working on the physiological processes of energy production and cell regeneration in the body. Adaptogenic herbs are held sacred in Ayurvedic tradition, where they are considered "rasayana," or rejuvenating. In Chinese traditions, they are thought of as energy tonics, helping the flow of chi—or energy—through the body. Adaptogens should be used sparingly for a short period of time to support a person at times of transition, such as during major life events or convalescence, or during a period of excessive stress.

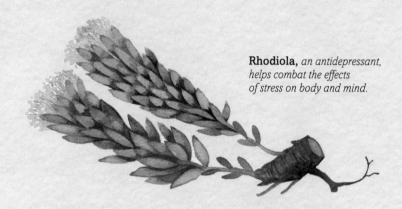

Rhodiola, *an antidepressant, helps combat the effects of stress on body and mind.*

Antioxidants improve cellular metabolism by reducing oxidative damage to cells so they work more efficiently, experience less wear and tear, and maintain vitality. Antioxidants play an important role in repairing damage from chronic inflammation. The effects of stress and systemic inflammation are very visible in the circulatory system, causing symptoms such as high blood pressure. Inflammation in the brain is harder to detect because there are no pain receptors to warn us, but signs such as "brain fog" and forgetfulness indicate chronic, low-grade inflammation. Medicinal antioxidant plants include cacao, rosemary, ginkgo, hawthorn, hibiscus, saffron, and turmeric.

Antispasmodic qualities in herbs such as California poppy, chamomile, lime flower, lemon balm, and mint relax smooth muscles and relieve tension. A state of tension, or unease, can be a hallmark of generalized anxiety disorder. These herbs help relax body and mind, ease headaches and stomach pain, and support a healthy gut–brain axis.

An anxiolytic, or anti-anxiety, action is present in many relaxing herbs, stemming primarily from their ability to reduce our fight-or-flight response and either increase the quantity or prolong the action of certain calming neurotransmitters. Key anxiolytic herbs are chamomile, lime flower, lemon balm, mint, motherwort, passionflower, and valerian.

Aphrodisiacal herbs, such as ashwagandha, cacao, damiana, Korean ginseng, and shatavari, help to promote libido, which plays a key role in relationships and sexual well-being, essential aspects of life. A healthy libido reflects a well-functioning hormonal system, as our reproductive hormones are directly linked with stress hormones via feedback mechanisms. When someone is under stress, the body reduces reproductive impulses, in turn creating tension and anxiety, which affect libido. Conversely, endorphins that are released during pleasurable moments have a positive effect on well-being.

"Herbal blends work together in synergy, using a range of actions to balance body, mind, emotions, and spirit."

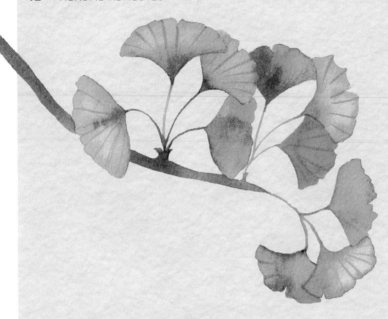

Ginkgo *is rich in flavonoids, protecting against inflammation.*

Bitter properties are found in many herbs. Vervain and motherwort are key bitters in this chapter. These work on bitter receptors in the gut and help balance the action of the vagus nerve, which runs from the brainstem to the colon and is linked with conditions such as stomachaches. Bitter herbs help regulate the gut–brain axis, improving the gut's bacterial composition. This increases serotonin and neurotransmitter levels that impact mood and energy.

Sedative herbs, also called relaxants or hypnotics, include chamomile, California poppy, lime flower, lemon balm, valerian, and passionflower. These calm and relax, helping the body switch to the "rest and digest," or healing mode, of the parasympathetic nervous system, which replenishes energy and supports healthy sleep.

Tonic herbs boost energy. There are various types of tonics. Nervine tonics, such as lime flower, hyssop, milky oats, wood betony, and reishi, work on the nervous system and are nutritive and restorative. Adrenal tonics such as licorice can be used to offer prolonged support, for example, when convalescing. Tonics to support cognition include bacopa, cacao, ginkgo, Korean ginseng, and skullcap. Lemon balm, St. John's wort, rhodiola, and damiana are antidepressant, while the mint family, such as hyssop, mint, lemon balm, vervain, and sage are uplifting tonics that improve mood without overstimulating. Circulatory tonics such as ginkgo, cacao, hawthorn, lime flower, and motherwort also offer support when grieving or in emotional pain.

CHOOSING HERBS

To select herbs, herbalists may consider if symptoms suggest a "hot" or "cold" condition or person. Lack of energy, fatigue, and depression are "cold" conditions, needing warming, nourishing herbs. For "hot" conditions, such as hot flashes, overstimulation, and being excessively energetic, cooling herbs such as sage and mint are chosen.

" Herbal blends can be used to nourish and warm where energy is lacking, or to cool and calm where there is overstimulation."

Blend three or four herbs to start with. If stressed, adding warming licorice (avoid with high blood pressure) gives adrenal support and harmonizes a blend. Herbs can also be used throughout the day. For example, for exhaustion, sedative herbs may be given in the evening and nutritive tonics in the morning; the aim is to restore sleep and give adrenal support, potentially building energy reserves before using stimulating tonics. Generally, stimulants—most adaptogens and tonics—should be taken before 2pm.

USING HERBS SAFELY

Start with one herb in a low dose to check tolerance and observe its effects. Nutritive tonics, such as lime flower, chamomile, licorice, and reishi, also used as food, can be good herbs to start with. Avoid taking herbs for a long period of time unless advised by a qualified herbalist. Cautions on specific herbs are given in this chapter and safety guidelines on all herbs are on page 242.

HOW HERBS ARE TAKEN

Herbs are prepared in infusions, decoctions, tinctures, and capsules. Powders can also be added to drinks. The following chapter gives step-by-step guidance on preparations.

Infusions *are used for leaves and flowers. See "How to Make a Herbal Infusion" on pages 46–7.*

Decoctions *are for mushrooms, roots, berries, and bark. See "How to Make a Decoction" on pages 52–3.*

Tinctures *provide a concentrated dose. Blends should be done by a professional. For single herb tinctures see "How to Make a Tincture" on pages 60–61.*

Capsules *are easy to take and give a therapeutic dose. See "How to Make Herbal Capsules" on pages 66–7.*

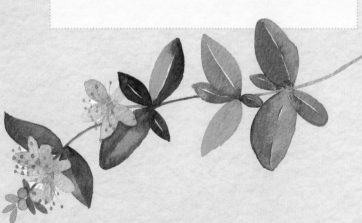

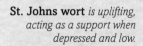

St. Johns wort *is uplifting, acting as a support when depressed and low.*

HERBS

Aromatic herbs and plants have been used for both culinary and medicinal purposes for millennia. Medicinal herbalists combine the knowledge and insights gleaned from modern medicine with respected herbal folklore to provide holistic remedies that employ the synergy of plant compounds to treat body, mind, and spirit simultaneously.

SHATAVARI
Asparagus racemosus

This rejuvenating plant is known as "the Queen of herbs." It is held in high esteem in the Ayurvedic tradition, where it is seen as one of the most valuable medicinal plants, linked with restoring youth, vitality, and preventing disease.

BENEFITS

Shatavari is an adaptogenic nerve tonic with a broad spectrum of restorative properties that act on the nervous, hormonal, and immune systems, enhancing quality of life. Studies suggest that this very potent antioxidant plant can reduce the impact of oxidative damage in the body caused by chronic stress.

" Shatavari has potent antioxidant and neuroprotective properties."

Shatavari's adaptogenic properties help to regenerate neural tissue, supporting memory and impacting the aging process in the brain.

The herb's potent antioxidant and neuroprotective actions can help to counter damaging low-grade inflammation, which can affect memory and cognition and lead to feelings of confusion, or "brain fog."

Studies show that shatavari has a significant antidepressant activity. It has a balancing effect on the levels of the "feel-good" chemical serotonin, which, together with antioxidants, acts directly on our fight-or-flight reaction, helping to reduce stress. One study reported improved mood, less fatigue, and better sleep and stamina.

Its phytoestrogens and antioxidants help make this a useful reproductive tonic, mitigating the effect of stress on the reproductive system.

HOW TO USE

The root is used in powders, capsules, and tinctures.

Blend with reishi in equal parts to reduce anxiety and improve sleep.
➡ *For mild symptoms, add ½–1 tsp powder to a cup of warm milk. For more severe anxiety and insomnia,* take 1–2 500mg capsules 1–2 times a day, including before bedtime.

Take on its own to lift a low mood.
➡ *Take 1–2ml tincture in a little water 1–2 times a day.*

Blend in equal parts with cacao, nettle, and ashwagandha for a tonic.
➡ *Add ½–1 tsp powdered herb blend to a cup of warm milk.*

OTHER COMBINATIONS

Take with bacopa and holy basil to aid memory.

CAUTION

Seek professional help before blending with other adaptogens. Avoid during pregnancy, unless under supervision.

MILKY OATS
Avena sativa

Nourishing and soothing, oats are considered a sacred plant in many traditions of the Northern hemisphere. As well as milky oats, the green oat tops, where seeds produce a milky sap when squeezed, there is also oat straw, which refers to the green, unripened oat stems used in herbal preparations.

BENEFITS

Oats nourish the nervous system. They restore and tonify when someone is frail, exhausted, or lacks stamina, acting like a cushion around the nerves.

Milky oats ease anxiety accompanied by exhaustion, often from overworking. They also help tackle insomnia.

Oats support recovery from long-term conditions such as fibromyalgia, which increases the risk of depression, and are supportive with other neuro-degenerative conditions.

Oats can aid recovery after difficult emotional events, or from addictions such as smoking or drug use.

Milky oats can help with exhaustion, tension, headaches, and nausea linked to PMS, and during menopause with symptoms such as fatigue and palpitations linked to anxiety.

Milky oats can be a tonic for low libido or male sexual dysfunction that is linked to stress and exhaustion.

HOW TO USE

Milky oats are most potent medicinally, while seed and straw are rich in nutrients. Decoctions and tinctures are most efficient.

Blend equal parts with lime flower, mint, motherwort, and hawthorn for emotional recovery.
➡*Make a decoction with 1 tsp dried herb blend and 9fl oz (250ml) boiling water to drink 3 times daily.*

Milky oats make a soothing, restorative bath for stress-related eczema.
➡*Put 1–2 handfuls organic pin-rolled oats in a sock or muslin bag. Place in the water for 15 minutes prior to a bath; gently squeeze to release the sap.*

OTHER COMBINATIONS

Milky oats can be added to any blend to build a nutritive foundation.

BACOPA
Bacopa monnieri

Bacopa, also known as brahmi, grows widely in tropical areas. It is often called an "herb of grace," as it is used to support the declining cognition that comes with age.

BENEFITS

Bacopa is rejuvenating and revitalizing and a nervous system tonic. It supports neural cell communication, stimulates serotonin, and helps eliminate toxins.

Bacopa aids memory. Research shows that when taken over a period of time, it helps retain newly acquired information longer.

Bacopa is helpful when the ability to think clearly is impaired by stress or previous trauma, and when it is hard to concentrate, making it helpful for ADHD in children and adults.

Chemical compounds called saponins in bacopa are thought to reduce neural inflammation, which can help ease anxiety. It can be supportive where mental distress is severe and affects the ability to function in everyday life.

HOW TO USE

The dried herb makes a pleasant infusion. Or take in capsules, tinctures, or powders.

Take as capsules or a tincture to counter long-term anxiety.
➡*Take 1–2 500mg capsules, or 1–2ml of tincture with water 3 times a day, for 1–3 months.*

Blend equal parts bacopa with ashwagandha and gotu kola for a strengthening tonic to boost mental performance. Or with Siberian ginseng and ginkgo (avoid ginkgo if taking blood-thinning medication), and a little ginger for cognitive

support when older.
➡*Infuse 1–2 tsp dried herbs with 6fl oz (175ml) boiling water. Drink 3 times a day.*

OTHER COMBINATIONS

Bacopa works with many blends to aid mood and cognition. Try infusing with holy basil, milky oats, skullcap, and rose.

CAUTION

Avoid during pregnancy, unless under supervision of a herbalist.

REMEDY

Uplifting oat blend

To alleviate depression, infuse 1 tsp of a blend of milky oats, St. John's wort, vervain, and skullcap in equal parts in 6fl oz (175ml) boiling water. Drink 3 times daily.

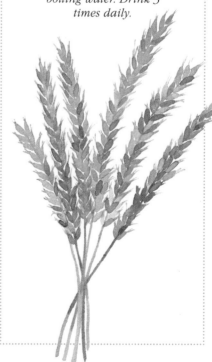

HOW TO MAKE
AN HERBAL INFUSION

Hot or cold infusions are a quick and effective way to create therapeutic herbal remedies. They are made with the delicate parts of a plant, such as the leaves and flowers. The method below can be used as a standard measure of herbs to water, but quantities may vary depending on individual herbs.

Makes 1 cup, or multiply ingredients for a larger batch

INGREDIENTS

1–2 tsp dried herbs, or 3–4 tsp fresh herbs (or recommended quantity)

6fl oz (175ml) freshly boiled water

½ tsp honey (optional)

EQUIPMENT

Teapot, or tea-ball infuser

Tea cozy (optional)

Strainer

Teacup

Jug, if refrigerating

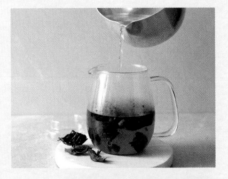

1 Warm the teapot. Place the herbs in the teapot together with the freshly boiled water. If you want to make enough for a day's dose of up to three cupfuls, triple the ingredients. If using a tea-ball infuser, place the herbs in the ball and steep in a cup of freshly boiled water.

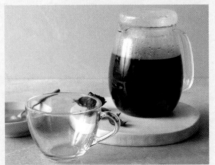

2 Place the lid on the teapot, which helps to prevent the volatile oils from escaping, and let the herbs infuse for 10–15 minutes. If you wish, use a tea cozy to keep the teapot warm.

STORAGE

The strained infusion can be stored in the fridge for up to one day. Gently reheat or drink cold, as required.

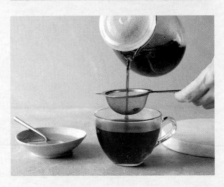

3 Strain the herbs, pouring the infused water into a cup. Drink warm or let cool, as prescribed. Add the honey for sweetness, if desired.

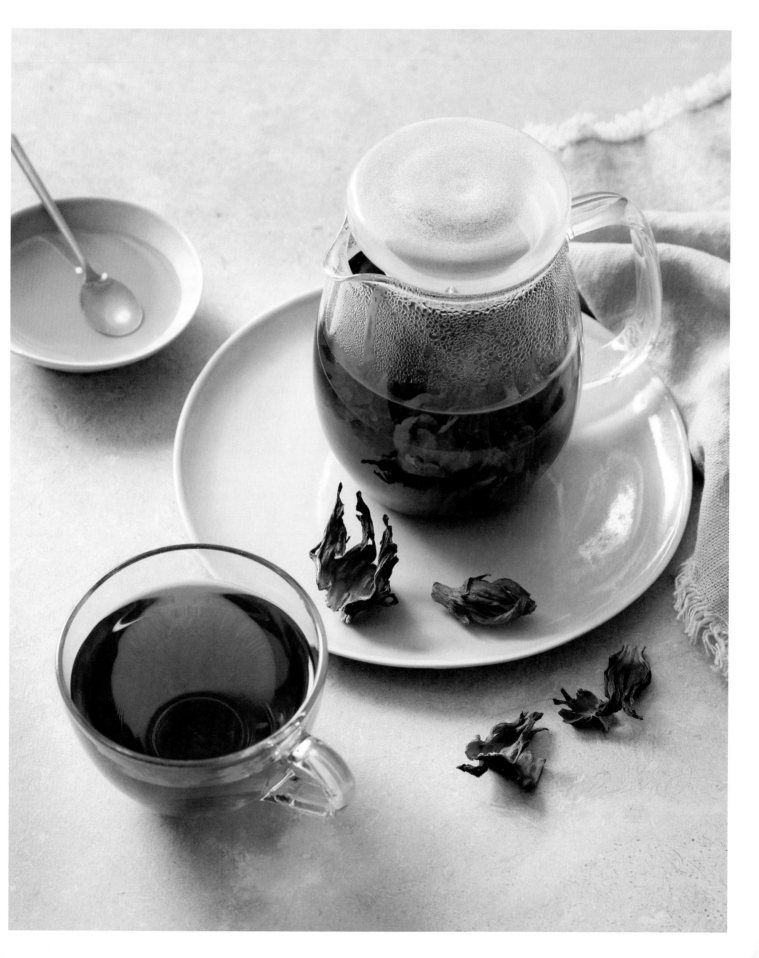

HAWTHORN
Crataegus monogyna

Hawthorn grows worldwide and species such as *C. monogyna*, *laevigata*, **and** *oxyacantha* **can be used interchangeably. In the West, it is traditionally thought of as a heart-strengthening herb, while Chinese herbalists use it to calm the spirit.**

BENEFITS

As an anxiolytic herb—one that reduces anxiety—hawthorn helps us to cope with overwhelming emotions caused, for example, by relationship breakup, trauma, or bereavement. It is also a very safe and effective remedy for protecting the aging heart, as well as supporting overall well-being.

As an antioxidant herb, hawthorn has heart-protecting properties. A growing body of research around "heart intelligence" highlights the connection between the emotions we experience and their impact on our physical health. One study found a correlation between heart disease and negative emotions.

Studies show that hawthorn can play a role in balancing blood pressure, which is negatively impacted by stress. Antioxidants in hawthorn also support artery health, offering protection from the effects of cholesterol and calcium deposits.

Hawthorn relaxes nerves, helping to calm restlessness where there is an inability to sit still and concentrate.

Hawthorn's calming properties help to combat insomnia linked to overstimulation or weakness, for example, during convalescence.

Hawthorn improves circulation and oxygenation of the muscles, making it useful for combatting exercise fatigue that can be common in perimenopause.

HOW TO USE

Both berries and flowering tops are used in powders, capsules, and tinctures. The berries also make decoctions and the flowering tops infusions.

Blend with other anxiolytic herbs such as California poppy, or with ashwagandha for menopausal symptoms such as anxiety, mood swings, palpitations, and insomnia.
➡ *Take 1–2 500mg capsules with water 1–3 times a day.*
Create an herbal synergy for well-being. Blend equal parts with liver-supporting schisandra and rejuvenating rosehip.
➡ *Make a decoction with 1 tsp dried herb blend and 9fl oz (250ml) boiling water to drink 3 times daily.*

OTHER COMBINATIONS

Try with turmeric or milky oats.

CAUTION
Consult a medical herbalist if taking with heart medication.

SAFFRON
Crocus sativus

Saffron, a sacred flower of Crete, has culinary and medicinal uses. The stigmas are removed by hand, a labor-intensive method that makes saffron the world's most expensive spice. Its Latin name "sativus" refers to qualities of positivity, serenity, balance, and spiritual purity.

BENEFITS

Saffron provides carotenoids, responsible for its color. These powerful antioxidants reduce the impact of stress and neuro-inflammation, supporting DNA repair and detoxification and stimulating nerve growth.

Saffron is thought to aid learning and memory. It also supports brain health during the aging process.

Its antidepressant and antianxiety qualities are helpful during postnatal depression. It helps reduce levels of stress hormones, slows the breaking

FOCUS ON

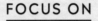
Hawthorn

PROFILE
This spring-blooming plant is native to North America and other temperate zones.

PROPERTIES
Hawthorn supports efficient oxygenation in the body. It has a reputation as a cooling and calming herb.

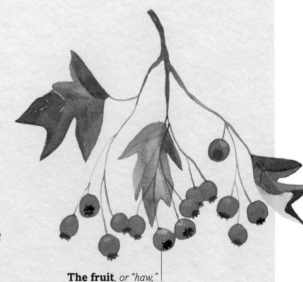

The fruit, *or "haw," resembles a berry.*

> " *Turmeric is powerfully antioxidant, supporting memory, cognitive processes, and learning.* "

down of the neurotransmitter dopamine, and supports the recycling of the feel-good chemical serotonin.

Its antioxidant capacities help to reduce inflammation in the body, supporting brain health.

Prolonged treatment can positively impact sleep. A 2018 study found it enhanced deep sleep, the key factor defining sleep quality, and reduced wakening episodes, ensuring sleep continuity so participants felt rested.

It has a long history as an aphrodisiac for men and women.

Saffron has been shown to alleviate PMS symptoms and hot flashes.

HOW TO USE

Use the stigma in powders, or in capsules or tinctures for a therapeutic dose. Sparing doses of this precious herb are advised.

Make a mood-lifting blend with St. John's wort, lime flower, and milky oats.
➥ *Infuse several dried stigmata and 1 tsp herb blend with 6fl oz (175ml) boiling water and drink 3 times daily.*

Try a vitality-boosting tincture.
➥ *Take 1–2ml tincture with water 1–2 times a day, including before bedtime.*

OTHER COMBINATIONS

Combine with valerian and chamomile to promote sleep. Or with turmeric to reduce neuro-inflammation and support vitality.

CAUTION

Enjoy in food during pregnancy, but avoid therapeutic doses.

TURMERIC
Curcuma longa

Turmeric is one of the most widely used plants in the Indian Ayurvedic tradition. Often called "Indian saffron," its orange color has been associated with the sun and the sacral chakra. It is widely used in ceremonies symbolizing spiritual connection with the earth, fertility, abundance, and purity. Today, its key uses include reducing inflammation, detoxification, and liver support, all of which support mental well-being.

BENEFITS

Turmeric, a calming plant, is also a potent antioxidant and anti-inflammatory, providing protection for the nerves. Some antioxidant constituents in turmeric are thought to help reduce neuro-inflammation and toxicity.

Turmeric aids circulation to the brain. This, along with its antioxidant activity, supports memory, cognitive processes, and learning. Several studies show that turmeric can be used as a preventative and supportive therapy for Alzheimer's disease and other brain-degenerative conditions.

Taken over a period of time, it can help to combat fatigue, especially when associated with chronic stress, and improve general levels of energy and well-being.

Curcumin, one of the active ingredients in turmeric, has been shown to help

balance neurotransmitters and modify the stress response, which in turn helps with symptoms of depression such as low mood, sadness, loss of energy, inability to concentrate, and anxiety.

HOW TO USE

Fresh turmeric root or dried and powdered turmeric can be added to smoothies or used regularly as a spice. For more severe or chronic symptoms, a capsule provides a therapeutic dose. Often curcumin, one of the constituents in turmeric, is available as an independent product; in this case, its bioavailability is enhanced with piperine from black pepper and quercetin, an antioxidant available in foods such as onions and broccoli.

Turmeric "golden milk' latte is a comforting, calming bedtime drink. Make with a plant-based milk such as coconut or oat, or with dairy.
➥ *Add 1 heaping tsp turmeric powder or freshly grated root to 9fl oz (250ml) warm milk. Strain if using fresh root. Add a little maple or agave syrup if desired, to sweeten.*

Make an energy-boosting blend. Try with equal parts schisandra and ginger, or combine with ashwagandha and reishi to restore energy when fatigued.
➥ *Take 1–2 400mg capsules with water 2–3 times a day, including pre-bedtime.*

OTHER COMBINATIONS

Blend with rosemary, holy basil, and bacopa to support cognitive processes and memory. In powder form, turmeric blends well with many herbs; however, for some, large doses can be too drying.

CAUTION

Doses of more than 10g a day should be taken under professional supervision. Enjoy in food during pregnancy, but avoid therapeutic doses.

SIBERIAN GINSENG
Eleutherococcus senticosus

Ginseng root comes from the thorny shrub, which grows in Northeast Asia. In Chinese tradition, Siberian ginseng is seen as a remedy to balance "the five elements"—wood, fire, metal, earth, and water—believed to be fundamental forces of nature that help to prolong life.

BENEFITS

Siberian ginseng is an adaptogenic or "harmonizing" remedy. Its balancing effect comes from the regulation of the nervous, hormonal, and circulatory systems. It has a variety of benefits, including supporting recovery from fatigue and exhaustion.

Siberian ginseng stimulates the metabolism. As a result, DNA is replicated more efficiently and blood is better oxygenated. In addition, its action on cells helps energy to be used more efficiently, building up stamina and improving vitality.

As an adaptogen helping the body cope with external stressors, it helps the chronically stressed, where the adrenal glands are overworked, marked by dark under-eye circles. One study found it helped mitigate the impact of psychological and physiological stress from night shift work.

Siberian ginseng acts as a brain tonic, helping to lift "brain fog," improve focus, and support memory.

There is evidence that Siberian ginseng supports male sexual function and is a gentle relaxant for women.

Siberian ginseng acts as a tonic remedy to alleviate depression and anxiety, especially when accompanied by symptoms such as palpitations. It helps calm the heart, reduce anxiety, and improve symptoms of low mood.

HOW TO USE

The root is used in powders, capsules, and tinctures. Slow acting, it can be used for a long period of time, unlike stimulating Korean ginseng (see p.63),

Blend with St. John's wort to alleviate mild to moderate depression.
➡ *Take 1–2 500mg capsules 1–3 times a day.*

OTHER COMBINATIONS

Blend with rhodiola and schisandra for a nerve tonic to combat fatigue, especially when linked to menopause.

CAUTION
Combine with other adaptogens under professional supervision. Avoid during pregnancy, unless under supervision.

CALIFORNIA POPPY
Eschscholtzia californica

California poppy, also called gold poppy, has bright orange flowers, forming a delicate, silky goblet. Initially grown mainly in California in the US, it is now cultivated all around the world. Its profoundly calming, almost hypnotic, effects are ideal for those who get easily overexcited and distracted, then have trouble settling back down to everyday life.

BENEFITS

California poppy is a sedative, antispasmodic remedy, with pain-relieving properties. Unlike other members of the poppy family, it is not addictive or toxic, so is safe to use.

The herb is a useful support for anxiety, restlessness, and where there is a tendency to dwell on everyday troubles or fret over possible scenarios in the future.

Its sedative action makes this a good choice for a sleep remedy. It is used to help fall asleep, support staying asleep, and avoid waking up too early. It is also helpful for children who are prone to nightmares, overexcitability, restlessness, and bedwetting, which may be stress-related.

As a pain-reliever, California poppy can be helpful for headaches and migraines, which may be caused by or lead to stress.

"Deeply calming, California poppy is an ideal herb for those who get overexcited and easily distracted."

REMEDY

Nerve tonic

For a nerve tonic to strengthen and support fatigue during convalescence or with post-viral fatigue, infuse 1 tsp equal parts California poppy, milky oats, and lime flower in 6fl oz (175ml) boiling water. Drink 3 times a day.

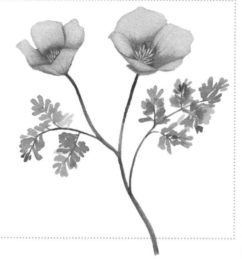

HOW TO USE

The aerial parts—the flowers, leaves, and stems—are used in infusions, powders, capsules, and tinctures.

For a soothing sleep remedy, blend California poppy in equal parts with passionflower and valerian, adding a pinch of nutmeg. If insomnia is linked to menopause, blend with ashwagandha, motherwort, and sage.
➡️*Infuse 1 tsp dried herb blend with 6fl oz (175ml) boiling water and drink 3 times daily. Or for chronic insomnia, take the blend in 1–2 500mg capsules 3 times a day.*

Make a nerve tonic blend.
➡️*See remedy, above.*

Take a tonic for chronic or acute anxiety.
➡️*Take 1–2ml California poppy tincture in a little water 3 times a day.*

OTHER COMBINATIONS

California poppy has a pronounced bitter taste. When using it in an infusion, adding pleasant-tasting herbs such as chamomile, mint, and lime flower can help to make it more palatable.

CAUTION
Best avoided during pregnancy.

REISHI

Ganoderma lucidum

Reishi is a type of fungus native to Asia, referred to as the "mushroom of immortality." In ancient Taoist literature, it is described as part of the "elixir of eternal youth" and is mentioned in the first book of Chinese herbal medicine 2,000 years ago. Its reputation is explained by its potent antioxidant properties that make it a tonic for heart and brain.

BENEFITS

Reishi is an adaptogen that helps our bodies to manage stress. It is used to aid memory and mental functioning, promote restful sleep, strengthen the heart, and bring vitality. It also plays an important role in immunity and the balancing of blood sugar levels, and is used as a support during cancer treatment.

Traditionally, reishi "calms the spirit," being a heart and brain tonic. Its balancing action is believed to support the connection between the heart and brain. In traditional healing, the heart energy is thought to govern our mental processes and vitality.

It has a protective action on the nervous system and can be used as a supportive therapy for Alzheimer's disease and neuromuscular degenerative conditions.

Reishi is used to relieve symptoms of fatigue and exhaustion that occur, for example, after a debilitating illness.

Its calming properties can help to combat insomnia. Research into the fungus has identified 300 molecules that play a role in improving the duration and quality of sleep.

HOW TO USE

Reishi can be taken over a long period of time to provide ongoing support. Its spores, fruiting body, and underground part of the mushroom can be used in tinctures, capsules, powders, and decoctions. The powder can also be added to stews, soups, and drinks.

When used in a tincture, reishi, like most other medicinal mushrooms, needs to undergo a double extraction, first boiled in water then steeped in alcohol, to maximize its active ingredients.

For insomnia, make an antioxidant latte with equal parts reishi, ashwagandha, and turmeric plus a pinch of saffron. Take before bedtime to promote restful sleep.
➡️*Add ½–1 tsp of the herb blend to 9fl oz (250ml) hot milk.*

For a potent brain tonic to support memory, combine equal parts reishi, ginkgo, bacopa, and rosemary.
➡️*Make a decoction with 1 tsp dried herb blend and 9fl oz (250ml) boiling water. Drink 3 times daily.*

OTHER COMBINATIONS

Blend with other supporting, nutritive herbs such as milky oats, lime flower, and shatavari; with adaptogens such as Siberian ginseng and rhodiola; and with tonics such as cacao and damiana.

HOW TO MAKE

A DECOCTION

Decoctions, like infusions, are herbal water extracts, but made with the harder parts of herbs, such as the berries, roots, bark, and seeds. These more fibrous ingredients are boiled and simmered in water to extract their active constituents. Both fresh and dried herbs can be used in this herbal preparation.

Makes 1 large cup, or multiply ingredients for a larger batch

INGREDIENTS

1 tsp dried herbs, or blend of herbs, or 3 tsp fresh herbs
9fl oz (250ml) water, tap or filtered

EQUIPMENT

Saucepan with lid
Strainer or sieve
Teacup
Jug, if refrigerating

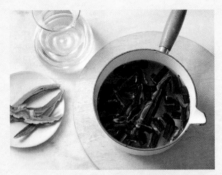

1 Place the dried or fresh herbs in a saucepan with the measured water. If you wish, triple the ingredients to make enough for a day's dosage of three cups. Cover the saucepan to stop water from evaporating, which can lead to active constituents being lost in the steam. Bring to a boil.

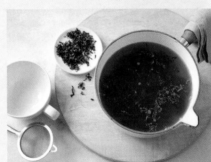

2 Reduce the heat and simmer for 15–30 minutes, covered, until the water is infused with the herb. Hard materials such as bark take the longest. If adding soft herbs, do this once you have removed the pan from the heat. Place the lid back on and allow them to infuse for 10 minutes.

STORAGE

If making up a day's batch, cool, then refigerate the decoction for up to 24 hours. Reheat gently if required before drinking.

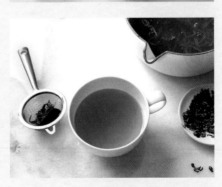

3 Strain into a teacup, or jug if storing a batch, and drink warm or cool, as required.

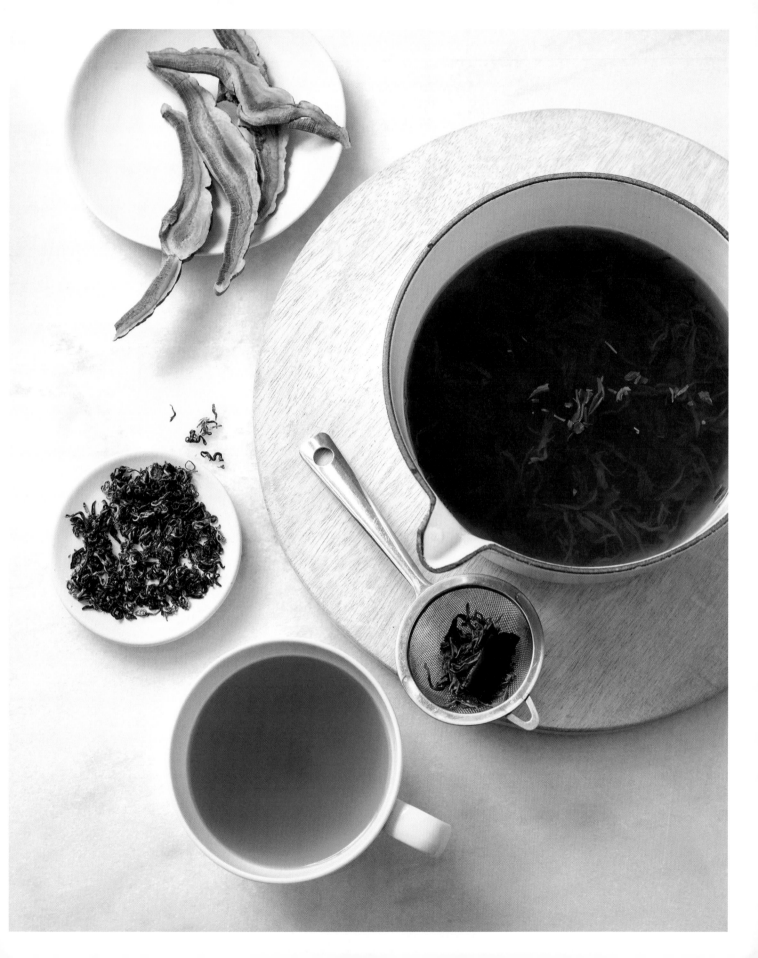

GINKGO
Ginkgo biloba

At over 150 million years old, ginkgo is the oldest tree on the planet. Its fanlike leaves, separated into two lobes, are thought to resemble the human brain, providing a visual metaphor of its potential effects on cognition.

BENEFITS

Ginkgo supports blood flow to the brain, helping to relieve symptoms that can be linked to circulation, such as dizziness, headaches, and "brain fog." Historically, ginkgo was used as a brain tonic to support the decline in cognitive function that occurs with age, improve mental agility, and support short-term memory.

Ginkgo is rich in flavonoids, which protect the body from free radical toxins and reduce levels of chronic inflammation, improving brain function and promoting clear thinking.

Ginkgo is restorative for nervous tissues, promoting the renewal and increasing the activity of brain cells.

By supporting circulation and oxygenation to the brain, ginkgo can play a therapeutic role in relieving anxiety, depression, and headaches.

Ginkgo has a calming action where stress from allergies leads to fatigue and foggy thinking.

" As a brain tonic, ginkgo supports mental agility."

HOW TO USE

The dried leaves are used for decoctions, powders, capsules, or tinctures.

Take on its own as a restorative tonic.
➥ *Take 1–2 500mg capsules, or 1–2ml tincture with water, 3 times a day for no longer than 6 weeks.*
Blend equal parts with bacopa to support mental performance. For the elderly, add Siberian gingseng and a pinch of ginger.
➥ *Make a decoction with 1 tsp dried herb blend and 9fl oz (250ml) boiling water. Drink 3 times daily.*

OTHER COMBINATIONS

Blend with other circulation-supporting herbs such as hawthorn and rosemary.

CAUTION

Avoid with blood-thinning medication. Avoid, too, during pregnancy, unless under the supervision of a professional medical herbalist.

FOCUS ON
Hibiscus

PROFILE
This flowering plant is native to warm, temperate, and tropical regions.

PROPERTIES
As well as protecting the body from oxidative damage, the high levels of antioxidant vitamin C in hibiscus support the immune system, promoting physical and mental wellness.

LICORICE
Glycyrrhiza glabra

Traditionally, herbalists called licorice "a root of great virtues." This highly regarded herb probably originated from China where it is called "the grandfather of herbs" and is thought to provide strength and endurance. Roman physicians used licorice extensively in medicine. With its sweet taste, it is often added to blends to harmonize the taste of other bitter herbs.

BENEFITS

Sweet, warming, mucilaginous, and nutritive, licorice is used as an adrenal tonic and a protective remedy for the gut and lungs.

Licorice helps to gently restore adrenal function when the adrenal glands, which regulate stress hormones in the body, are affected

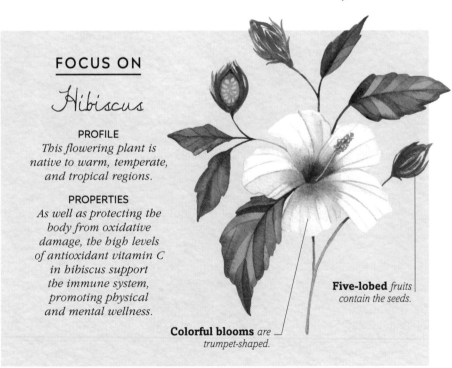

Five-lobed *fruits contain the seeds.*

Colorful blooms *are trumpet-shaped.*

by chronic stress. Licorice acts as a tonic, enabling the adrenals to cope more easily with daily stresses. This is especially helpful where exhaustion is experienced and there is a feeling of "running on empty."

Licorice has been found to be successful in treating chronic fatigue. It prolongs the action of cortisol, our natural restorative and healing hormone, while offsetting some of its side effects, such as mood swings and irritability.

Some studies show that licorice can be successfully used as a restorative and mucous-protecting herb. This can be helpful where prolonged stress damages the stomach lining, especially when this is caused by excessive alcohol consumption, which is used as a way of coping with stress.

Licorice is often used as part of a detox program, where it can help to improve bowel function, in turn supporting the gut–brain axis—the interconnection between the gut and the brain whereby a healthy gut supports cognitive function.

HOW TO USE

The licorice root can be used in decoctions, powders, capsules, and tinctures.

Blend licorice in equal parts with ashwagandha and a pinch of ginger for a blend to support adrenal health and circulation, and to improve resistance to stress.
➡️*Take a 300mg capsule 1–3 times a day.*

OTHER COMBINATIONS

Licorice can be used to "harmonize" other herbal blends. Thanks to its sweet taste it is particularly useful in herbal preparations for children.

CAUTION

Avoid with high blood pressure; deglycyrrhized root extract (where the compound triterpenoid glycyrrhizin, which can have side effects, has been removed) is considered safe, but it is best taken under professional supervision. High doses should not be taken for a prolonged period of time. Also do not take during pregnancy.

HIBISCUS
Hibiscus sabdariffa

Also called roselle or karkade, this beautiful shrub with exotic flowers is much loved across the globe. High in protective antioxidants, it is generously used to flavor cooling drinks and sweets and scent cosmetic products. Hibiscus is a very safe herb that can be taken for a prolonged period of time.

BENEFITS

Hibiscus is rich in vitamin C and other antioxidants, helping to protect the body from damage caused by free radicals, support healthy blood circulation, and improve vitality.

Numerous studies show that hibiscus can play a role in helping to lower high blood pressure, in turn protecting the body against the effects of chronic stress.

The cooling properties of hibiscus are very useful during menopause, particularly for hot flashes, which can lead to stress. Its gentle hormonal-regulating mechanisms can also be beneficial for PMS.

There is growing evidence that hibiscus can play a role in weight management. A study that used a combination of hibiscus and lemon verbena demonstrated a reduction

SUMMER BLOSSOM

Hibiscus typically flowers throughout August. The pod, known as the calyx, is used to make the cooling tea.

in appetite in overweight patients, together with positive changes in other health parameters such as high blood pressure and a healthy heart rate, all of which has a domino-effect benefit for mental wellness.

An infusion has a calming effect, helping to support deep, prolonged, restful sleep and reducing anxiety.

HOW TO USE

The flower buds are dried and used in infusions, powders, capsules, or tinctures.

Try a cooling infusion with hibiscus only to soothe hot flashes. Or blend hibiscus with rose petals and lemon verbena or mint for a refreshing drink to cool, hydrate, and calm. For a tea infusion to calm anxiety, blend hibiscus with lemon balm and skullcap.
➡️*Infuse ½–1 tsp dried herb, or herb blend, in 6fl oz (175ml) boiling water and drink 1–3 times a day.*

OTHER COMBINATIONS

Hibiscus can be used widely with other herbs, adding a slightly sour taste and a beautiful pink color.

CAUTION

Enjoy in food during pregnancy, but avoid therapeutic doses.

ST. JOHN'S WORT
Hypericum perforatum

St. John's wort was used in the Middle Ages for "driving away evil influences." Flowering around the midsummer solstice, in mythological thinking it helped to illuminate dark places in the soul, linking with its use today as an antidepressant. Its leaves contain translucent oil-filled sacks. When crushed, the active constituents photosensitize in the presence of light and turn red.

BENEFITS

St. John's wort is anti-inflammatory and antiviral, with an affinity for the nerves. Modern use evolves around its antidepressant effect.

Over 30 studies support its use for mild to moderate depression. Effects were noticed in 4–6 weeks, with more profound effects over several months.

It is supportive for obsessive-compulsive disorder (OCD) and social anxiety—excessive worries and fears linked with potential embarrassment in public or social situations.

St. John's wort helps to lift spirits with seasonal affective disorder (SAD) linked to the winter months, characterized by low mood, excessive sleepiness, and increased appetite.

Its antiviral properties make it very helpful for post-viral fatigue and fibromyalgia. It can also offer support for neurodegenerative disorders such as Alzheimer's and Parkinson's.

Its soothing properties are helpful for tackling insomnia.

It strengthens the autonomic nerves involved in digestion. It can help when stress causes persistent, mild indigestion, sluggish digestion, and discomfort. It is also supportive for "nervous bladder," where there is a frequent urge to urinate without an infection, a condition that can be caused by emotional stress.

It can be useful where repetitive thoughts lead to negativity.

HOW TO USE

The flowers and leaves are used in infusions, powders, capsules, and tinctures.

Take as a mood-lifting tonic.
➥ *Take 1–2ml tincture in a little water 1–3 times a day.*

Blend equal parts with passionflower, vervain, and skullcap to stop negative thoughts. For insomnia, with valerian, California poppy, and a little saffron.
➥ *Infuse 1 tsp dried herb blend in 6fl oz (175ml) boiling water. Drink 1–3 times a day.*

OTHER COMBINATIONS

For low mood, try blending with hawthorn, hibiscus, and rose, or with damiana and ashwagandha.

CAUTION

Avoid during pregnancy unless under supervision. Caution is required with medication. St. John's wort speeds up processes in the liver and makes some medications less efficient. It can increase photosensitivity.

A NATURAL HEALER

Traditionally, St. John's wort was used to dress wounds thanks to its anti-inflammatory healing action.

HYSSOP
Hyssopus officinalis

Hyssop has been used as a holy herb in several traditions, playing a role in purifying and cleansing rituals. Its antiseptic properties and the high content of antibacterial components in the essential oil would be used to help purify the air. A beautiful plant with a fresh, minty scent that is much loved by bees, it is used to lift the spirits.

BENEFITS

Though hyssop's main medicinal use is for respiratory complaints such as coughs and throat infections, its antispasmodic, relaxing action means it is used widely as a calming remedy and a tonic for recovery after illness.

Hyssop is a nerve tonic that is particularly helpful during convalescence, especially where there is post-viral fatigue.

Its antispasmodic and calming properties make hyssop a useful herb for relieving tension and anxiety and helping to cope with stress.

Some recent studies indicate that hyssop can help to increase the duration of sleep.

HOW TO USE

Hyssop is usually taken as an infusion. Because of its volatile oil content, infuse under a lid. Taking in a tincture should be done with professional supervision due to the potentially high content of a neurotoxic component.

One of the traditional uses is in a bath.
➥ *See remedy, opposite. Alternatively, add a strained infusion right into the bath.*

Try a blend with ashwagandha, milky oats, and lime flower to support convalescence.
➡️*Infuse 1 tsp dried herbs in 6fl oz (175ml) boiling water and drink 1–3 times a day.*

OTHER COMBINATIONS

Hyssop is a part of the mint family and blends well with many herbs in a tea such as chamomile, wood betony, and skullcap.

CAUTION

A truly warming remedy, avoid with hot flashes. Also avoid during pregnancy. It should not be taken over a long period of time.

REMEDY

Calming bath

Place a handful of dried hyssop in a muslin cloth and add to a hot bath while it fills. Steep for 15–20 minutes before taking the bath.

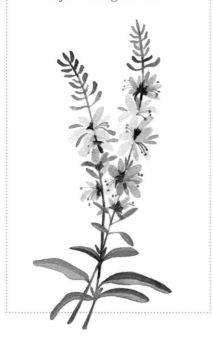

MOTHERWORT
Leonurus cardiaca

This hardy herb, which is part of the mint family, is native to Europe and Asia. Its use is documented as far back as the ancient Greeks. The English name, motherwort, suggests the traditional use of this plant for female health, while the Latin meaning "lion's heart," links to its heart-supporting properties.

BENEFITS

Motherwort is used as a calming remedy for heart palpitations. This balancing plant is also used to support and regulate female hormones, particularly after giving birth and during menopause.

Motherwort can help to calm and strengthen the heart. It can be supportive where, for example, a mild functional disorder causes palpitations and an increased heart rate, or where there is high blood pressure or stress, both acute and chronic. It is also often used in herbal blends for an overactive thyroid, characterized by palpitations, and it is very helpful during menopause when symptoms include palpitations, general anxiety, and insomnia.

As a balancing herb for female hormones, it can be helpful for postnatal "baby blues."

HOW TO USE

The aerial parts of the plant are dried and used mainly in capsules or as a tincture. A tincture provides a therapeutic dose if a remedy is needed quickly.

Blend with hawthorn and lime flower to soothe general anxiety, or for more acute episodes of anxiety, combine with passionflower and skullcap.

Use 20 percent motherwort with 40 percent each hawthorn and lime flower. Or combine with ashwagandha to alleviate menopausal symptoms, particularly palpitations, mood swings, anxiety, and insomnia.
➡️*Try as a blend in a capsule or on its own in a tincture. Take a 500mg capsule or 1–2ml tincture in a little water 1–3 times a day.*

OTHER COMBINATIONS

Blending motherwort with valerian and California poppy makes an effective support for insomnia. Or combine with vervain and St. John's wort for supporting a low mood that is linked to the menstrual cycle. Motherwort is an extremely bitter herb, so if using in an infusion or decoction, add pleasant-tasting herbs such as lime flower and mint.

CAUTION

Avoid during pregnancy.

CHAMOMILE
Matricaria recutita

Chamomile is often called a "hug in a mug." The soothing properties of this herb balance the signaling, or interaction, between the central nervous system and enteric nervous system—which is located in the gut and forms the "gut–brain axis"—to relieve the impact of stress. The word chamomile comes from Greek "earth-apple," because of the applelike scent of the plant.

BENEFITS

Chamomile is especially useful for those who internalize worries, feel fragile, turn to comforting sugary food, or who feel the effects of stress in their stomach.

➤ CONTINUED...

Studies show that chamomile's calming properties can help relieve symptoms of anxiety.

A gently sedative and anxiety-relieving herb, chamomile helps to improve sleep when taken 1–2 hours before bedtime.

It is antispasmodic, making it useful for abdominal pain, especially when linked to stress.

Chamomile infusions have been found to help reduce blood glucose levels, which in turn helps to control sugar cravings.

It can soothe irritability where allergies cause agitation due to the effect of histamine, released during an allergic reaction.

When children are under stress, they tend to feel it more in their bodies, particularly as abdominal discomfort. Chamomile can help to calm children and settle stomach upset that is linked to stress.

FOCUS ON

Chamomile

PROFILE

This perennial plant with daisy-like flowers is a popular addition to gardens.

PROPERTIES

Traditionally, chamomile was used for its analgesic and healing antiseptic properties and would be applied directly to the skin.

Blooms *are made up of delicate white or yellow flowers.*

HOW TO USE

The flowering heads of the chamomile plant can be used in various preparations. Most typically, chamomile is taken in a gentle infusion; it is also used in tinctures for a therapeutic dose of the plant. The plant is rich in volatile oils so an infusion is best prepared under a lid. For more chronic complaints, a chamomile infusion should be taken 3 times a day for several weeks to achieve a sustained result.

Try blending chamomile with a pinch of ground cinnamon bark to help manage swings in blood sugar levels that can lead to irritability and a feeling of being "hangry."

➽ *Infuse 1 tsp dried herb in 6fl oz (175ml) water and take 1–3 times a day. Or take on its own in 1–2ml tincture in a little water 3 times a day for a stronger dose.*

To relieve the symptoms of an irritated stomach, particularly where the cause is likely to be nervous tension, add to a licorice root decoction.

➽ *Make a decoction with 1 tsp dried herb blend (use 3g chamomile with 2g licorice root) and 9fl oz (250ml) boiling water. Drink 3 times a day.*

OTHER COMBINATIONS

Chamomile blends well with many other herbs, where it can improve the taste of an infusion, making it particularly useful for children. Try combining with lime flower and rose, mint, lemon balm, milky oats, or passionflower.

CAUTION

Caution needs to be taken if there is a known allergy to the daisy (*Asteraceae*) family of plants. If using in a licorice decoction, note that licorice is contraindicated where there is high blood pressure, so avoid if this is the case.

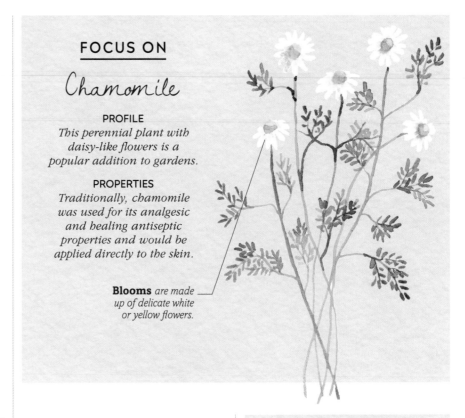

LEMON BALM

Melissa officinalis

Lemon balm, a beautiful plant that is grown widely in gardens and on windowsills, was used traditionally to lift melancholic feelings. The Greeks called this melissa, meaning a honey bee, and the plant is widely used to attract bees. It has a long history of use in Europe for its sedative properties.

BENEFITS

Lemon balm, part of the mint family, is a nervine tonic. It relaxes muscles to ease spasms and cramps, relieves nervous tension, and elevates mood. It is useful for anxiety-induced indigestion.

Lemon balm supports the action of the limbic system in the brain. This system is involved in our emotions and fight-or-flight response. When imbalanced, it can cause restlessness, anxiety, and difficulty sleeping. Lemon balm helps to regulate this system, reducing feelings of stress and calming, and increasing focus and the ability to process and memorize information.

Its calming action can help with heart palpitations linked to anxiety, nervousness, and constant worrying.

Lemon balm is antispasmodic, making it helpful for relieving headaches and migraines, which may be stress-related or lead to stress.

Several studies show its sedative effect is useful for treating insomnia, increasing sleep quality and duration.

Lemon balm lifts the spirits and can be a support for mild depression.

HOW TO USE

Lemon balm is a very safe herb that can be given to children. Rich in volatile oils, it is advisable to prepare infusions under a lid. It is one of the herbs best used fresh in infusions and tinctures.

Use dried leaves in a "sleep" pillow to keep close by at night. Add lavender and chamomile to increase its effects.
➡️*Put 2–3 tbsp dried herb, or blend of dried herbs, in a muslin sachet.*

Blend two parts lemon balm, milky oats, and skullcap with one part motherwort, for anxiety.
➡️*Infuse 1 tsp dried blend with 6fl oz (175ml) boiling water. Drink 3 times a day. Or make a tincture of lemon balm only for more severe symptoms: take 1–2ml in a little water 3 times a day.*

OTHER COMBINATIONS

Lemon balm blends well with many herbs. It improves the taste of infusions, so is helpful for children. Other useful blends include with chamomile for PMS; with vervain and sage for hot flashes; with lime flower, motherwort, and hawthorn for palpitations; or try with chamomile, licorice, and mint for a nervous stomach.

CAUTION

Avoid prolonged use and high doses of lemon balm if thyroid function is low.

PEPPERMINT
Mentha piperita

Peppermint is an ancient herbal remedy, rooted in mythology and folklore. In Greek mythology, the nymph, Minthe, governed rivers; when she was present the air was fresh. Widely used today as a culinary and medicinal herb, its calming properties explain its traditional use as a digestive remedy. It was also used by early philosophy scholars to help clarify thoughts.

BENEFITS

Peppermint has antimicrobial and muscle relaxant properties that can help to relieve nausea. The compound menthol and other ingredients also act as natural pain relievers, as well as helping to reduce anxiety, lift spirits, and improve memory and levels of alertness.

Mint extracts have been shown to have neuroprotective effects that may be supportive in brain-degenerating conditions such as dementia.

Its potent antioxidant properties are thought to help revert cellular damage and protect neurons. This in turn aids memory, learning, and mental performance in highly demanding tasks, and reduces mental fatigue.

Mint lifts the spirits and eases stress and anxiety, thanks to its ability to modify neurotransmitters, reduce levels of stress hormones, and improve serotonin metabolism.

Mint calms muscle spasms, inhibits the release of inflammatory chemicals, and acts on pain receptors locally and in the brain. These actions help ease anxiety- and stress-related symptoms such as tension headaches, stomach cramping, and shortness of breath.

Because of its capacity to promote deep relaxation, mint can be supportive after trauma and psychological shock.

Menstrual pain is significantly aggravated by stress and lifestyle factors. When taken over several cycles, mint's antispasmodic action gradually reduces the pain experienced.

HOW TO USE

The flowers and leaves are used in infusions, powders, capsules, and tinctures.The best way to use peppermint is fresh in food or added to drinks.

Try a stress-busting blend with equal parts lemon balm and verbena, and a little licorice. Or try with hibiscus and sage for hot flashes.
➡️*Infuse 1 tsp blended herbs with 6fl oz (175ml) boiling water. Drink 3 times daily.*

OTHER COMBINATIONS

Peppermint can be added to most blends to help improve taste.

"Lemon balm can help to reduce feelings of stress, bringing a sense of calm and renewed focus."

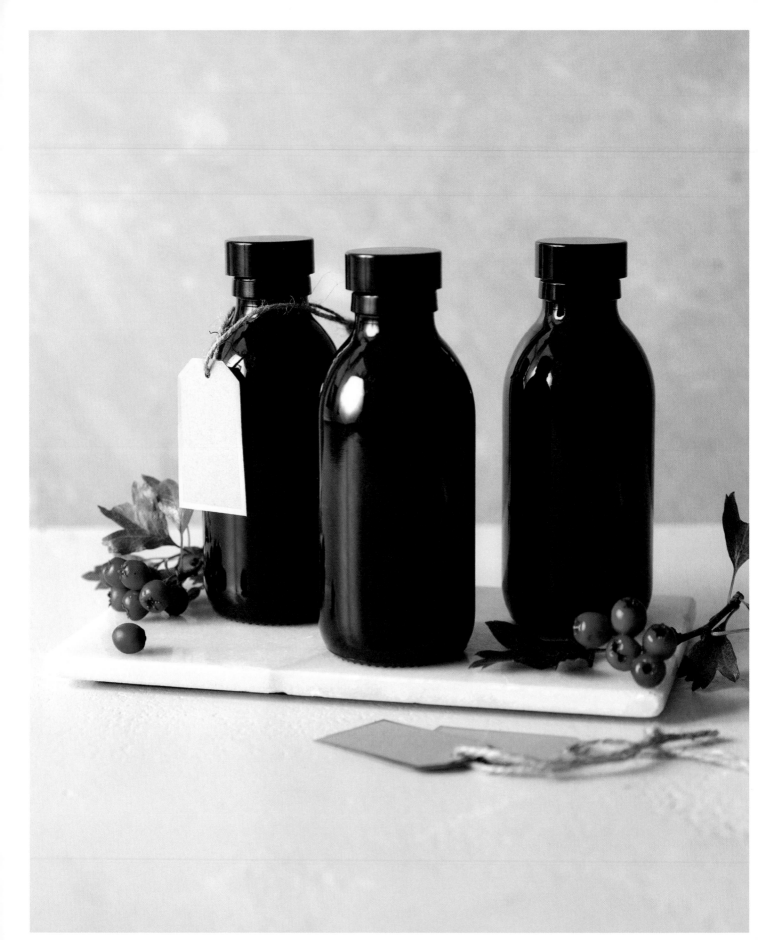

HOW TO MAKE
A TINCTURE

Tinctures combine alcohol with herbs to extract the herb's active constituents for use in remedies. Alcohol also extends a tincture's shelf life. The dose below comprises one part fresh herb to three parts vodka, or one part dried herb to five parts vodka. For a stronger tincture, consult a professional herbalist.

Makes approximately 1³/₄ pints (1 liter)

INGREDIENTS

7oz (200g) dried herbs,
or 11oz (330g) fresh herbs, chopped
1¾ pints (1 litre) 37.5% vodka

EQUIPMENT

Kilner or fermentation jar,
plus pouring jar, if needed
Labels
Dark glass bottles with screw tops
Large bowl
Sterile gloves (optional)
Muslin cloth
Fine mesh strainer
Fruit/wine press (optional)
Paper coffee filter (optional)

STORAGE

*Store in a cool, dark place.
Tinctures can be stored for
at least 12 months and
for up to four years.*

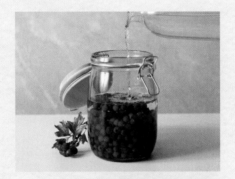

1 Sterilize the jars: wash these thoroughly then dry in an oven at 275°F (140°C), or in a microwave for 35–40 seconds. Place the herbs in the jar and pour in the vodka to cover them fully. Seal, shake well, label, and store in a cool, dark place for 2–3 weeks. Shake every other day.

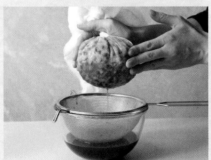

2 Sterilize the storage bottles and bowl (see method, above). Using clean hands or sterile gloves, strain the herbs into the bowl through a muslin-lined strainer. Gather the herbs in the cloth to squeeze out any remaining liquid. Alternatively, use a fruit press.

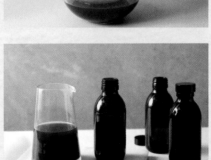

3 Pour the liquid into dark glass bottles, seal, and label with the herbs' names and the date.

HOLY BASIL

Ocimum sanctum/tenuiflorum L.

Also known as tulsi, this is a sacred plant from the Indian Ayurvedic tradition. A member of the mint family, there are two types of holy basil, one with green leaves called Rama tulsi, and one with purple leaves called Krishna tulsi. Holy basil is mentioned in ancient texts as a rejuvenating elixir known as rasayana, which today is referred to as an adaptogenic herb.

BENEFITS

Holy basil is an adaptogen and a potent antioxidant that helps to manage our response to physical and psychological stress; it calms the mood, supports a positive emotional outlook, enhances intellectual work, and is a general nerve tonic. It is widely used as an antidiabetic remedy, immune tonic, and as a support in cancer therapy, particularly postradiation therapy, helping the body to cope and thereby reducing stress.

Extensive studies show that holy basil has a tonifying effect that helps to relieve stress. It is thought to enhance mental capacities and help recovery

" *A potent antioxidant and calming herb, holy basil helps manage the body's stress response.* "

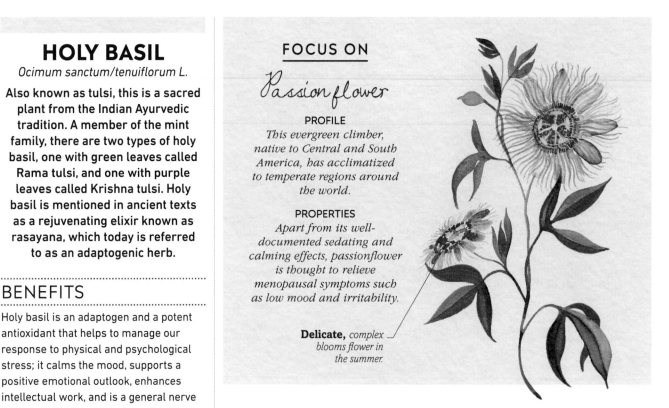

from chronic tiredness. The tonifying effect is achieved without the help of stimulant components but via its antioxidant activity and by acting on neurotransmitters, managing stress hormones, stimulating insulin activity, and supporting the action of enzymes.

Its antioxidant properties support brain health, offering some protection against age-related deterioration. The antioxidants improve cell metabolism, optimize mineral turnover, and protect against oxidative damage to DNA and some lipids. This is especially helpful for the brain, which has a high lipid content—the building blocks of cells—and is at high risk of oxidation.

HOW TO USE

The flowers and leaves are used in infusions, powders, capsules, and tinctures. If you have access to the fresh herb, the best way to use it is as with other mints, adding it to drinks and using it in cooking.

It can also be made into a "tulsi chai tea" with favorite spices.

Blend with hibiscus, passionflower, and sage for menopausal hot flashes and mood swings. Or with lemon balm and California poppy to ease headaches that may be stress-related. ➥*Infuse 1 tsp blended herbs, equal parts, in 6fl oz (175ml) boiling water. Drink 3 times daily. Or for a stronger dose, take 1–2ml tincture in water, or 1–2 500mg capsules, 1–3 times a day.*

OTHER COMBINATIONS

Holy basil also blends well with ginkgo and bacopa to act as a brain tonic.

CAUTION
Holy basil has been found to reduce male fertility in therapeutic quantities. Consult a trained herbalist if needed. Enjoy in food during pregnancy, but avoid therapeutic doses.

KOREAN GINSENG
Panax ginseng

Ginseng, native to the mountains of East Asia, is called the king of tonics. Its Latin name comes from panacea, or "cure all."

BENEFITS

Ginseng is a key adaptogen. It is used as a vitality tonic, restoring life's energy chi to promote health and longevity.

Ginseng's key adaptogenic action is in supporting the adrenal glands. It helps them to adapt to chronic stress and increases resilience, maintaining or restoring well-being.

It helps revitalize when there is exhaustion and feelings of faintness. This is especially helpful when illness leads to restlessness, insomnia, and irritability. Traditionally, it has been used as a tonic to restore depleted energy levels in old age.

Ginseng helps combat and support symptoms of anxiety, especially heart palpitations, stress-linked stomach upsets, and addictive behaviors.

Traditionally, it is a male tonic, supporting blood circulation to the genitals, so increasing libido.

Studies show that saponins in ginseng aid learning and memory. Improvements are noted in one week and sustainable results in two months.

Ginseng supports exercise, which has a measurable impact on mental health. It helps increase muscle strength and endurance, and reduces recovery time.

HOW TO USE

Ginseng is a precious root, best taken in a capsule or a tincture, though the root can be decocted in a blend. Blending in a tincture should be done by a professional herbalist to avoid contraindications.

Blend with ginkgo to aid cognition. Or with hawthorn as a tonic when older.
➡ *Take 1–2 500mg capsules (1:2 parts ginseng to ginkgo; or 1:3 parts ginseng to hawthorn) 1–2 times a day.*

OTHER COMBINATIONS

Blend with nutritive herbs such as milky oats, reishi, or licorice. Combine with other adaptogens under supervision.

CAUTION

A strong stimulant, it should be taken in the morning and at lunch for no longer than 3 months at a time. Avoid during pregnancy, with hot flashes or warm weather, or if overstimulated, for example, from caffeine.

PASSIONFLOWER
Passiflora incarnata

Passionflower is a prolific vine with exotic, bright flowers, used traditionally by Native Americans as food, medicine, and as a sedative. Source by its botanical name, as another genus, *Passiflora edulis*, has no effects on the nervous system.

BENEFITS

Passionflower has a history of use for the treatment of insomnia and anxiety. It is also antispasmodic and pain-relieving.

A range of active constituents act as sedatives. Studies show it has a positive impact on sleep duration and quality. It is also thought to modulate the calming neurotransmitter, gamma aminobutyric acid (GABA), which promotes sleep and relaxation.

Its calming properties can relieve anxiety, enabling individuals to distance themselves from worries and stop overthinking. Physiologically, it can help reduce stress hormones, which in turn slows the heart rate and lowers blood pressure.

Passionflower's sedative, anti-anxiety, and anticonvulsant properties can be a support when withdrawing from alcohol or drugs, helping to reduce addictive patterns and withdrawal symptoms such as anxiety and pain.

Its calming and relaxing effects can act as an aphrodisiac in lower doses.

HOW TO USE

Use the flowers and leaves in infusions, powders, capsules, and tinctures. Studies show its active constituents need to be metabolized by gut flora, signaling the importance of a healthy gut microbiome.

It is used in anxiety-provoking situations, such as public speaking or traveling, that may trigger a panic attack.
➡ *Take 1–2 500mg capsules 1–3 times a day.*

OTHER COMBINATIONS

Blend with bacopa and ginkgo to aid focus; with St. John's wort to uplift in menopause; and with valerian to promote restful sleep.

CAUTION

Avoid during pregnancy unless under supervision of an herbalist.

THE PASSION

Passionflower's Latin name is from Spanish missionaries who linked its complex structure to Christ's "passion," or suffering.

RHODIOLA
Rhodiola rosea

Rhodiola, otherwise known as Arctic rose or golden root, is grown in boreal forests and in high altitudes and is a valuable plant in Chinese, Tibetan, and Russian pharmacopeia.

BENEFITS

Rhodiola is a true adaptogenic plant and is a tonic and stimulant. It supports the immune system, boosting physical endurance and enhancing resistance to stress, and can be supportive in cancer therapy. As well as aiding cognition, it is helpful with depression, anxiety, fatigue, nervous system disorders, and headaches. Studies also show it can improve anaerobic exercise capacity, which in turn promotes mental well-being.

Rhodiola extract has a calming and tonifying effect. When taken for 8–12 weeks, it has been shown to help significantly alleviate symptoms of stress such as exhaustion, fatigue, irritability, anxiety, low mood, and a feeling of losing control.

Rhodiola extract is used in traditional Chinese medicine to reduce inflammation, helping to support the nervous and cardiovascular systems from the effects of stress.

Rhodiola is strongly antidepressant, especially when lethargy is brought on by intellectual or physical strain.

Studies indicate rhodiola might help to balance estrogen, making it useful as a support during menopause for fatigue, stress, and low mood.

Research suggests that rhodiola improves concentration, increasing accuracy and quality of work when performing stressful cognitive tasks. It can also help to support recovery from night shifts.

HOW TO USE

Use the root in powders, capsules, and tinctures. Can take over a period of time. If over-stimulating, take in the morning only.

Enjoy a daily latte tonic.
➥*See remedy, opposite.*
Blend equal parts with ashwagandha and reishi if "burned out," or with St. John's wort, passionflower, and skullcap for low mood and anxiety.
➥*Take 1–2 500mg capsules, or 1–2ml tincture with water, 1–2 times a day.*

OTHER COMBINATIONS

Use with damiana, schisandra, and cacao for a vitality tonic or with ashwagandha and sage during menopause; or with ginkgo, bacopa, and rosemary for cognition.

CAUTION
Avoid during pregnancy unless under supervision of an herbalist.

ROSEMARY
Salvia rosmarinus

Rosemary, a popular culinary herb and member of the mint family, is a widely grown Mediterranean shrub with beautiful flowers—much loved by bees—and a highly fragrant aroma. Strongly antioxidant, it is associated with areas known as "blue zones," where people live longer and experience less impact from aging.

BENEFITS

As well as being antibacterial and anti-inflammatory, this potent antioxidant and nervine tonic supports blood flow to the brain and protects against oxidative damage to the brain and heart. Increasingly, research links it with mental capacities and its ability to aid learning.

"Rhodiola acts as an antidepressant, easing anxiety and lifting mood."

Research shows that rosemary can improve the speed of recall—how quickly something is remembered—one of the signs of cognitive decline linked to an aging brain.

Its antioxidant action stimulates genes that regulate key neurotransmitters, protecting against damaging stress hormones and providing support for depression and anxiety.

By supporting a healthy blood supply to the brain, it protects against damaging inflammation.

HOW TO USE

As a valuable culinary herb, one of the best ways to use it preventatively is to add fresh to meals. The leaves, flowers, and young twigs are used in infusions, decoctions, powders, and tinctures.

Combine equal parts with ginkgo and reishi for a tonic for intellectual aid.
➥*Take 1–2 500mg capsules 1–2 times a day.*

OTHER COMBINATIONS

Blend with passionflower, rhodiola, and hawthorn for a heart tonic to cope with emotional stress.

CAUTION
It can suppress iron absorption; if taking iron supplements, take 2 hours apart from rosemary. Enjoy in food during pregnancy, but avoid therapeutic doses.

SAGE
Salvia officinalis

The 11th-century herbalist, Hildegard von Bingen, claimed sage "heightened perception and intuition." Its botanical name, salvia, comes from the Latin "to save," and in the Middle Ages, sage tea was used as a tonic for many ailments.

BENEFITS

Sage is a nervine tonic, protecting the nerves and brain. It is anti-inflammatory and antimicrobial and contains potent antioxidants that promote mental wellness.

A high content of phenolic compounds and flavonoids support menopausal symptoms such as hot flashes, sleep disorders, palpitations, depression, anxiety, brain fog, and forgetfulness. A 2020 study showed that sage could reduce menopausal symptoms by up to 40 percent within 3 weeks.

It has been shown to support the capacity to retain information and improve cognition.

Its anti-anxiety actions are well-documented. It has been shown to boost mood over a short period of time.

HOW TO USE

Use in cooking, for a refreshing infusion, or medicinally in tinctures.

Combine equal parts with hibiscus and a few threads of saffron as a menopause support.
➡ *Infuse 1 tsp in 6fl oz (175ml) boiling water and drink 3 times daily. Let cool before drinking for hot flashes.*

Take in a tincture to lift a low mood.
➡ *Take 1–2ml in water 3 times daily.*

OTHER COMBINATIONS

Blend with skullcap and milky oats for emotional fatigue and worry. Or with St. John's wort for menopausal low mood.

CAUTION

Enjoy in food if pregnant or breastfeeding, but avoid therapeutic doses.

SCHISANDRA
Schisandra chinensis

Schisandra fruits have been part of traditional pharmacopeia in the Far East for millennia. In Chinese medicine, it is linked to the Five Elements, representing the forces governing nature and our lives. It is therefore considered a key plant, helping to balance the elements, keep the spirit intact, and bring harmony.

BENEFITS

Its antioxidant properties reduce nerve damage caused by stress, improving cell renewal and cognition. A strengthening tonic, it is antiviral and anti-inflammatory.

Schisandra aids learning and eases fatigue and absentmindedness.

It is used as an antidepressant. Its calming effect soothes acute anxiety.

It can be an aid in menopause, helping to ease hot flashes, excessive sweating, and palpitations. It also helps soothe perimenopause hormonal fluctuations, reducing mood swings and fatigue.

Its aphrodisiac properties increase libido and support natural lubrication.

Schisandra has been found to support muscle volume and strength and reduce muscle fatigue after exercise, boosting mental wellness.

HOW TO USE

Berries are made into decoctions or the powder used in capsules and tinctures.

Blend equal parts with Siberian ginseng, reishi, and rhodiola to combat fatigue.
➡ *Make a decoction with 1 tsp dried herb blend and 9fl oz (250ml) boiling water. Drink 3 times daily.*

OTHER COMBINATIONS

Blend with holy basil, rosemary, and ginkgo to support intellectually demanding tasks. Blend schisandra, cacao, and damiana for their aphrodisiac qualities.

CAUTION

Avoid during pregnancy.

REMEDY

Rhodiola tonic

Start the day with this soothing tonic latte to build resistance to stress and lift spirits. Mix ¼–½ tsp rhodiola powder with 9fl oz (250ml) warm oat milk and rooibos tea combined. Add a little agave syrup and a sprinkle of cinnamon.

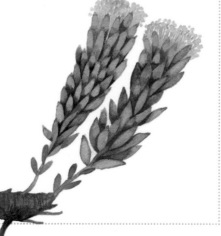

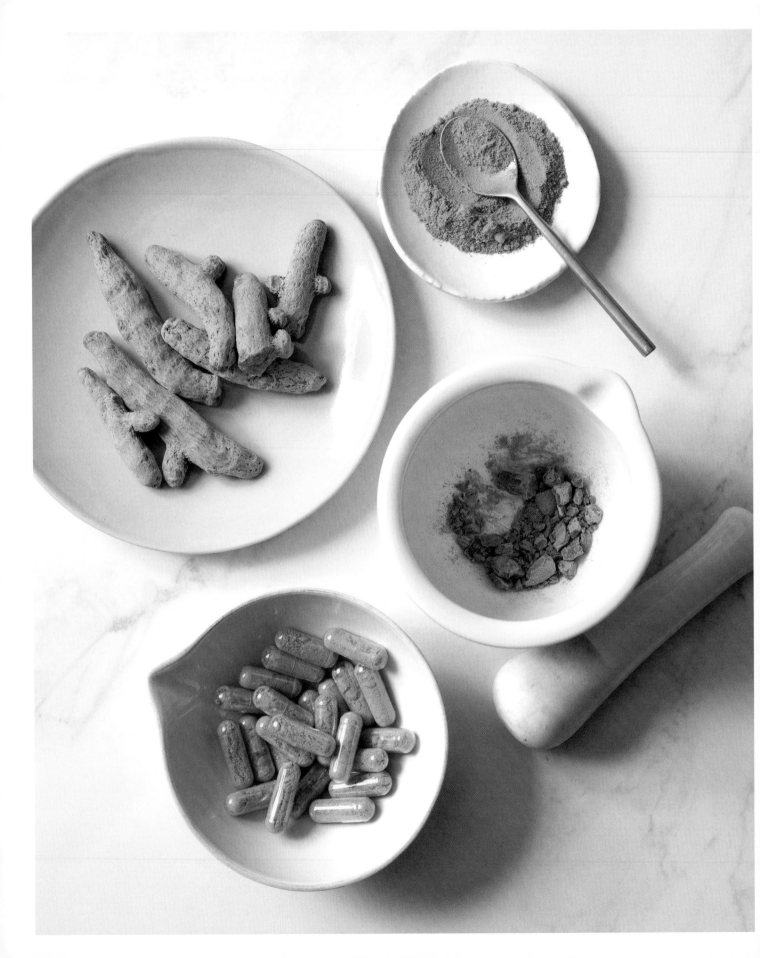

HOW TO MAKE
HERBAL CAPSULES

Dried herbs can be ground into powders to make herbal capsules using simple capsule-making equipment. When herbs are ground down into small particles it increases their surface area, making it easier for the body to absorb active constituents. Powders can also be blended into smoothies or sprinkled over food.

Makes approximately 45 capsules

INGREDIENTS

3 tbsp dried herbs

EQUIPMENT

Mortar and pestle or spice grinder
Fine sieve
Sterile gloves
Capsule-making machine with capsules
(either 735mg or 500mg)

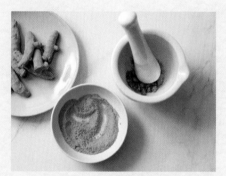

1 Grind the herb in batches with a mortar and pestle, making a fine powder. Using a mortar and pestle produces evenly sized particles that fill capsules densely and prevents herbs from overheating. You can also use a spice grinder if available. Sieve the powder to make sure it is as fine as possible.

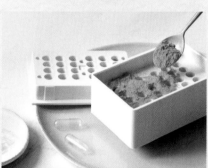

2 Wearing sterile gloves, weigh an empty capsule and note its weight. Separate the two ends of each of the capsules and place in the machine as instructed. Sprinkle the powder evenly over the capsules according to the manufacturer's instructions.

STORAGE

Store capsules in an airtight container in a cool, dry cupboard for three to six months.

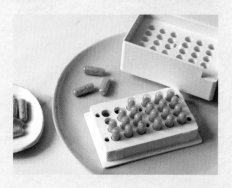

3 Remove the capsules from the machine. Weigh a filled capsule and subtract the weight of the empty capsule to ensure the correct dosage. A full capacity "00" capsule is 735mg, and a "0" capsule is 500mg. Many find "0" capsules easiest to swallow.

SKULLCAP
Scuttelaria lateriflora

This widely used medicinal plant mentioned in Cherokee medicine received its common name from its helmet-shaped blue flowers.

BENEFITS

Skullcap is a key herb for hyper-aroused, anxious states, especially useful if there is a tendency to overthink and an inability to switch off. As a restorative nervine tonic that supports the adrenals, it revives where there is exhaustion or depression.

Skullcap helps to reduce anxiety through its balancing action on neurotransmitters such as serotonin and GABA. Its potent antioxidant effect protects the brain and nervous system.

In a sleep blend it can support deep, restorative, and healing sleep.

It is calming for tension headaches and nerve pain. It also aids memory and focus, helpful for anxiety during exams.

It can be supportive for stress-linked palpitations and agitation, coupled with anxiety.

As a nerve tonic and muscle relaxant, it helps when an urge to urinate, not linked to an infection, leads to anxiety.

HOW TO USE

The fresh or dried plant can be used in infusions, capsules, and tinctures.

Blend with equal parts milky oats and Siberian ginseng for mental fatigue.
➡ *Infuse 1 tsp dried blend in 6fl oz (175ml) boiling water. Drink 3 times daily. For acute symptoms, take 1–2 300g capsules, or 1–2ml tincture (skullcap only) in water, 1–3 times a day.*

OTHER COMBINATIONS

Try with valerian and California poppy for restful sleep; or with vervain, saffron, and schisandra for anxiety in perimenopause.

CAUTION
Avoid in pregnancy unless supervised.

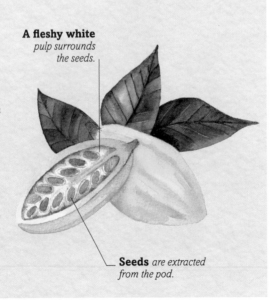

FOCUS ON

Cacao

PROFILE
Native to the Amazon basin, cacao beans form the basis of chocolate.

PROPERTIES
This strong antioxidant ingredient increases the bioavailability of iron in the body, helping to combat fatigue, especially due to menstruation.

A fleshy white *pulp surrounds the seeds.*

Seeds *are extracted from the pod.*

WOOD BETONY
Stachys betonica, betonica officinalis

Also called bishop's wort, this mint family herb is documented as a headache remedy as far back as the ninth century and was used for a range of psychiatric ailments.

BENEFITS

This mild nerve tonic is antioxidant-rich. Like many mint plants, it calms and uplifts. It is anti-inflammatory and antibacterial.

Wood betony is thought to help regulate the brain–gut axis—the link between gut and brain whereby the health of the gut can impact brain health.

Supportive for emotional shock and grief, it counters a tendency to introspection.

Its tonifying effect supports the stomach, especially in times of stress.

As an anxiolytic herb (anxiety easing) it calms and relaxes nervous tension.

It enhances focus and memory.

It stimulates appetite when older or recuperating. It can also signal fullness if there is a tendency to overeat.

HOW TO USE

Dried leaves and flowers are used in infusions, powders, capsules, or tinctures.

Blend equal parts with skullcap and valerian to ease anxiety and nerves.
➡ *Infuse 1 tsp in 6fl oz (175ml) boiling water. Drink 3 times a day.*

OTHER COMBINATIONS

Blend with milky oats, licorice, and hawthorn for a supportive tonic when older or convalescing. Or with chamomile and lime flower for digestion.

CAUTION
Avoid in pregnancy unless supervised.

CACAO
Theobroma cacao

Cacao is one of the cornerstones of Mayan culture: traces were found in drinking vessels as early as 1900BC. The terms "yollotl" (heart) and "eztli" (blood) were synonymous with the Aztec terms for chocolate, which studies show has the capacity to build up endurance and fight fatigue.

BENEFITS

Both acute and chronic stress can harm cardiovascular health. Cacao has been shown to have a significant cardio-protective effect by helping to reduce inflammation and having an impact on blood pressure and blood vessel health.

Flavonoid-rich cacao has a powerful antioxidant action. Several studies show that dark chocolate can increase resistance to oxidative damage, improving oxygenation, cellular metabolism, and, in turn, moderating the stress response. Flavonoids are also thought to support blood flow to the brain, reducing stress or injury-related degeneration and inflammation.

Cacao supports the bioavailability of iron, which can help to alleviate anemia and, in turn, fatigue, particularly due to heavy periods.

Research shows that people who eat dark chocolate report feeling happier and less lonely and depressed.

Historically, chocolate is an aphrodisiac. Chemically, cacao stimulates phenylethylamine, which is naturally released when "in love," and in turn triggers the release of endorphins.

HOW TO USE

The seed is dried, fermented, and crushed into nibs to make powders and tinctures.

Make a strengthening tonic latte.
➡*Add 1 tsp organic, raw powder to 9fl oz (250ml) warm milk. Enjoy daily instead of a morning coffee.*
Take a tincture for more acute or chronic symptoms.
➡*Take 1–2ml tincture in a little water 3 times a day.*

OTHER COMBINATIONS

Cacao can be combined with many herbs, especially as a powder. Try with milky oats, ashwagandha, or turmeric. For a heart-protecting remedy, add powder to a hawthorn berry and schisandra decoction.

CAUTION

Exercise caution if prone to migraines. Enjoy in food during pregnancy, but avoid therapeutic doses.

LIME FLOWER
Tilia cordata

Native to Europe and Asia, species include *Tilia europaea, platyphyllos,* and *americana.* In herbal lore, this majestic tree was thought to "soften wounds" and was seen as a symbol of love and happiness, which can be attributed to its uplifting effect.

BENEFITS

Lime flower is helpful for easing tension, whether in the form of a headache, muscle discomfort, or as anxiety or irritability.

Lime flower is an important cardio-tonic herb, helping to reduce palpitations. Its calming effect helps to settle restlessness and anxiety.

A relaxing herb, it is very helpful for insomnia, promoting restful sleep and helping to feel refreshed on waking.

Its relaxing effect and high flavonoid content help with tension headaches.

As it is gently sedative and has a pleasant taste, lime flower is very useful for restless, overactive children.

HOW TO USE

The infusion and decoction are very different: when brewed longer, the brew turns a rich red and is deeply nourishing, useful for nervous exhaustion, fatigue, and convalescence. A tincture is also potent. This is a safe herb for children—– a bath with a tea can be used for babies.

Make an uplifting blend, equal parts vervain, chamomile, and peppermint.
➡*Infuse 1 tsp dried herb blend in 6fl oz l (175m) boiling water and drink 3 times daily.*
Blend with valerian and California poppy for insomnia. Or with hawthorn and motherwort for a gentle heart tonic for anxiety and restlessness.
➡*Make a decoction with 1 tsp herb blend and 9fl oz (250ml) boiling water to drink 3 times daily.*

OTHER COMBINATIONS

Lime flower improves bitter herbs such as motherwort. Try with chamomile and rose for PMS-linked tension; with motherwort for menopausal-linked anxiety; or in a cold infusion with hibiscus for hot flashes.

DAMIANA
Turnera diffusa

This small, woody shrub is native to central and South America. The ancient Maya used damiana for treating nervous exhaustion, while traditional Mexican herbalists added it to blends for muscular weakness, nervous exhaustion, and over-tiredness, enjoying it as a revitalizing tonic drink after long marches.

BENEFITS

This strengthening herb has aphrodisiac and stimulant properties, providing a euphoric and relaxing effect.

Considered a restorative, nervine tonic, damiana can be supportive for mild depression.

Damiana is used for low libido. Its testosterone-boosting qualities and antioxidative properties support blood circulation to the pelvic area. In women, it stimulates the uterus, which can increase orgasmic ability.

It can be indispensable for working parents, especially for perimenopausal women or women taking the contraceptive pill, when the level of natural testosterone is low.

Damiana has a protective effect on the stomach lining, which is supportive when stress disturbs normal digestion.

" *Restorative damiana can be supportive for mild depression.* "

HOW TO USE

The aerial parts are used dried for infusions, powders, capsules, or tinctures.

Blend with ginseng and ginkgo for sexual dysfunction.
➥*Take 1–2 500mg capsules 3 times a day.*
Make a restorative blend with equal parts milky oats for nerves. Or blend equally with schisandra and ashwagandha for menopausal fatigue.
➥*Infuse 1 tsp dried herb blend with 6fl oz (175ml) boiling water. Drink 3 times daily.*

OTHER COMBINATIONS

Try with verbena, skullcap, or mint.

CAUTION
Avoid during pregnancy.

VALERIAN
Valeriana officinalis

The name valerian is derived from the Latin term "valere," which means "strong" or "healthy." It was a known remedy for shell-shocked war veterans of World War I to help reduce the strain on their nerves. Valerian has an unmissable, archetypal acrid smell and taste.

BENEFITS

With more than 150 constituents, valerian is rich in antioxidants. Its sedative action eases anxiety and accounts for its use as a traditional sleep remedy. It also relieves spasms, helping to reduce pain.

Valerian helps to fall asleep and stay asleep. Its sedative effect is from its ability to interact with sedative neurotransmitters in the brain via multiple pathways. It also supports metabolism of the neurotransmitters GABA, dopamine, and serotonin.

Valerian helps with hypochondria, restlessness, and with mental fixation. It can reduce overstimulation from external factors, promoting calmness.

High in antioxidants, it supports brain health, reducing the impact of stress hormones and improving learning. It shares some chemical constituents with lemon balm, chamomile, and lavender, all of which ease anxiety.

Reduction of anxiety is coupled with pain reduction. Valerian has been used to calm patients prior to dental and hospital procedures.

It relieves spasms, such as period pain, and "nervous" bladder. It also eases the severity of tension headaches to improve quality of life.

HOW TO USE

The root is used in decoctions or, when cut finely, infusions, or made into capsules and tinctures. The tincture is best in low-drop doses, as, rarely, an opposite, albeit temporary, hyper-stimulatory effect develops with a high single dose.

Make a sleep blend with equal parts California poppy and passionflower.
➥*Infuse 1 tsp dried blend in 6fl oz (175ml) boiling water. Drink 30–60 minutes before bed as part of a wind-down routine.*
Make a blend for anxiety.
➥*See remedy, opposite.*

OTHER COMBINATIONS

This blends well with most herbs. Use less in blends due to its prominent taste, adding nicer-tasting herbs. Try with lemon balm and skullcap for anxiety, or with vervain and damiana for nervous bladder.

CAUTION
Avoid during pregnancy.

VERVAIN
Verbena officinalis

A gentle tonic, this is seen as an herb to strengthen the liver, spleen, and heart. In North America, the variety *hastata* is used interchangeably.

BENEFITS

With anti-anxiety and sedative actions, it lifts spirits, calms, and eases anxiety. It is also an anti-inflammatory support for asthma and soothes menstrual spasms, tension headaches, and nervous bladder.

Its grounding properties help to let go of unrealistic expectations that can frustrate and drain mental energy.

It is an antioxidant, nervine tonic that helps to protect brain health.

As a tonic, it is used to calm anger. In children and teenagers, depression can manifest as irritability and even aggression; vervain can be a support while seeking professional help.

HOW TO USE

Aerial parts are used in infusions, capsules, and tinctures.

Blend equal parts with St. John's wort and milky oats for a low mood and with passionflower for anxiety.
➡ *Infuse 1 tsp dried herb blend in 6fl oz (175ml) boiling water. Drink 3 times daily.*

OTHER COMBINATIONS

Try with chamomile, wood betony, and licorice for nervous digestion.

CAUTION

Get professional help if taking a tincture with blood-thinning medication. Take 2 hours apart from iron supplements. Avoid if pregnant or breastfeeding.

REMEDY

Nerve-calming blend

Try this infusion to calm nerves and reduce anxiety. Infuse 1 tsp equal parts dried valerian, lemon balm, and skullcap in 6fl oz (175ml) boiling water. Drink when required.

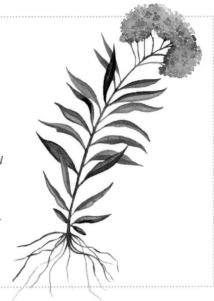

ASHWAGANDHA
Withania somnifera

Also called Indian ginseng, this is an adaptogenic, rejuvenating plant. Its botanical name, *somnifera*, means sleep-producing.

BENEFITS

Ashwagandha is a unique adaptogen because it combines two distinctive properties: it is tonic and sedative, bringing energy and inner calm.

Ashwagandha can help when someone is "wired and tired," too stressed and preoccupied with worries, constantly ruminating over events, and unable to fall asleep. Unlike most adaptogens, it can be taken pre-bedtime to promote sleep.

In Ayurveda, the plant has many uses, including as a nervine tonic, improving stamina and strengthening memory.

It helps improve the absorption of iron.

It is used broadly in debilitating conditions where it can help to gain weight during recovery when someone is fatigued, losing weight under stress, or needs support to build a healthy muscle mass.

It is attributed with aphrodisiac properties and is widely used for improving libido in women and men.

Rich in iodine, it helps to support a healthy thyroid function and maintain optimal energy levels.

HOW TO USE

The root is used in powders, capsules, and tinctures.

Take as a general tonic.
➡ *Add 1 tsp to warm milk, or for more severe symptoms, take 1–2 500mg capsules, or 1–2ml tincture with water 1–2 times a day.*

OTHER COMBINATIONS

Combine with licorice root and ginger to support the adrenals' response to stress, or with shatavari or sage for mood swings.

CAUTION

Avoid if pregnant and with known sensitivity to the *Solanaceae* family of plants. Combine with other adaptogens under professional supervision.

AROMATHERAPY

INTRODUCTION

THE ROLE OF OILS

Aromatherapy is a type of herbal medicine that uses plant extracts called essential oils, found in some plants, whose primary function in plants is protective, to stop microbial infection or attack by predators. Essential oils are complex; an individual oil can have hundreds of components. This chemical complexity means that each oil has a range of potential therapeutic uses that can be beneficial to the body, mind, and emotions.

HOW DO ESSENTIAL OILS WORK?

Most essential oils are extracted by steam or water distillation of the plant material. Essential oils from citrus peels are extracted by a cold-pressing process called "expression," while some delicate florals produce aromatic extracts that are obtained by solvent extraction. These are referred to as "absolutes" rather than essential oils. The highly concentrated oils then need to be diluted carefully for safe application. The three main ways in which essential oils enter the body are by absorption through the skin; by steam inhalation into the lungs; and via the olfactory receptor cells in the nose, to reach the brain.

OILS FOR MENTAL WELLNESS

The stress response is complex, driven by the autonomic nervous system responding to danger, or a perceived danger, and is expressed slightly differently in each individual, according to character, life experience, and individual constitution, including the influence of genetic and environmental factors.

Our emotions manifest physically, and, in turn, symptoms we feel in our bodies affect our emotions. Each of us has areas of fragility, and when we are under stress, the effects reflect in that particular area. Oils are therefore chosen for their range of actions. So a calming oil that is chosen to ease anxiety may also have uplifting effects or specific properties that are helpful for the effects of stress on the skin, the lungs, or other parts of the body.

The following actions are found in the essential oils listed on pages 78 to 101 and also referenced below.

Calming, sedating, and balancing essential oils include lavender, Roman chamomile, neroli, petitgrain, bergamot, mandarin, coriander, palmarosa, melissa, clary sage, geranium, and sweet marjoram. These help to moderate our response to external threats.

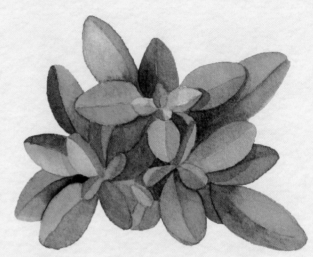

Sweet marjoram *is deeply relaxing and fortifying when feeling overwhelmed.*

High-arousal fight-or-flight responses can be expressed emotionally as anger, irritability, terror, or fear. The overreaction to outside stimuli, or to the perceived threat of outside stimuli, affects our core inner stability. Calming essential oils help to rebalance our responses to stress and provide support for symptoms. The relaxing properties of these oils also help to tackle sleep problems, in particular where the mind is unable to switch off.

Uplifting, antidepressant essential oils that are opening, stimulating, and expressive, are helpful when emotions feel frozen. Just as an animal may avoid danger from a predator by freezing, when we experience traumatic stress, we can go into an emotionally frozen, numb state, internalizing, rather than releasing, our emotions. Uplifting oils are also helpful with depression, typified by a state of underarousal to the outside world leading to a feeling of despair. Some of the citrus oils profiled in the following chapter—lime, grapefruit, sweet orange, petitgrain, lemon, and bergamot—are powerful here, helping to uplift and energize. Many oils from flowers such as ylang ylang, jasmine, neroli, and rose are also useful; as are may chang, melissa, thyme, cinnamon, and cardamom.

Grounding and meditative oils, particularly ones from the wood of trees, are helpful if there is a feeling of disassociation. This can be the way in which extreme, often traumatic, stress manifests, leading to a feeling of not being in the here and now. Oils such as frankincense, sandalwood, and cedarwood Atlas bring us back to ourselves. Other oils, such as jasmine and patchouli, can reconnect us to a sense of safety because they connect us to a feeling of being fully embodied.

Nervines, or nerve tonics, such as melissa, thyme, and patchouli, support the nerves and have a balancing and strengthening effect on the autonomic nervous system.

"Oils are chosen for their range of actions. So an oil for anxiety may help with stress-related skin problems, too."

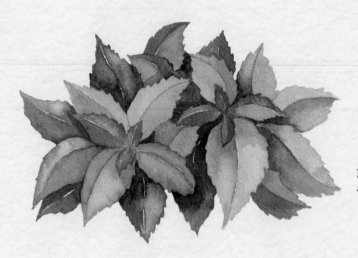

Patchouli *acts as a tonic to support the nervous system.*

Focusing and stimulating oils, such as rosemary, juniper, cardamom, lemon, and grapefruit increase alertness and concentration. These can be helpful when there is a tendency to introspection.

Antimicrobial oils, such as lemon, lime, cinnamon, lavender, thyme, and juniper, support the immune system, which can be negatively impacted by depression and depleted by chronic stress.

Anti-inflammatory oils, such as Roman chamomile and palmarosa, can help where chronic stress has a tendency to manifest in inflammatory skin conditions such as eczema.

Essential oils that help when stress negatively impacts digestion include the antispasmodic oils neroli, patchouli, Roman chamomile, coriander, sweet orange, and mandarin. When appetite is lost through stress, rosemary, grapefruit, and cardamom can help to awaken this.

CHOOSING ESSENTIAL OILS

While a single, well-chosen oil can be effective in treating or supporting simple acute physical complaints, when dealing with the complexity of the stress response, a blend of oils is usually more effective, enabling a more nuanced, comprehensive approach. A few oils may be complex enough in their actions to be used on their own in certain situations, but this is rare.

To understand how a blend might work, consider how symptoms are experienced emotionally and physically and choose oils that supports the physical area where stress is manifesting. For example, commonly, stress may be felt as discomfort in the throat, heart, lungs, solar plexus (diaphragm), or the gut.

If emotional responses are all quick and reactive, or all heavy and stuck, blending all calming or all stimulating oils can be useful. However, if anxiety and depression coexist, a balancing oil may be blended with calming, uplifting ones.

"When dealing with the complexity of the stress response, a blend of oils, giving a more nuanced approach, is often more effective."

When choosing oils for well-being, their therapeutic effectiveness is not the only consideration. How we respond emotionally and aesthetically to aromas is hugely important. If an oil's odor triggers a stressful memory or is not liked, its objective actions will be overridden. Blending can help to change a disliked aroma into a harmonious aesthetic.

USING ESSENTIAL OILS SAFELY

General advice for safe usage of these highly concentrated oils is to not use them undiluted on the skin or ingest them. The information given for usage in this chapter is for adults. Page 81 gives a guide for safe percentages when blending, but for blends used regularly long term, such as in a body lotion, a more diluted blend is advisable. Cautions on specific oils, and on certain oil blends, are given in this chapter. When using oils during pregnancy or with babies and infants, seek professional guidance. Additional general safety guidelines on using oils are on page 243.

HOW OILS ARE APPLIED

The primary methods of application for essential oils are directly to the skin in lotions, massage blends, and wash-off bath and shower blends.

Oils are also used in facial spritzers, or sprays, and in rollerball pulse-point applicators, which can be purchased to add oil blends to. Essential oils are also inhaled from diffusers and tissues.

The following chapter gives step-by-step guides on preparations.

Essential oil blends *are used in all of the applications above. See "How to Make an Essential Oil Blend" on pages 80–81.*

Facial spritzers *can be prepared and carried around to use when needed. See "How to Make an Essential Oil Spray" on pages 92–3.*

Palmarosa *produces a cooling essential oil that helps combat feelings of irritability.*

ESSENTIAL OILS

These complex compounds found in plants—the simplest has more than 80 chemical components and the most complex more than 400—have a range of therapeutic applications that have beneficial effects on the body, mind, and emotions. Some essential oils are effective used on their own, while many work best in combination with other essential oils to provide a more nuanced approach.

ROMAN CHAMOMILE

Anthemis nobilis/Chamaemelum nobile
Steam-distilled from the flowers, this daisy family member has a sweet and fruity aroma, reminiscent of apples and pears. Soothing and comforting, Roman chamomile is a helpful remedy for calming irritable feelings and inflamed skin that is caused or intensified by stress.

BENEFITS

Roman chamomile's calming, sedating action makes it a classic remedy for anxiety, panic attacks, tension, and agitation, particularly where these are linked to sleeping difficulties.

It has an antispasmodic effect on involuntary smooth muscle, which makes it especially useful where anxiety manifests in the digestive system as irritable bowel syndrome (IBS), and in the respiratory system as shallow breathing and asthma.
Its anti-inflammatory properties are helpful for inflammatory skin conditions such as psoriasis and eczema that are provoked or intensified by stress.

HOW TO USE

Inhaling this oil, whether from pulse points, or in a bath, lotion, or massage blend, helps bring calmness.

Use in a rollerball applicator.
➡ *Add 1 drop Roman chamomile, 3 drops cedarwood Atlas, 1 drop lavender, and 10ml of your chosen carrier oil to a rollerball. Apply to the wrist pulse points to inhale, or dab between the upper lip and nose, to ground yourself when feeling panicky.*
Enjoy a soothing bedtime bath soak.
➡ *Dissolve 6 drops in 10ml of unscented bubble bath, dispersant, or carrier oil.*

OTHER COMBINATIONS

Blends beautifully with other florals and calming, herby aromatics, such as clary sage and sweet marjoram, to quell anxiety.

FRANKINCENSE

Boswellia carterii/sacra/serrata/thurifera
This aromatically complex oil, steam-distilled from the tree's resin, has been used therapeutically since antiquity. It has medicinal, piney notes and a sweet spiciness.

BENEFITS

Frankincense uplifts and stills the mind, and deepens and steadies the breathing.

Its meditative quality makes it a powerful tool for calming anxious thoughts and panic attacks where there is shallow, fast breathing.
Tonic and strengthening, it is used where long-term emotional stress leads to a sense of depletion, fatigue, and hopelessness.
Long used in skin care, it is especially helpful in skincare blends with stress-related eczema or psoriasis.

HOW TO USE

This can be used as a conscious accompaniment to meditation. It is also helpful blended with calming oils to slow and deepen shallow breathing during anxiety spikes.

Add to a diffuser during mindful meditation practice, yoga, or other focused relaxation exercises.
➡ *Add 6–8 drops to a diffuser.*
Use in a rollerball applicator when feeling panicky. The association of the aroma with conscious mindfulness and relaxation makes the effects even more powerful.

"Frankincense has a meditative quality that helps to quell anxiety."

➡ *Add 3 drops frankincense, 1 drop ylang ylang, 1 drop lavender, and 10ml of your chosen carrier oil to a rollerball. Apply to wrist pulse points to inhale, or dab between the upper lip and nose, when panicky or overwhelmed by anxiety. Ylang ylang and lavender gently calm a rapid heartbeat.*

OTHER COMBINATIONS

Frankincense is aromatically harmonious with many oils. For a low mood, blend with uplifting, stimulating oils such as may chang and cardamom. For anxiety, try calming oils such as palmarosa and Roman chamomile.

HOW TO USE

Carry this with you to use when feeling low and apathetic. It can also be blended with other joyous, uplifting oils for use at the start of the day.

Use in a rollerball applicator with other relaxing oils to heighten its calming effects.
➡ *Blend 2 drops ylang ylang, 2 drops clary sage, 4 drops lavender, and 10ml carrier oil to use in a rollerball. Apply to a pulse point to inhale, or dab between the upper lip and nose, when anxiety is making the heart race.*

Make a morning shower gel or post-shower body lotion with zingy, refreshing grapefruit and bergamot.
➡ *Add 2 drops ylang ylang, 6 drops grapefruit, and 4 drops bergamot to 50ml of unscented shower gel or unscented body lotion.*

Create an uplifting spritzer.
➡ *Add 5 drops ylang ylang to 10ml of vodka or glycerine, then add this to a 50ml spray bottle, topping up with water. Spritz a mist in front of the face, keeping the eyes closed.*

OTHER COMBINATIONS

Ylang ylang also blends well with sweet marjoram essential oil to help settle and calm the mind.

CAUTION

The powerful scent can provoke headaches where there is a tendency for these to be induced by strong odors, so use at a low dosage.

YLANG YLANG

Cananga odorata

Steam-distilled from the flowers of the tree (see right), this has an almost hypnotically sweet, thick, floral aroma, so it is best used sparingly.

BENEFITS

Its uplifting and balancing properties have notable mental health benefits.

Ylang ylang imbues a sense of safety that can play a supportive role where anxiety and the "freeze" response may be associated with past trauma.

Its uplifting properties make this a useful oil for alleviating depression and anxiety.

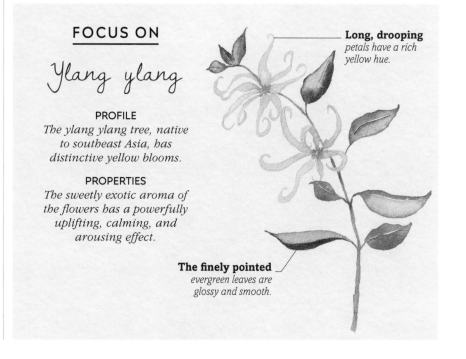

FOCUS ON

Ylang ylang

PROFILE
The ylang ylang tree, native to southeast Asia, has distinctive yellow blooms.

PROPERTIES
The sweetly exotic aroma of the flowers has a powerfully uplifting, calming, and arousing effect.

Long, drooping *petals have a rich yellow hue.*

The finely pointed *evergreen leaves are glossy and smooth.*

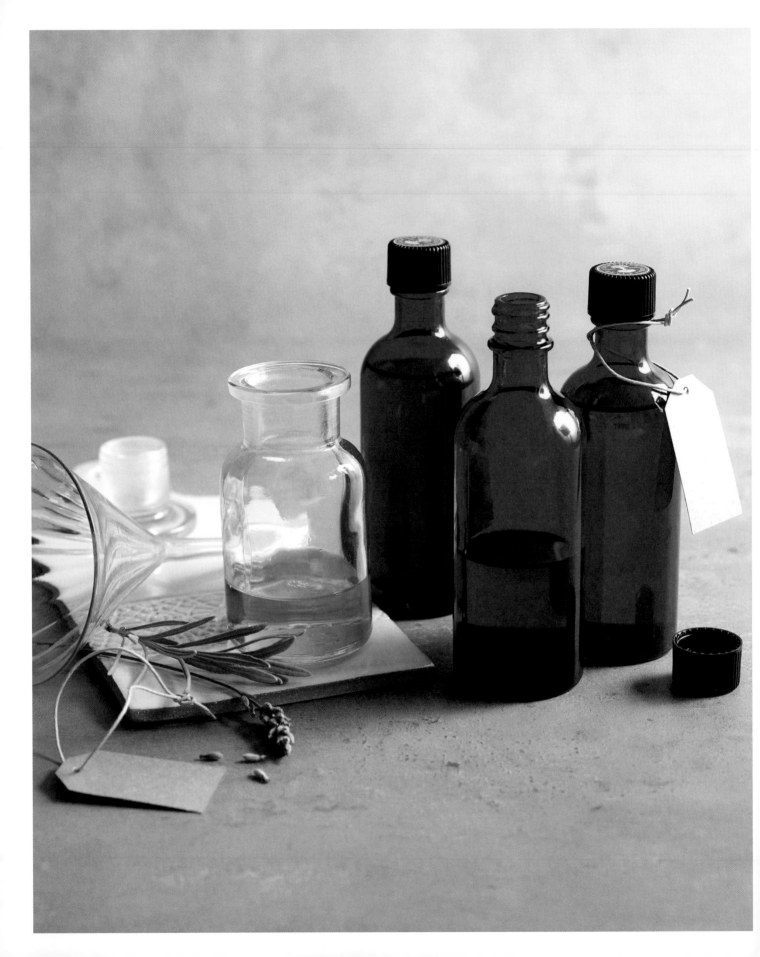

HOW TO MAKE

AN ESSENTIAL OIL BLEND

Before essential oils are used next to the skin, most of these highly concentrated substances need to be diluted in a base, or carrier, oil. Most carrier oils have no therapeutic value—they simply provide a neutral base. Dilutions vary depending on the essential oil, its properties, and its intended use.

Makes 1½–2½ tbsp

INGREDIENTS

Essential oil drops—either one oil or a blend of oils; the number of drops depends on the oil and its usage
1–2 tbsp base oil

EQUIPMENT

Small beaker, cup, or bottle
Dark glass bottle
Label

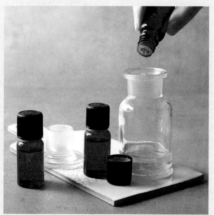

1 Combine the essential oil drops with the base oil in a beaker, saucer, or bottle. Typical dilutions are: for a bath blend, 4–6 drops essential oil to 1 tbsp base oil (or other bath dispersant); for a body massage blend, 7–15 drops essential oil to 1–2 tbsp base oil; and for a facial blend, 3 drops essential oil to 1 tbsp base oil (a 1 percent dilution of essential oils to base).

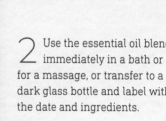

2 Use the essential oil blend immediately in a bath or for a massage, or transfer to a dark glass bottle and label with the date and ingredients.

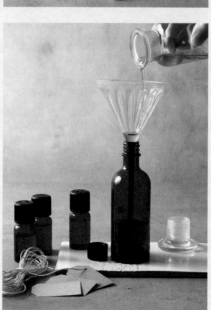

STORAGE

Store bottled blends in a cool, dark place to keep them away from the damaging effects of light and heat. Blends can be kept for up to three months.

CEDARWOOD ATLAS

Cedrus atlantica

This essential oil, steam-distilled from the wood of the magnificent tree, has a complex aroma—slightly sweet, soft, and woody. Cedarwood Atlas promotes a sense of stability and of being grounded.

BENEFITS

This strengthening and grounding essential oil is particularly useful when emotions are overstretched and a feeling of being exhausted sets in.

Cedarwood Atlas is helpful during focused meditative practice, where it helps to still the mind and deepen the breath.

It is seen as a remedy that tonifies and strengthens, helping us to be steady and present in the here and now. It is especially suited for providing emotional support where traumatic past events cause us to "freeze" when faced with a trigger.

HOW TO USE

To increase the positive effects of cedarwood Atlas, use it as a conscious accompaniment to yoga and meditation, rather than just as a "background" scent.

Use in a diffuser during meditative practice.

➽ *Add 6–8 drops to a diffuser as part of a conscious practice of mindful meditation or during focused relaxation exercises.*

Use in a rollerball applicator.

➽ *Add 3 drops cedarwood Atlas, 1 drop rose otto or absolute, 1 drop jasmine, and 10ml of your chosen carrier oil to a rollerball. Apply to the wrist pulse points to inhale, or dab between the upper lip and nose, when overwhelming emotion leads to feelings of faintness, shakiness, and a sensation of being disconnected.*

OTHER COMBINATIONS

Use with other woody oils such as frankincense and sandalwood to help you feel centered and grounded, and aware of your core strength and resilience.

FOCUS ON

Cedarwood Atlas

PROFILE

This ancient species, native to the Atlas mountains of Morocco, is endangered so should be bought from a reputable supplier.

PROPERTIES

The evocative woody aroma of cedarwood Atlas is deeply grounding and strengthening.

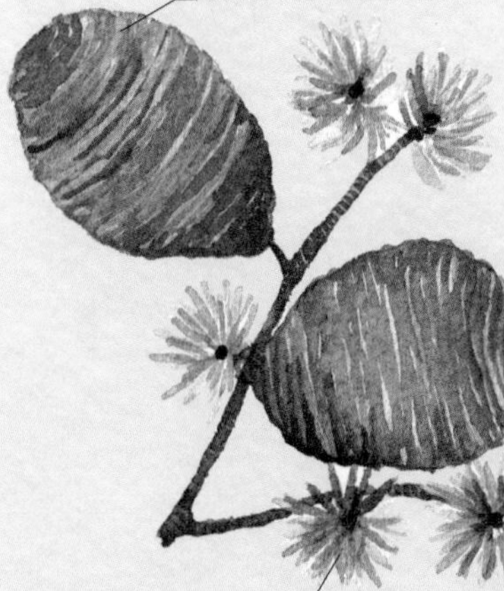

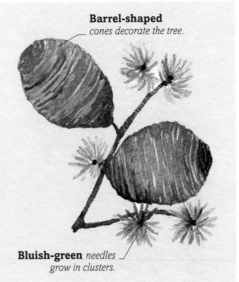

Barrel-shaped *cones decorate the tree.*

Bluish-green *needles grow in clusters.*

> "Cedarwood Atlas brings a sense of stability that helps to calm the mind when emotions are stretched."

CINNAMON (LEAF)

Cinnamomum zeylanicum/C. verum

This fiery essential oil is steam-distilled from the leaves of the cinnamon tree. A favorite massage oil of the ancient Egyptians, cinnamon's popularity has endured over the centuries. This powerfully warming oil has comforting associations with its culinary use and holiday connections.

BENEFITS

The complex sweet and spicy aroma of cinnamon essential oil is both comforting and uplifting.

Cinnamon is a wonderful oil for lifting a low mood, supporting the grieving process, and soothing feelings of anxiety or despair. Its superb uplifting effects can be particularly useful in the winter months for those affected by seasonal affective disorder (SAD).

It is a strongly fortifying and powerfully antimicrobial oil, useful for those who are depleted by the

long-term effects of stress on the adrenal glands, which can lead to extreme fatigue and a greater susceptibility to infection.

HOW TO USE

The essential oil should be used cautiously for skin application and should be avoided, including in the bath, with sensitive skin. It is best used in a diffuser, or in the lowest dilution of 1 drop in a rollerball for the wrist pulse only.

Use in a diffuser to lift the spirits.
➡️*Add 2 drops cinnamon, 2 drops may chang, and 4 drops sweet orange to a diffuser.*

Use in a rollerball applicator to help lift the spirits and promote calm.
➡️*Add 1 drop cinnamon, 2 drops rose otto or absolute, 4 drops clary sage, and 10ml of your chosen carrier oil to a rollerball. Apply this to the wrist pulse points to both uplift and calm. This blend is particularly helpful when a racing pulse and feelings of panic are associated with menopause, as rose and clary sage are widely used in aromatherapy during this time.*

OTHER COMBINATIONS

Like other culinary herbs and spices, cinnamon blends well in a diffuser with other appetite stimulants, such as cardamom, coriander, and mandarin, acting as a support for those who lose their appetite due to ongoing anxiety, grief, or despair.

CAUTION
Cinnamon essential oil should be sourced carefully from a reputable supplier. Make sure that the oil is from the plant leaf, not the bark, as the bark yields an essential oil that is a strong skin irritant, unsuitable for use in aromatherapy.

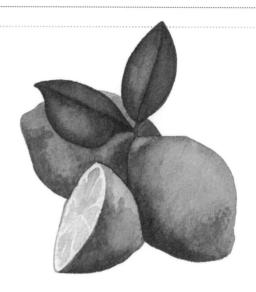

REMEDY

Grounding inhalation

Add 3 drops lime, 2 drops jasmine absolute, 5 drops clary sage, and 10ml of your chosen carrier oil to a rollerball to apply to the wrist pulse points and inhale when panicky.

LIME (DISTILLED)
Citrus aurantifolia

Lime essential oil is extracted from the fruit peel. It is steam-distilled or expressed, but the expressed oil can be phototoxic so should be avoided. The aroma is clean, sweet, sherbet citrussy, and powerfully uplifting.

BENEFITS

Lime is energizing and motivating. It lifts the spirits and promotes a sense of happiness, where there is a low mood.

Its uplifting and vitalizing properties make lime essential oil perfect to use at the start of the day when motivation is needed.

Lime has antimicrobial properties, beneficial for those who are prone to stress-related outbreaks of acne and boils. A recent study of its antimicrobial actions also showed its effectiveness against several strains of viruses. Immunity to infection is often lowered when stress is ongoing, so the antimicrobial properties of lime essential oil are doubly helpful here.

HOW TO USE

Blend with other stimulating oils for a feeling of freshness and vitality at the start of the day. Or combine with hypnotic, grounding oils to use in the moment when feeling anxious.

Make an energizing shower gel or body lotion.
➡️*Blend 3 drops lime, 2 drops rosemary, and 5 drops grapefruit in 50ml unfragranced shower gel or body lotion.*

Use in a rollerball applicator to ground you when you feel overwhelmed and are in a panicky state, experiencing shallow breaths.
➡️*See remedy, above.*

OTHER COMBINATIONS

Blend with exotic florals and tree oils such as cedarwood Atlas and sandalwood to lift spirits and ground.

CAUTION
Source this essential oil carefully. The expressed oil can be phototoxic and should be avoided.

NEROLI

Citrus aurantium var. amara (flos)

Also referred to as orange blossom, this profound essential oil is water-distilled from the flowers of the bitter orange tree. Regarded as the "rescue remedy" of essential oils, its layered aroma has floral, green, citrus, and deep molasses notes.

BENEFITS

Neroli is uplifting—helping to combat a low mood. It also calms anxious feelings and can be a supportive remedy where past trauma causes feelings of being emotionally paralyzed.

Its settling, calming effects on the autonomic nervous system make neroli particularly helpful for intense emotional distress that impacts the heart—causing a rapid, irregular pulse—or the digestive system.

Neroli supports where long-term stress leads to adrenal fatigue, affecting the function of the hormone-producing adrenal glands, leading to symptoms such as tiredness.

Some studies show that sniffing neroli may be particularly effective for women experiencing a rapid pulse and anxiety during menopause.

HOW TO USE

Neroli is an oil that can be used on its own but also combines beautifully with other essential oils. Its intensity and potency mean it is best served by conscious, thoughtful use during meditative practice, rather than diffused as a background scent.

Make a calming face spray.
➥*Add 5 drops neroli to 5ml vodka or glycerine, then add to a 50ml spray bottle and top up with water. Spritz a*

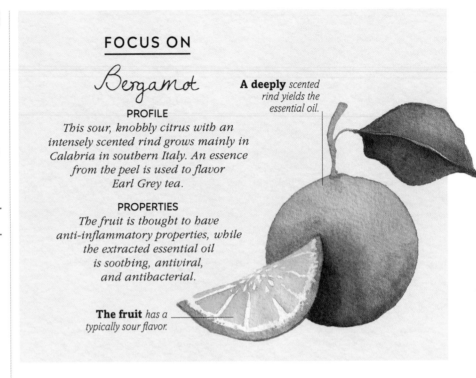

FOCUS ON

Bergamot

PROFILE
This sour, knobbly citrus with an intensely scented rind grows mainly in Calabria in southern Italy. An essence from the peel is used to flavor Earl Grey tea.

PROPERTIES
The fruit is thought to have anti-inflammatory properties, while the extracted essential oil is soothing, antiviral, and antibacterial.

A deeply *scented rind yields the essential oil.*

The fruit *has a typically sour flavor.*

mist in front of the face, keeping the eyes closed, when feeling faint and shaky from stress and anxiety.

Use in a rollerball applicator.
➥*Add 5 drops neroli and 10ml of your chosen carrier oil to a rollerball. Inhale from the wrist pulse points, or dab between the upper lip and nose, to uplift or ground you when a low mood or panicky feelings overwhelm.*

Make a winding-down bath blend for the end of the day.
➥*Add 2 drops neroli, 3 drops lavender, and 1 drop vetiver to*

10ml of unscented bubble bath, dispersant, or your chosen carrier oil and add to a relaxing bedtime bath to promote restful sleep.

OTHER COMBINATIONS

Neroli's calming effect on the heart rate is enhanced when used alongside essential oils that help to deepen breathing, such as frankincense or cedarwood Atlas. Such blends are beneficial when anxiety is felt most intensely in the heart and lungs, as is often the case with panic attacks.

"An uplifting essential oil, neroli is particularly effective for lightening a low mood."

PETITGRAIN

Citrus aurantium var. amara (fol)

The leaves and twigs of the bitter orange tree are steam-distilled to produce petitgrain essential oil, a lighter aromatic than the flower oil and less profound in its actions. This balancing, refreshing oil has a fresh, lightly floral, green aroma.

BENEFITS

Petitgrain has a sedating action, making it a useful essential oil to help dispel feelings of bubbling irritability and emotional volatility that are part of the stress response.

A less intense oil than neroli essential oil (see opposite), petitgrain is more suited for settling everyday tension to help keep emotions on an even keel, especially when feeling irritable and snippy.

Petitgrain's sedating properties are helpful for calming a racing pulse when this is brought on by anxiety.

The balancing effects of petitgrain make it suitable both for daytime use when blended with stimulating oils, to energize and support mental focus, and for evening use when blended with sedating oils, to promote sleep.

HOW TO USE

Petitgrain can be used safely on the skin, for example in massage or a spray, and is also effective in a diffuser.

Make a balancing facial spritz.
➡*Mix 2 drops petitgrain, 2 drops lemon, and 1 drop rosemary in 5ml of vodka or glycerine. Add to a 50ml spray bottle and top up with water. Spritz a mist in front of the face, keeping the eyes closed, when feeling flat, low, and unmotivated.*

Enjoy a sedating bedtime soak.
➡*Add 3 drops petitgrain, 3 drops lavender, and 1 drop vetiver to 10ml of unscented bubble bath, dispersant, or carrier oil to disperse in the bath.*

OTHER COMBINATIONS

Blend petitgrain with sedating essential oils such as sweet marjoram, lavender, or palmarosa to help calm feelings of acute anxiety when these are experienced as palpitations.

BERGAMOT

Citrus bergamia

Bergamot is expressed from the fruit of the bergamot tree, a close relative of bitter orange, and has a sweet and fruity odor. It is an uplifting and balancing essential oil.

BENEFITS

Many studies conducted with bergamot show that the oil has positive mental wellness outcomes, easing anxiety and increasing focus and positivity.

Bergamot is a euphoric oil, helping to profoundly lift the spirits.

The oil's calming properties help promote a feeling of being alert and vibrant, rather than on edge.

Studies show that bergamot reduced anxiety in cancer patients and improved mild symptoms of stress.

The skin-kind rectified oil (see caution, right) is helpful where stress provokes irritable skin conditions such as eczema and psoriasis.

HOW TO USE

The rectified oil is safe to use in normal dilutions for skin applications and is also calming in a diffuser.

Make an uplifting facial spritz to raise the spirits.
➡*Add 5 drops bergamot to 5ml vodka or glycerine, then add to a 50ml spray bottle and top up with water. Spritz a mist in front of the face, keeping the eyes closed, for a sense of relief when feeling low and overwhelmed.*

Use in a rollerball applicator.
➡*Add 6 drops bergamot, 4 drops sandalwood, and 10ml of your chosen carrier oil to a rollerball. Apply to the wrist pulse points and inhale, or dab between the upper lip and nose, to center and ground you when you are feeling panicky.*

OTHER COMBINATIONS

Aromatically harmonious, bergamot blends well with stimulating oils such as rosemary for morning showers or with deeply calming oils such as lavender and vetiver for a winding-down evening bath.

CAUTION

Source bergamot essential oil carefully from a reputable supplier as it is strongly phototoxic. Look for rectified, FCF (furanocoumarin-free) essential oil, as this has had a particular chemical removed that can cause skin irritation when exposed to UV rays.

REMOVING CHEMICALS

Rectified oils undergo an additional process after distillation to remove skin-irritating or other problematic components.

LEMON
Citrus limonum

Lemon essential oil is expressed from the fruit peel. The aroma is a vibrant, lemony one—true to the fruit—and is intensely uplifting.

BENEFITS

Emotionally, lemon essential oil is incredibly effective at lifting a feeling of fogginess to bring clarity and a sense of "light" to the mind.

Lemon's focusing properties— helping to concentrate and clear the mind to lift brain fog—make it particularly suited for daytime use, especially when the heaviness of depression seems hard to lift.

A small study of a group with depressive symptoms in a clinical setting found that the diffused essential oil improved mood and raised the immune response, and that, subsequently, lower doses of pharmaceuticals were needed.

HOW TO USE

An aroma most enjoy, lemon essential oil is ideal for using in shared spaces. Try incorporating it into your morning routine, too, to enhance well-being.

STRESS REDUCTION

Studies suggest that the component S-limonene in lemon essential oil can ease physical and psychological stress.

Use in a diffuser to create an uplifting environment that encourages optimism and vibrancy. Diffusing lemon essential oil can also be helpful in a work space to counter post-lunch energy dips.
➡ *Add 6 drops to a diffuser.*

Inhale the oil from a tissue.
➡ *Place a drop on a tissue to inhale if you feel faint, or not quite present.*

Enjoy in a morning shower gel or post-shower body lotion.
➡ *Add 5 drops lemon, 3 drops petitgrain, and 2 drops rosemary to 50ml unscented shower gel or body lotion for a zingy and energizing start to the day.*

OTHER COMBINATIONS

If exotic floral essential oils seem overpowering, in aroma or effect, blend them with lemon—its lightness, both in aroma and mood, helps to lessen the intensity of other oils so that they are not overwhelming.

CAUTION

Lemon essential oil is slightly phototoxic, so it should not be used in dilutions of more than 2 percent (2 drops to 5ml of carrier oil). Care should be taken when blending with grapefruit oil (see right) because both have phototoxic properties. If the two are used together, the combination of both oils should not exceed 2 percent.

" Cooling and refreshing grapefruit helps to overcome feelings of heaviness and lethargy."

GRAPEFRUIT
Citrus paradisi

Grapefruit essential oil is expressed from the peel of the fruit and, like most citrus oils, it is vibrantly uplifting. The aroma of grapefruit oil is a zesty, bittersweet citrus—as with lemon, true to the fruit.

BENEFITS

Grapefruit's intensely joyous and sweetly refreshing aroma makes it a natural choice when seeking a remedy to help tackle dark moods and a feeling of depleted energy. Its uplifting properties mean that the oil is best suited for daytime use.

Grapefruit is a cooling essential oil, which makes it a wonderful choice to help combat general feelings of lethargy and heaviness, particularly during the height of summer, when the heat may feel mentally depleting.

Its uplifting properties also make grapefruit a welcome essential oil to use during the shorter, darker days of the winter months, especially for those who suffer from seasonal affective disorder (SAD), which can cause lethargy, oversleeping, feelings of irritability, and changes in appetite, typically leading to overeating and, in turn, weight gain.

HOW TO USE

Use grapefruit essential oil alone or together with other vibrant oils to stay refreshed throughout the day, or enjoy its uplifting effect for a burst of energy first thing in the morning.

Make a revitalizing shower gel to help create a feeling of positivity for the day ahead. You can also add this blend to an unscented body lotion.
➡*See remedy, right.*

Use in a diffuser throughout the day to create an environment that enhances focus and injects energy.
➡*Add 6 drops grapefruit and 2 drops cardamom to a diffuser to help focus thoughts when you are feeling overwhelmed with work deadlines.*

OTHER COMBINATIONS

Grapefruit's light-bringing qualities are usefully blended with the deeply hypnotic floral essential oils for rollerball pulse point use, when moods swing between anxiety and depression.

CAUTION

Grapefruit is a mildly phototoxic oil so it should not be used in dilutions of more than 4 percent (4 drops to 5ml of carrier oil) for application to the skin. Particular care should be taken if blending with lemon essential oil (see opposite) as both oils are phototoxic—when used together, the combination should not be above 2 percent.

MANDARIN
Citrus reticulata

Like other citrus oils, mandarin essential oil is expressed from the peel of the fruit. Mandarin has a sweet, soft citrus aroma, which tends to settle rather than rise.

➡*See remedy, right.*

REMEDY

Zesty shower gel

Enjoy an energizing start to the day with this citrus shower gel. Add 6 drops grapefruit, 3 drops rosemary, and 3 drops may chang to 50ml unscented shower gel.

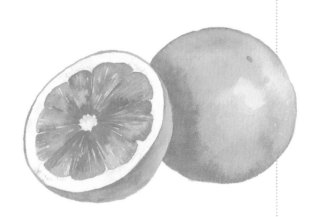

The gentle mellow softness lacks the vibrancy of the more stimulating citrus oils, giving mandarin a calming, restful effect.

BENEFITS

This oil is the Roman chamomile of the citrus family, being comforting and nurturing and bringing a sense of peace by calming anxious thoughts.

Mandarin is a good choice of oil for children and speaks to the inner child within all of us, gently soothing fretfulness and anxiety, suggesting hope and optimism, and dispelling feelings of gloom.

This relaxing oil is particularly helpful when stress is felt in the digestive system, for example, with conditions such as irritable bowel syndrome (IBS), where stress can exacerbate the condition, or with bloating and constipation. In this case, mandarin acts as a digestive tonic.

Using mandarin around bedtime can help to still an overactive and anxious mind that can make it hard to switch off and sleep.

HOW TO USE

Using this essential oil in a blend during the evening is particularly helpful when winding down before going to bed. Blend with other relaxing essential oils as part of a sleep management plan to help tackle insomnia.

Enjoy a relaxing bathtime soak.
➡*Dissolve 3 drops mandarin, 3 drops lavender, and 1 drop vetiver in 10ml unscented bubble bath, dispersant, or your chosen carrier oil for a relaxing soak in the evening.*

Diffuse in the bedroom around bedtime.
➡*Diffuse 2 drops mandarin and 2 drops Roman chamomile before bedtime. This gentle blend is helpful in a child's bedroom before settling them down, to help a fretful child sleep more soundly.*

OTHER COMBINATIONS

Try blending mandarin with rose and patchouli essential oils to use in a rollerball application—this is especially beneficial during times of anxiety and when you need grounding.

SWEET ORANGE
Citrus sinensis

Expressed from the fruit peel, this essential oil has a sweet and smooth citrus odor, strongly reminiscent of the fruit. Though this is an uplifting essential oil, it is more of a calmative than a stimulant, useful in settling intense emotional states, for example, where there is a general sense of anxiety without any clear trigger.

BENEFITS

Though this oil is similar to mandarin, sweet orange brings more of a joyful burst, rather than the feeling of calm happiness that is associated with mandarin. The greater vitality that sweet orange promotes makes this one of the more helpful citrus oils for lifting dark thoughts and a low mood.

Sweet orange has a physiological effect on the digestive system, especially where this is impacted by stress, which can lead to complaints such as irritable bowel syndrome (IBS). It is helpful when painful emotions lead either to a loss of appetite entirely, or to the need to suppress emotions by comfort eating.

This oil is comforting when used in a diffuser for older people suffering mental confusion with dementia. Several studies in clinical settings indicate that sweet orange's gently calming properties are beneficial for supporting dementia and helping to alleviate depression and general feelings of anxiety. Its stimulating properties also make it useful for helping to lift stuck, heavy feelings experienced with depression.

It has antimicrobial properties that are helpful when the immune system is depleted by long-term stress.

FOCUS ON

Coriander

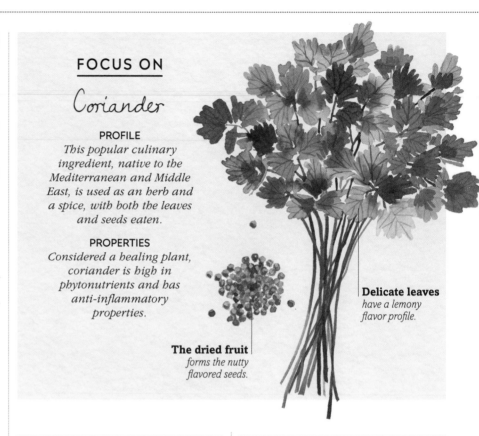

PROFILE
This popular culinary ingredient, native to the Mediterranean and Middle East, is used as an herb and a spice, with both the leaves and seeds eaten.

PROPERTIES
Considered a healing plant, coriander is high in phytonutrients and has anti-inflammatory properties.

The dried fruit *forms the nutty flavored seeds.*

Delicate leaves *have a lemony flavor profile.*

HOW TO USE

This easily vaporized oil is well tolerated, making it suitable for use in care settings, where its antimicrobial actions would be beneficial. It is also suitable for use on the skin, for example in massage or a spray.

Use in a diffuser to dispel low mood.
➡*Add 6–8 drops to a diffuser to lift your mood while staying calm.*
Make an uplifting facial spritz.
➡*Add 3 drops sweet orange and 2 drops geranium to 5ml vodka or glycerine, then add to a 50ml spray bottle and top up with water. Spritz a mist in front of the face, keeping the eyes closed, to bring a sense of optimism when overwhelmed.*
Make a relaxing massage blend.
➡*Add 3 drops sweet orange, 3 drops lavender, and 1 drop vetiver to 15ml of your chosen carrier oil for a massage to promote restful sleep.*

OTHER COMBINATIONS

Like most of the citrus oils, sweet orange is harmonious both aromatically and therapeutically with many other essential oils. Try with cardamom or rosemary to energize and motivate.

❝ *Sweet orange's vitality makes it a key citrus for helping to dispel dark thoughts.* ❞

CORIANDER
Coriandrum sativum

The essential oil is steam-distilled from the crushed seeds of the coriander plant. A leaf oil, cilantro, also exists. The aroma of coriander essential oil is fresh and spicy–sweet. Coriander is sometimes referred to as "the lavender of the seed oils," because it is a more calming oil than most.

BENEFITS

Coriander is both calming and uplifting and is helpful where stress impacts the digestive system, for example with irritable bowel syndrome (IBS), where its beneficial tonic effects are strong.

Coriander, in common with other culinary herbs and spices, stimulates the appetite, often something that is disrupted in times of stress, where some find that appetite completely vanishes, and others that emotional stress leads to comfort eating in an attempt to quell emotional pain. As stress interrupts digestive secretions, pain and discomfort in the digestive tract are common experiences.

HOW TO USE

Coriander is an effective deodorizer, useful when anxiety provokes sweating. It also helps to stimulate appetite that is lost due to stress.

Make a refreshing deodorant for times when you feel likely to perspire because of stress.
➡*Add 3 drops coriander and 2 drops lime to 5ml vodka or glycerine, then add to a 50ml spray bottle and top up with water. Spritz to dispel the odor of stress-induced perspiration.*

Diffuse to calm and stimulate.
➡*Add a few drops each of coriander and sweet orange to a diffuser to calm, uplift, and trigger the release of digestive enzymes when appetite is lost.*

OTHER COMBINATIONS

Coriander also blends well with sedating essential oils. Try an evening bath blend with Roman chamomile and lavender to help improve sleep.

PALMAROSA
Cymbopogon martinii

Steam- or water-distilled from the leaves and flowering tops of this tall grass, palmarosa is aromatically subtle with grassy, lemony–rose notes and is refreshing and uplifting. This safe, cooling oil can be freely used at all times of the day, on its own, or blended with other oils.

BENEFITS

Palmarosa calms feelings of pent-up irritability and the sensation of being a coiled spring of anxiety or tension. It is particularly helpful for emotional and physiological relief during menopause.

Physiologically, this oil is used in cooling blends to calm stress-related irritation and itchiness in the skin, particularly in a lotion or spritzer.
Palmarosa is useful where anxiety and panicky feelings result in a rapid pulse, or, during menopause, when stress increases the incidence of hot flashes and palpitations. This combination of how emotions and body can connect during menopause make it useful at this time.
It is helpful where tension may lead to a feeling that you might erupt or lash out. The combination of being an

especially safe oil to use and its ability to gently balance volatile emotions make this a helpful essential oil for coping with anxiety and feelings of being overwhelmed in pregnancy.

HOW TO USE

Use the oil on its own to help calm in the moment. It can also be blended with a carrier oil for use in the day or evening.

Make a refreshing and calming spray.
➡*Add 5 drops to 5ml vodka or glycerine, then add to a 50ml spray bottle and top up with water. Spritz a mist in front of the face, keeping the eyes closed, to alleviate irritability and anxiety.*
Create your own uplifting shower gel or body lotion.
➡*Make a morning shower gel or post-shower body lotion with 3 drops palmarosa and 3 drops lemon added to 50ml unscented gel, bubble bath, or body lotion to help calm and keep the spirits lifted for the day ahead.*

OTHER COMBINATIONS

Palmarosa blends well with lavender, where it might be used in a rollerball to apply to the temples when tension causes headaches.

SKIN PROTECTION

A synergy of compounds in palmarosa, including geraniol, promote cell growth, helping to make it a skin-nourishing oil.

"Jasmine's calming effects can be supportive where there are symptoms of anxiety and depression."

CARDAMOM
Elettaria cardamomum

Cardamom essential oil is steam-distilled from the dried seeds. The complex aroma of cardamom is fresh and spicy–sweet with citrus and floral notes. A powerfully uplifting oil, cardamom helps to clear the mind and invigorate.

BENEFITS

A major culinary spice, cardamom is particularly useful where stress impacts the digestive system, both for physiological and psychological reasons. It is also an uplifting oil. It is especially beneficial when used in the morning to energize mind and body for the day ahead.

Cardamom's settling action on the involuntary smooth muscle of the gut helps to ease digestion that has become uncomfortable or painful due to stress. The oil's uplifting emotional effects also help to counter disruptions to appetite that are common when suffering from anxiety and depression, as well as from the trauma of past experiences that may lead to post-traumatic stress.

Uplifting cardamom helps clear the mind, motivate, and lift a low mood, encouraging a feeling of optimism and greater vitality.

HOW TO USE

Use cardamom essential oil, either on its own or in a blend with other stimulating essential oils, to help you stay focused throughout the day. Refreshing and deodorizing, it is also useful when added to a shower gel or body lotion.

Use in a diffuser to enhance focus.
➡*Add a few drops each of cardamom, may chang, and rosemary to a diffuser when overwhelmed by deadlines and needing to keep alert and focused.*

Use in a shower gel or body lotion for an uplifting start to the day.
➡*Make a morning shower gel or post-shower body lotion for a burst of energy first thing. Add 3 drops cardamom, 4 drops bergamot FCF, and 6 drops grapefruit to 50ml unscented shower gel, bubble bath, or body lotion.*

Enjoy an invigorating and refreshing massage blend.
➡*Add 2 drops cardamom, 2 drops juniper, and 3 drops lemon to 15ml of your chosen carrier oil.*

OTHER COMBINATIONS

Uplifting cardamom blends exceptionally well with hypnotic florals such as jasmine or rose otto or absolute, where it is especially useful in a rollerball to apply to a pulse point to both lift the spirits and calm when feeling anxious.

JASMINE
Jasminum officinale/J. grandiflorum

Jasmine absolute is solvent-extracted from the flowers, which are too delicate to yield an essential oil from distillation. The powerful, sensuous floral aroma is heady, sweet, and musky, making it both uplifting and hypnotic. Because jasmine is such a powerful oil, it is best used in small quantities.

BENEFITS

Jasmine connects us to our physical being. Calming and uplifting, it is useful for both anxiety and depression. It can also be used as an emotional support where traumatic past events result in a feeling of being disconnected.

Responses to jasmine can vary between individuals, with some finding it sedating and helpful with sleeping difficulties, while others find it stimulates and increases feelings of wakefulness and of being alert and present.

Used in massage blends and body lotions, jasmine can be helpful where there has been a tendency to self-harm or use alcohol or drugs in a medicating way to release or numb painful, intense emotions.

ANCIENT HEALING

Ayurvedic and Chinese medicine traditions both use cardamom to address digestive complaints.

Its sensuous aroma helps couples relax where stress affects intimacy.

HOW TO USE

Jasmine's heady aroma can overpower, so use sparingly.

Use in a diffuser to calm and uplift.
➡*Add a few drops to a diffuser.*
Enjoy in a relaxing massage to help let go of stress between you and your partner and encourage intimacy.
➡*Add 4 drops jasmine, 7 drops sandalwood, and 4 drops cardamon to 30ml of your chosen carrier oil.*
Enjoy a relaxing evening bath blend to help promote restful sleep.
➡*See remedy, right.*

OTHER COMBINATIONS

Try blending with frankincense and clary sage to ease anxiety, panic, or a low mood.

CAUTION

Use with caution on sensitive skin. Jasmine is best avoided in pregnancy.

JUNIPER (BERRY)
Juniperus communis

Juniper can be steam-distilled from a blend of twigs, leaves, and berries, but the preferred source is from the berries alone. The oil's piercing aroma is fresh, warm, and piney. Several "juniper" essential oils exist, some of which are less safe than others, so source with care by its botanical name.

BENEFITS

Juniper is a cleansing, no-nonsense oil. Its invigorating properties make it useful for supporting depression and helping combat exhaustion and a loss of purpose.

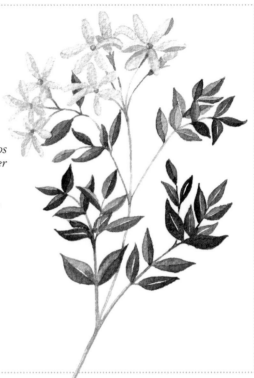

REMEDY

Unwinding bath blend

Add 2 drops jasmine, 2 drops vetiver, and 4 drops lavender to 10ml bubble bath, dispersant, or your chosen carrier oil. Add to the bath water for a sleep-inducing bedtime bath blend.

Juniper has an antimicrobial effect. Many studies show that depression weakens the immune system, so this strongly antimicrobial and stimulating oil is useful for those suffering from depression and low mood, helping to uplift and support immunity. Being prone to infection in itself lowers mood further, so the double action of this oil is beneficial.

HOW TO USE

Juniper is an effective background aroma, especially in the winter cold and flu season. As a stimulating oil, it is best used during the daytime, especially in the morning to lift spirits and motivate.

Use in a diffuser to promote a feeling of positivity.
➡*Add 4–8 drops to a diffuser, either on its own, or in a blend with lemon, which is both energizing and positive, as well as antimicrobial.*

Make an invigorating shower gel.
➡*Add 4 drops juniper, 4 drops lemon, and 6 drops bergamot FCF to 50ml unscented shower gel, bubble bath, or body lotion for a fresh start to the day.*
Use in a rollerball application.
➡*Add 3 drops juniper, 3 drops cedarwood Atlas, and 2 drops rose otto or absolute to a rollerball to apply to a pulse point on the wrist. (Use rose otto instead of absolute in the case of skin sensitivity.) This is a surprisingly steadying application when feeling overwhelmed, alone, or "lost," or when experiencing stress-related menopause symptoms.*

OTHER COMBINATIONS

Try blending juniper essential oil with soothing frankincense and focusing, stimulating rosemary.

CAUTION

Avoid juniper oil in pregnancy.

HOW TO MAKE
AN ESSENTIAL OIL SPRAY

Adding essential oils to water, or floral water, for use in a spray atomizer provides an effective way to use essential oils in the moment wherever you are. The essential oils need to be dissolved first in alcohol, such as 90 percent proof ethanol alcohol. Lower percentages will produce a cloudier liquid.

Makes 3½ tbsp

INGREDIENTS

Essential oil drops—as specified
1 tsp ethanol alcohol,
vodka, or glycerine
3 tbsp water, floral water (such as
rose), or a combination of water
and floral water

EQUIPMENT

Bottle with a spray atomizer

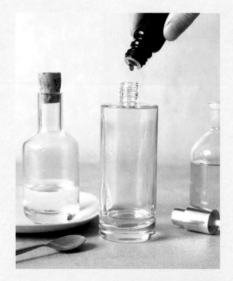

1 Sterilize the spray bottle (see p.53). Add the essential oil drops and the alcohol to the bottle. Allow to sit for a little while at room temperature until the drops have dissolved.

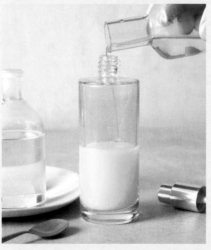

2 Top up with the water, floral water, or combination of the two, to fill the spray bottle. Seal with the atomizer lid, and it is ready to use.

STORAGE

Sprays are ideal for carrying around. When not using, keep the spray in the fridge, where it can be stored for up to three months.

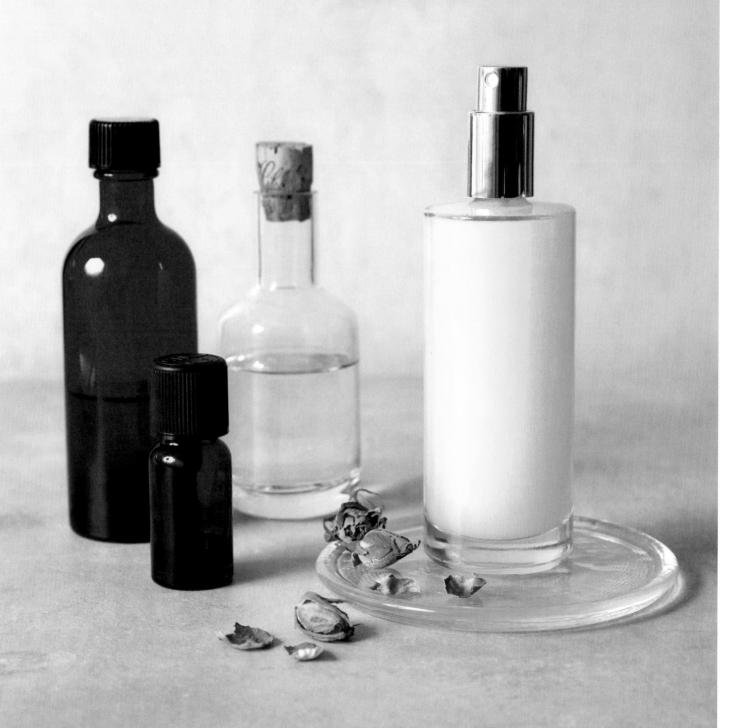

LAVENDER

Lavandula angustifolia/officinalis/vera

This well-known garden plant and medicinal herb needs careful sourcing by botanical name, as often lavender essential oil is not true lavender, but a less safe hybrid, lavandin. The essential oil is steam-distilled from the flowering tops. The familiar, bittersweet, comforting floral aroma is heady and relaxing.

BENEFITS

With its calming, balancing action on the body and mind, lavender is particularly helpful when emotions are volatile and overcharged, and normal rhythms in the body and behavior are disrupted, especially when suffering with anxiety.

Lavender's calming and sedative actions, whether as a herb or an essential oil, are well-documented, making it an extremely effective oil for sleeping disorders and anxiety. It is well known for helping to settle disturbed sleeping patterns.

The oil is especially supportive where stress impacts the body—in the heart as palpitations and raised blood

" Relaxing and sedative, lavender is a deeply supportive oil for sleep complaints."

FOCUS ON

Melissa

PROFILE

Documented in use since classical times, melissa, or lemon balm, is native to central and southern Europe. Its highly aromatic leaves release a sweetly tart scent when rubbed.

PROPERTIES

Melissa is a soothing, calming, and cooling essential oil.

The leaves *are a popular culinary ingredient.*

pressure; in the respiratory system as asthma; in the digestive system; and with skin conditions such as eczema and psoriasis.

Lavender is analgesic, relieving problems such as tension headaches, which can cause stress, or exacerbate it. It is also antimicrobial.

Several clinical studies have shown that this humble plant is an astonishingly effective remedy with wide medicinal application in a number of conditions. Because emotional stress always expresses itself via the body, and lavender is extremely effective in supporting every system and function in the body, this is an especially useful oil.

HOW TO USE

Lavender's sedative action means it is best used in the evening, when it can help

achieve calmness. As well as the methods below, use in a massage oil or body lotion.

Inhale the aroma at bedtime.
➡️*Sprinkle 2–3 drops on the pillowcase to quiet mental chatter before sleep.*

Make a relaxing bedtime bath blend.
➡️*Blend 3 drops lavender, 3 drops mandarin, and 2 drops vetiver with 10ml unscented bubble bath, dispersant, or your chosen carrier oil as part of a sleep-inducing routine.*

OTHER COMBINATIONS

Lavender has a complex fragrant profile, which makes it aromatically harmonious with most other essential oils. Therapeutically, it is best blended with other calming or balancing oils, such as Roman chamomile or geranium, rather than stimulating ones.

MAY CHANG
Litsea cubeba

This uplifting oil is steam-distilled from the peppercornlike fruits of the small tropical tree. Aromatically it is reminiscent of lemon sherbet, with sweet and zingy notes. Where skin is sensitive or damaged, application to the skin is best avoided (see caution, right).

BENEFITS

A vibrantly uplifting oil, may chang also has a calming action when anxiety may lead to stress-related palpitations or provoke stress-related asthma.

This oil has a joyous, optimistic effect, bringing a sense of vitality, helpful where low mood and depression make everything feel stuck and heavy.

The "sunburst" effect of inhaling may chang makes it a particularly welcome oil in the darkness and gloom of winter for those who suffer with seasonal affective disorder (SAD).

HOW TO USE

Properly diluted, paying attention to any cautions imposed by stress-related skin conditions such as eczema, this is a good choice of oil to use in the morning.

Use in a body lotion for an optimistic and energetic start to the day.
➡ *Add 4 drops may chang, 6 drops bergamot (FCF), and 3 drops rosemary to 50ml unscented body lotion for application after a morning shower.*

Diffuse the oil as a background scent, which is particularly helpful during the working day when energy and motivation tend to slump in the afternoon.
➡ *Diffuse 2 drops may chang, 4 drops bergamot, and 2 drops rosemary.*

OTHER COMBINATIONS

Blend may chang with lavender and frankincense if you swing between anxiety and depression for a sense of calm and balance. Take care when blending with melissa (see below) as this blend can irritate skin. Combined, the oils must not be above 2 percent.

CAUTION

May chang should not be used at more than 2 percent dilution (2 drops to 5ml carrier oil) as it can be a skin irritant.

MELISSA
Melissa officinalis

Melissa is a garden herb also known as lemon balm, used since classical times. Steam-distilled from the leaves and flowering tops, its aroma is herby, lemony, and haylike. The essential oil is often adulterated, as it has a very low yield, making it a costly oil. Avoid inexpensive "nature identical" melissa, which will be a blend of oils without therapeutic value. Do not use on broken or damaged skin (see caution, below).

BENEFITS

Melissa's folk name—Heart's Delight—indicates one of its major therapeutic actions, to promote a sense of calm. Melissa also helps to focus the mind and support cognitive function. The oil is used widely across an entire range of mental and emotional symptoms, as it is both extremely powerful and very gentle (other than its potential skin cautions).

Melissa both sharpens mental acuity and has a calming effect on the autonomic nervous system, particularly on the fight-or-flight response that comes with high anxiety levels, which in turn affects the heart and lungs.

There is now particular interest in using this essential oil to help Alzheimer's sufferers, when emotional distress and memory loss feed negatively into each other.

Uplifting and calming, melissa is helpful when emotional stress causes mental confusion and with anxiety, depression, mood swings, and sleeping problems.

HOW TO USE

Because of its calming action, melissa is best used later in the day to help promote restful sleep. It is also effective in times of anxiety.

Use in a diffuser to help wind down.
➡ *Add 2 drops melissa and 4 drops lavender to a diffuser an hour before bedtime as part of a conscious sleep management wind-down routine.*

Inhale to quell anxiety quickly.
➡ *Add a drop of a frankincense and melissa blend to a tissue. Cup it in the hand, hold loosely over the nose and mouth, and inhale during a panic attack as a rapid way to stop shallow breathing and ground yourself.*

OTHER COMBINATIONS

Combine melissa with uplifting, stress-relieving oils such as neroli and clary sage, dabbed on pulse points, if prone to anxiety. Or blend with vibrant, stimulating oils such as rosemary and grapefruit to help with low mood and feelings of hopelessness. Take care if blending with may chang (see above)—the combination of both oils must not exceed 2 percent.

CAUTION

Melissa should not be used a more than 2 percent dilution (2 drops to 5ml carrier oil) as it can be a skin irritant. Do not use on broken or damaged skin.

MARJORAM
Origanum marjorana

Sweet, or French, marjoram is a sedating and restorative essential oil. It is steam-distilled from the fresh or dried flowering tops and has a warm, herby, spicy, bittersweet aroma. Marjoram is a useful remedy for anxiety, but it is too sedating to use long-term for depression. Source the oil carefully by its botanical name because some oils are incorrectly named marjoram and are unsafe for use in aromatherapy.

BENEFITS

This somewhat emotionally numbing oil is a potent one for hyper-aroused, overreactive states, particularly when anxiety and panic affects the heart and lungs in the form of palpitations and shallow breathing.

Sweet marjoram is a deeply relaxing essential oil, which makes it a fortifying oil for when there is a feeling of being exhausted by overstretched emotions.

Used in combination with other sedating oils, sweet marjoram helps to break a cycle of restlessness, an inability to sleep, and a mind that

SETTLING TEA

Marjoram tea, made from the fresh or dried leaves, is a popular remedy for soothing stress-related digestive complaints.

cannot switch off, when prolonged nervous tension puts a strain on the adrenal glands, leading to adrenal burnout, thus perpetuating the cycle of fatigue.

HOW TO USE

Sweet marjoram is best used late in the day, and can be diffused or blended with other relaxing oils that are aromatically complementary. It is also a useful remedy to quell anxiety during panic attacks.

Enjoy a relaxing evening bath or wind-down massage.
➡ *Add 2 drops sweet marjoram, 3 drops lavender, and 1 drop neroli to 10ml unscented bubble bath, dispersant, or carrier oil for a bedtime soak. Or use this blend in a relaxing evening massage oil to help unwind.*
Use in a rollerball applicator.
➡ *Add 3 drops sweet marjoram, 2 drops ylang ylang, 5 drops cedarwood Atlas, and 10ml of your chosen carrier oil to a rollerball. Apply to the wrist pulse points and inhale, or dab between the upper lip and nose, to center and ground yourself when anxious feelings arise.*

OTHER COMBINATIONS

Sweet marjoram is a comforting aromatic combination when blended with hypnotic potent florals such as ylang ylang or rose essential oils.

"Geranium is balancing mentally and physically, making it a useful support for premenstrual symptoms."

GERANIUM
Pelargonium graveolens

The essential oil is steam-distilled from the leaves of the plant, which should properly be called a pelargonium, rather than a geranium, because it is not from the familiar garden plant, but a tropical species. Its powerful aroma is rosy, sweet, minty-fresh, and green.

BENEFITS

Geranium is an extremely balancing oil, both emotionally and physically. It is primarily used to alleviate some of the emotional symptoms associated with premenstrual syndrome and is also a major skincare oil.

As a hormonal balancer, geranium is particularly helpful where volatile mood swings, whether of anxiety, despair, irritability, rage, or weepiness, might be linked to the menstrual cycle.
With both antidepressant and calming properties, geranium is helpful in more general uses to alleviate anxiety and depression.
Geranium is an antimicrobial oil, sebum-balancing, and promotes skin health, making it useful when stress impacts the skin—whether the skin is dry or oily—leading to acne outbreaks or boils.

With its expressive, extrovert aroma, this is a remedy for those who take suffering inward and find it difficult to express their own emotional needs.

HOW TO USE

Geranium can be applied in many ways. As well as safe in a facial spritz and ideal to diffuse day or night, it can also be used in shower gels, a bath or massage oil blend, and is invaluable in a rollerball.

Use in a diffuser at any time to lift a low mood and feelings of despair.
➡️*Add 2–3 drops geranium and 4–5 drops sweet orange to a diffuser, for a powerfully uplifting blend.*
Make a refreshing facial spray.
➡️*Add 5 drops geranium and 5ml vodka or glycerine to a 50ml spray bottle and top up with water. Spritz a mist in front of the face, keeping the eyes closed, to cool, uplift, and refresh when hormonal fluctuations make you feel volatile and unsettled.*

OTHER COMBINATIONS

Blend with other balancing oils such as bergamot or frankincense in a rollerball to ground and settle. For anxiety, partner with lavender and clary sage essential oils; and to lift mood blend geranium with rosemary and grapefruit.

PATCHOULI
Pogostemon cablin

Steam-distilled from the lightly fermented dried leaves of the plant, this bushy tropical herb has a rich, sweet, musky, spicy, and earthy aroma. Grounding and revitalizing, patchouli is helpful for those who tend to "live inside their heads," which can lead to a feeling of being disconnected.

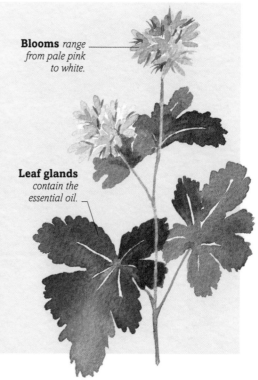

FOCUS ON

Pelargonium

PROFILE
Native to South Africa, this flowering shrub has pale pink to white flowers and deeply lined leaves, which hold the essential oil.

PROPERTIES
In addition to its balancing and antimicrobial properties, this geranium variety has astringent and anti-inflammatory actions, helping to combat the effects of stress on the skin and support the body and mind.

Blooms *range from pale pink to white.*

Leaf glands *contain the essential oil.*

BENEFITS

Patchouli is an antidepressant and tonic herb that is particularly helpful in supporting the nervous system.

Patchouli's grounding properties make it useful for alleviating symptoms of both anxiety and depression.
Patchouli can be used as a remedy to help reconnect to sensual enjoyment. It is also beneficial when emotional challenges lead to a more generalized loss of enjoyment in the physicality of existence—resulting, for example, in a loss of appetite for intimacy, food, or taking care of oneself, and in an inability to sleep.
Patchouli can be helpful for those whose experience of physicality is difficult and find that the body is a hard place to be—for example, those who live with chronic pain, or may have been through a very difficult and traumatic labor during childbirth.

HOW TO USE

This musky, peaty, sensual aromatic is particularly suited for intimate occasions in a massage oil blend, or in an evening bath to help relaxation before bed.

Use in a diffuser to relax and encourage feelings of intimacy.
➡️*Diffuse a few drops each of patchouli, jasmine, and sweet orange.*
Enjoy a relaxing bath blend.
➡️*Blend 2 drops patchouli, 3 drops lavender, and 1 drop geranium with 10ml of unscented bubble bath, dispersant, or carrier oil and disperse in a bath to unwind from the day's stresses and encourage restful sleep. Replace lavender with sandalwood for a sensual massage oil or bath blend.*

OTHER COMBINATIONS

Patchouli, neroli, and sandalwood make a helpful massage oil blend for those who are too stressed and exhausted to relax.

ROSE ABSOLUTE AND OTTO

Rosa centifolia/damascena

This long-venerated medicinal and garden plant yields two aromatic extracts from the handpicked flowers. Rose absolute is solvent extracted, usually from the *Rosa centifolia* variety. The essential oil, rose otto, is usually steam-distilled from *Rosa damascena*. Rose otto has a more ethereal, thinner, honey-soft aroma, whereas rose absolute contains much more of the flower's scent, true to the aromatic, musky, full-bodied depth of roses. The two oils can be used interchangeably, though rose otto is preferable with hypersensitive skin.

BENEFITS

Used since classical times as a heart remedy, both physically and emotionally, rose is powerfully comforting, soothing, and uplifting. Like other long-used aromatics with strong connections to sacred, meditative practice, its healing potential is intensified by conscious, mindful use and it is not an oil to be used liberally, without thought.

Rose is like a strong, steady "comfort blanket" for times when the spirit is wounded. Many experience the aroma as a release and softening of feelings that weigh heavily on the heart.

" Comforting rose can help release heavy emotions."

Soothing rose has long been used to support women with a difficult menstrual history—both physically and mentally, during the postnatal period, and, particularly, during menopause.

Rose evokes powerful positive associations in older people suffering with dementia, helping to lift mood and calm anxiety.

The oil can be very supportive alongside talking therapy, where the deep work involved can cause painful memories to resurface.

Used in aromatherapy massage with a sensitive practitioner, rose can help let go of difficult memories that get locked in the body, manifesting as physical and mental symptoms.

HOW TO USE

Only a few drops of this safe yet powerful oil are required when creating a blend. It is especially suited for use on its own when feeling overwhelmed.

Make a comforting facial spritzer to use when in a state of high anxiety or when you are experiencing heavy thoughts that feel overwhelming. This soothing facial spritz is also extremely helpful for hot flashes, where an adrenaline rush and racing heart induce anxiety.

➡ *See remedy, below.*

Use in a rollerball applicator.

➡ *Add 5 drops rose and 10ml of your chosen carrier oil to a rollerball. Apply the blend to the wrist pulse points and inhale, or dab between the upper lip and nose, to help center and ground yourself and lift the spirits when feeling low.*

OTHER COMBINATIONS

Rose partners with many essential oils, but is especially powerful with frankincense and sandalwood when consciously working to address long-standing emotional anguish.

REMEDY

Comforting facial spritz

Blend 5 drops rose otto or absolute with 5ml vodka or glycerine. Transfer to a 50ml spray bottle and top up with water. Spritz a mist in front of the face, keeping the eyes closed.

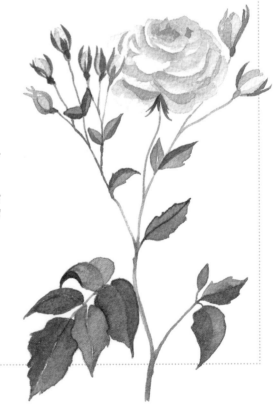

ROSEMARY
Rosmarinus officinalis

Rosemary is steam-distilled from the flowering tops. Its familiar odor is fresh, herby, and medicinal. Rosemary's chemistry can contain high levels of problematic compounds so the essential oil should be sourced carefully by its botanical name from a reputable supplier who trades specifically with practitioners.

BENEFITS

Rosemary's invigorating, stimulating actions make it most suitable for daytime use. It helps to motivate, lifts a low mood, and is useful for those who need a bit of help to get going in the morning. It can also be useful for reenergizing during the post-lunch slump.

Rosemary increases mental alertness and reactions, which means it is most useful for those prone to depression and over-introspection, but can be overly stimulating, rather than calming, for those who are hyper-aroused and prone to anxiety.

Rosemary sharpens thinking and alertness and is a useful essential oil for clearing fuzzy thinking—or brain fog.

HOW TO USE

Try using rosemary in combination with other uplifting and stimulating oils in the morning or use in the early afternoon to increase energy levels and stay alert.

Use in a diffuser to enhance focus.
➡ *Add 3 drops each of rosemary and juniper berry to a diffuser to freshen and cleanse stuffy environments to help promote clear thinking.*

Use in an invigorating shower gel or body lotion at the start of the day.
➡ *Add 4 drops rosemary, 2 drops cardamom, and 6 drops lime to 50ml unscented shower gel, bubble bath, or body lotion to energize body and mind.*

OTHER COMBINATIONS

For the most effective synergy, blend with other invigorating oils. Uplifting citrus oils pair particularly well, as do may chang, frankincense, and thyme linalool.

CAUTION

Avoid during pregnancy. Consult a trained practitioner before using with epilepsy.

CLARY SAGE
Salvia sclarea

Steam-distilled from the flowering tops, the tenacious aroma of clary sage is bittersweet, musky, and haylike. Calming and uplifting, this powerful oil has a traditional use as a support to spiritual practice. It can have a profound and sedating effect, leading some to feel spaced out, so should be used with caution. As several sages exist, some less safe than others, source by its botanical name from a reputable supplier.

BENEFITS

This intense oil is both uplifting and sedating. Blended with calming, sedative oils, it can be helpful for extreme anxiety; blended with uplifting and stimulating oils, it can be supportive with depression.

Clary sage is helpful, physically and emotionally, during menopause.

It can be an excellent oil for sleeping difficulties; however, some report vivid dreams after evening massage with this oil, so experiences can vary.

MEMORY BOOST

A 2016 study found that students who studied in a room scented with rosemary essential oil showed a 5 to 7 percent improvement in memory.

Its calming properties are especially helpful when anxiety affects the heart, in the form of palpitations and raised blood pressure, and the lungs, with shallow breathing and asthma.

HOW TO USE

Clary sage is helpful in the moment to quell anxiety and panic attacks. It is also useful when hot flashes trigger palpitations and anxiety.

Make a calming facial spritz.
➡ *Add 2 drops clary sage, 3 drops geranium, and 5ml vodka or glycerine to a 50ml spray bottle and top up with water. Spritz a mist in front of the face, keeping the eyes closed, to reduce anxiety linked to menopausal hot flashes.*

Inhale from a tissue.
➡ *Add a drop of clary sage to a tissue. When in a state of panic, cup the scrunched tissue in the hands, hold over the nose and mouth, and inhale.*

OTHER COMBINATIONS

Try with ylang ylang and cedarwood Atlas or frankincense to uplift and calm.

CAUTION

Avoid during pregnancy.

SANDALWOOD
Santalum album

Sandalwood has been used in Oriental medicines for thousands of years. Its aroma is unforgettable—soft, deep, and sweetly woody. This restorative and grounding essential oil is a major remedy for deep emotional trauma. Because it is steam-distilled from the felled tree, this precious oil should be used with respect, as the species is under threat. Source from an ethical supplier who is committed to sustainability.

BENEFITS

This, like other tree oils with connections to sacred and religious use, is most therapeutically helpful when used intentionally and mindfully to accompany practices such as yoga and meditation, rather than as a "quick fix" for symptoms.

Sandalwood is a deeply comforting support when undergoing times of immense challenge, and it is particularly indicated with those whose emotional challenges may be

" A deeply balancing oil, sandalwood can enhance meditative practice."

FOCUS ON

Thyme linalool

PROFILE
Native to the Mediterranean, thyme is now grown worldwide. Woody and strongly aromatic, this popular culinary plant thrives in dry, sunny climes.

PROPERTIES
As well as thyme linalool's supportive and fortifying properties, the plant is thought to be strongly antioxidant, helping to protect the body and mind against the damaging effects of long-term stress.

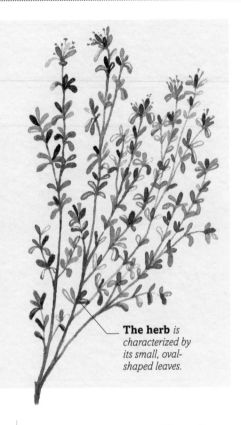

The herb *is characterized by its small, oval-shaped leaves.*

linked with the diagnosis of a progressive or terminal illness. **Energetically and spiritually,** sandalwood is seen as a supremely balancing remedy. It is an essential oil that can be helpfully and thoughtfully connected with for those who have suffered traumatic stress. Massage from a practitioner who is able to listen and respond sensitively can work well therapeutically alongside talking therapies or cognitive therapy work.

HOW TO USE

This is one of the few oils that is powerful enough to use on its own, for mental, emotional, and spiritual well-being, though there are other oils of similar depth with which it can be usefully combined.

Use in a diffuser as part of a conscious practice of mindful meditation or focused relaxation exercises.

➤*Add a few drops to a diffuser. To increase the positive effects of this oil, avoid vaporizing it just as a "background" aroma.*

Make a massage blend for massaging the hands of a loved one who is terminally ill.

➤*Add 2 drops to 5ml of your chosen carrier oil to use in a sensitive hand massage. Touch and the power of this oil combined are emotionally healing to both the giver and the receiver here.*

OTHER COMBINATIONS

The most powerful partners for sandalwood, which could be used in a massage or rollerball, are frankincense and rose. This is a helpful combination to have on hand when someone is engaged in deep work in talking therapy, particularly when used in a massage by a sensitive practitioner who is careful not to provoke a release of emotions too early.

THYME LINALOOL
Thymus vulgaris

Thyme is steam- or water-distilled from its leaves and flowering tops. Its aroma is warm, herby, spicy, floral, and somewhat medicinal. This strengthening, fortifying oil is useful for those who feel depleted by long-term stress. The essential oil must be sourced carefully because the same botanical can produce oils that vary in safety. Look for thyme linalool or thyme linalol, and avoid any essential oils that are identified as red or white thyme, which can provoke skin irritation.

BENEFITS

Uplifting and slightly bracing, thyme is also supportive for the nervous system.

Thyme linalool is helpful for lifting the spirits with depression.

The supportive properties of thyme linalool can be used where long-term anxiety has caused the adrenal glands to be overworked, leading to fatigue.

Thyme linalool can be useful when combined with more relaxing oils to help address sleeping difficulties; in particular, where the body and mind have become too exhausted and wired to relax properly.

As an antimicrobial and immune-stimulant remedy, thyme linalool is not only helpful in supporting those suffering from depression, but also in supporting the depleted immune system that is so often linked with chronic depression.

HOW TO USE

Use thyme linalool during the day with other stimulating and uplifting oils, or combine with restful essential oils when winding down in the evening.

Diffuse with other uplifting oils for an upbeat, spirit-lifting daytime blend.
➡*Add a few drops each of thyme linalool, may chang, and lime to a diffuser.*

Make a shower gel or body lotion.
➡*Add 3 drops thyme linalool, 5 drops bergamot (FCF), and 5 drops petitgrain to 50ml unscented shower gel, bubble bath, or body lotion for a refreshing blend that is uplifting and balancing.*

Enjoy in a relaxing bedtime bath.
➡*Add 4 drops thyme linalool, 3 drops neroli, and 1 drop Roman chamomile to 10ml of unscented bubble bath, dispersant, or your chosen carrier oil.*

OTHER COMBINATIONS

Use with ylang ylang and lavender to calm.

VETIVER
Vetiveria zizanoides

Vetiver is a tropical grass whose essential oil is steam-distilled from the dried roots. The tenacious aroma is smoky and sweet, earthy, rich, and textured. Vetiver is a helpful remedy for anxiety, though it can be too grounding and introspective to use long-term with depression. The plant itself is extremely strong, and has been widely used ecologically to help rectify soil erosion and contamination.

BENEFITS

Deeply sedating and restorative, this oil echoes the strength of the plant, helping us to hold on to our sense of identity.

Its restorative action is helpful when traumatic stress affects sleep and leads to a feeling of being spaced out, and where vitality is depleted by chronic anxiety.

Vetiver helps to contain emotions, useful when extreme panic and an overreactive state prevents us from accessing our core strength. Its restorative properties help us to rest and tap into our inner resources.

HOW TO USE

Vetiver is not an oil that is well-suited to daytime use, unless it is used in a rollerball pulse point application during a panic attack. The oil is effective when it is used with other calming, strong-smelling essential oils in a bath blend or late evening diffusion.

Enjoy a restful evening soak.
➡*Add 2 drops vetiver, 2 drops ylang ylang, and 3 drops lavender to 10ml of bubble bath, dispersant, or your chosen carrier oil for a bedtime bath.*

Use in a rollerball application.
➡*Add 2 drops vetiver, 4 drops neroli, 4 drops cedarwood Atlas, and 10ml of your chosen carrier oil to a rollerball to apply to the pulse points and inhale when feeling overwhelmed by anxiety.*

OTHER COMBINATIONS

Vetiver essential oil also blends well with patchouli and jasmine; this blend might be used in a sensual massage to help unwind from the stresses of the day.

POPULAR SCENT

Vetiver essential oil has a complex chemical composition with more than 100 compounds, making it a commonly chosen ingredient in perfumes.

FOODS AND SUPPLEMENTS

INTRODUCTION

THE ROLE OF NUTRIENTS

What you eat has a direct and long-lasting effect on your brain. Optimal mental health and well-being requires a diet with a wide variety of nutrient-rich foods. The following chapter explores a range of beneficial foods that support optimal brain function and help maintain energy, avoiding sugar dips to keep moods balanced and supporting concentration, focus, and memory.

FOODS FOR MENTAL WELLNESS

Each of us is unique, requiring different nutrients in varying concentrations depending on age, sex, lifestyle, genetics, culture, and ethnicity. There are also variations in the nutrients found in any one food: how it was grown, when it was picked, and how long it was stored all make a difference. Despite individual variations, there are key nutrients that are crucial for our bodies and brains.

Energizing foods are vital for the brain to work well. Our brains account for only about 2 percent of our total body weight, yet consume at least 20 percent of our daily energy supply, which comes from the food we eat. Sustained energy comes from a steady release of glucose from complex carbohydrates such as whole grains and legumes, which support alertness and balance mood. Complex carbohydrates also provide fiber to support the gut. Proteins are critical in delivering essential nutrients to the brain and optimizing cognitive function. Aim to eat a small amount of protein at each meal from a range of sources such as meat, fish, poultry, eggs, legumes, nuts and seeds, grains, and pseudo-grains, such as quinoa and wild rice.

Antioxidants prevent damage to the body's cells from highly reactive, unstable free radical molecules. Fruit and vegetables are packed full of antioxidants such as beta-carotene, vitamins C and E, copper, zinc, and selenium. They also contain phytonutrients, plant compounds that act as antioxidants. Lycopene in tomatoes, quercetin in onions, ergothioneine in shiitake mushrooms, and glutathione in asparagus are potent phytonutrients.

Hydrating foods play a role along with fluids in preventing loss of brain function. Water is critical for our brains, as it helps to form proteins, absorb nutrients, and eliminate waste. Just a 2 percent decrease in hydration

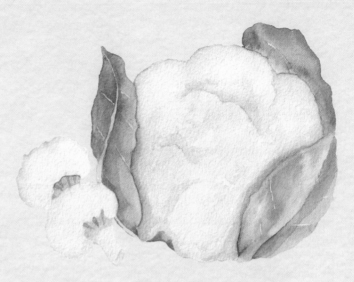

Cauliflower is an excellent source of fiber, supporting the gut and, in turn, the brain via the gut–brain axis.

can affect concentration, memory, mood, and emotions. Consume fruit and vegetables with high water content, such as oranges, grapefruit, and celery.

Gut-supporting foods are key for mental wellness. The foods we eat affect the diversity, quality, and quantity of healthy gut microorganisms. The gut and brain are linked via the gut–brain axis (see p.22), so a healthy gut microbiome can positively affect mental health. Two foods that increase beneficial bacteria are probiotics, which supply healthy bacteria, and prebiotics, nondigestible complex carbohydrates that ferment in the gut to produce energy and promote beneficial bacteria. Yogurt and kefir are probiotics. Prebiotics are found in foods such as onions and garlic, Jerusalem artichokes, and apples. Other pre- and probiotics are highlighted throughout this chapter. Fiber, soluble and insoluble, also supports the gut. Whole grains and most fruit and vegetables such as cauliflower are good sources.

Certain nutrients promote calm and relaxation. Magnesium is thought to support brain functions that help lower stress levels, and omega-3 fats are beneficial for calming the nervous system. In addition, the amino acid tryptophan is converted in the body to the soothing neurotransmitter serotonin, and choline is needed for the production of neurotransmitters that affect mood. Leafy greens, almonds, and pumpkin seeds are good sources of magnesium; salmon supplies omega-3 fats; oats provide tryptophan; and eggs are packed full of nutrients, including choline, which help keep us calm and relaxed.

Immune-boosting foods that help us ward off illness support our well-being. Key nutrients help our highly complex immune systems to function optimally. Beta-carotene, vitamin C, and vitamin E, found abundantly in vegetables and fruits, all boost immune function. Gut health, supported by probiotics and prebiotics (see opposite) also plays a major role in immunity.

" Foods with anti-inflammatory properties help to support healthy brain function."

Foods with anti-inflammatory properties, such as tomatoes, green leaves, olive oil, nuts, summer berries, and fruits, control chronic inflammation in the body. Eating the right fats is also key for healthy brain function. The fatty acid DHA (docosahexaenoic acid) promotes healthy brain functioning. DHA is found in fatty fish or is synthesized from plant-based sources of alpha-linolenic acid (ALA) found in hemp or linseed.

Mood-enhancing foods include vitamin C-rich vegetables and fruits, high-fiber whole grains and good-quality protein, especially from chicken, eggs, nuts, and seeds, high in tryptophan, the amino acid that triggers serotonin. B vitamins produce mood-regulating neurotransmitters; pulses are a good source. Prebiotics and probiotics create a healthy gut microbiome, linked with lower rates of mood disorders; and phytonutrients in raw chocolate are well known for enhancing mood. In addition, the deep connection of food with home and community nourishes well-being.

SUPPLEMENTS

Eating a range of wholefoods generally meets our nutritional needs. However, for different reasons, sometimes we do not get enough nutrients from the food we eat and need extra help. Pages 174–5 look at key mineral and vitamin supplements that can support diet if needed. High-quality supplements provide the most nutritional value, so look for the best you can afford that are free from additives.

WHAT TO AVOID

As well as ensuring we eat key nutrients for well-being, it is also important to know what to avoid, both in terms of damaging foods and cooking methods that leach nurients.

Refined carbohydrates can wreak havoc on brain health. A diet high in sugar and refined carbohydrates causes a rapid rise in blood sugar levels. To stop the level of

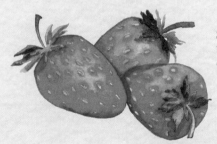

Strawberries *provide folate, which helps the body to make neurotransmitters such as dopamine.*

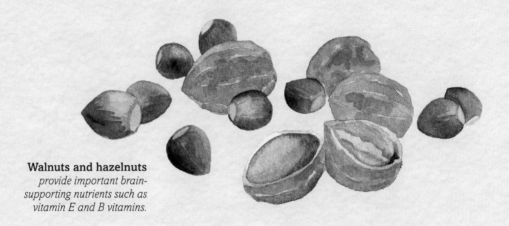

Walnuts and hazelnuts
provide important brain-supporting nutrients such as vitamin E and B vitamins.

glucose in the bloodstream spiraling, the pancreas releases insulin, sending a signal to muscle cells to take up excess sugar. In time, muscles become insulin resistant, negatively impacting cognitive function and increasing the risk of Type 2 diabetes, associated with a range of neurological diseases.

Altered fats are detrimental to brain health. Trans fats found in processed foods negatively affect mood and memory. Avoid cooking with polyunsaturated oils, as heat will create free radicals that can damage brain cells.

Avoid high-temperature cooking methods. If you boil vegetables, use the water as it contains valuable nutrients. To preserve nutrients, steam, steam–sauté, or bake.

Aluminum cookware has been linked to Alzheimer's disease. Also, many nonstick pans contain toxic compounds. Stainless steel, glass, and ceramic are the safest choices.

BOOSTING NUTRIENTS

While high-temperature cooking should be avoided (see opposite), practices such as soaking, sprouting, and fermenting can boost nutrients.

Soaking *grains and legumes pre-cooking reduces phytates, compounds that bind to minerals such as calcium, iron, and zinc, impairing absorption; and lectins, which damage the gut wall.*

Sprouting seeds *makes valuable nutritients more accessible. Most seeds, including grains and legumes, can be sprouted (p.170). After sprouting, cook red kidney beans before eating to destroy toxic phytohaemagglutinin.*

Lacto-fermenting *vegetables improves the bioavailabilty of nutrients and provides the gut with good bacteria. Fermented grains, legumes, and dairy are also easier to digest.*

LEAFY GREENS

Green leaves are brimming with nutrients and plant compounds that provide antioxidants, supporting our mental health and well-being. As well as being a natural and easy way to relieve stress and soothe the mind, an increasing amount of evidence suggests that regularly including leafy greens in our diets—ideally every day—can help to slow the decline in cognitive function that occurs with age.

CHARD

This slightly bitter vegetable has large, distinctive green leaves and an array of different-colored stalks, depending on the variety. Colors range from white (commonly known as Swiss chard) to yellow, pink, and red. Its bitter edge is lost during cooking, leaving an earthy, sweet flavor. Chard is a rich source of phytonutrients with antioxidant and anti-inflammatory properties.

BENEFITS

Chard is full of beneficial nutrients that support mental health and well-being. A good source of magnesium, vitamin E, and B vitamins, it also provides iron, potassium, beta-carotene, and vitamin C. It is an excellent source of fiber, helping to maintain gut health and, in turn, promote a healthy brain–gut connection.

Magnesium is a mineral fundamental to health and well-being, supporting a wide range of chemical reactions in the body. By assisting electrical activity in the brain, it helps us to have an effective recall of events and also promotes positivity and good-quality sleep. Magnesium is also key for the production of feel-good hormones such as serotonin in the brain. A lack of magnesium in the diet can contribute to symptoms of depression and other mood disorders.

Vitamin E is a potent, fat-soluble antioxidant that protects the fats that line cells throughout the body. In the brain, this vitamin protects neurons, which are made primarily of cholesterol and polyunsaturated fats and are highly susceptible to oxidative damage. Research suggests that eating foods high in vitamin E can reduce inflammation and help lower the risk of Alzheimer's disease and general cognitive decline.

B vitamins in chard work in synergy, playing an essential role in the brain, supporting the production of neurotransmitters to help regulate mood and promote positivity.

SUGGESTED SERVING

Aim to eat 7–10 portions of leafy greens, such as chard, a week. One portion is 3½–5½oz (100–150g).

HOW TO ENJOY

Add fresh young leaves to salads or cook lightly to preserve nutrients—vitamin E in particular is damaged by high heat.

RECIPE

Chard smoothie

Put a handful of chard stalks and leaves in a food processor or blender. Add 2 cored and chopped pears and a tablespoon of shelled hemp seeds and process to the desired consistency.

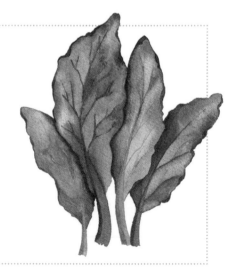

" Purslane has significant amounts of antibodies, B vitamins, and other brain-supporting nutrients. "

Rustle up a brain-boosting smoothie with chard, pear, and hemp seeds. The pear balances the bitterness and hemp seeds add essential fatty acids to help the absorption of fat-soluble vitamins.
➤ *See recipe, opposite.*

Make a simple chard pickle.
➤ *Pack chard stems into a jar with garlic, chili, mustard and fennel seeds, and peppercorns. Cover with brine (2 tbsp salt to 1¾ pints/1l water). Ferment at room temperature for a week. Seal and refrigerate for up to a month.*

WHEN TO AVOID

Avoid chard if you are at risk of kidney stones, as it contains oxalates, which can be stone-forming.

ENDIVE

Crisp Belgian endive is sweet with bitter overtones. The tightly packed heads of pale yellow leaves, or the alternative variety with red hues, are an excellent source of brain-protective nutrients. Because endive is grown in cool, dark spaces—often in cellars—it is available most of the year. When refrigerated, it remains fresh longer than other leafy greens.

BENEFITS

As well as providing folate, potassium, and manganese, slender endive heads are an excellent source of vitamin K, beta-carotene, and vitamin C, all potent antioxidants that help to neutralize damaging free radical toxins in the body. Endive also has a high water content, keeping the body and brain hydrated.

Folate (also known as vitamin B9) is needed to form red blood cells, which carry oxygen to the brain. It is also involved in neurone messaging. Research shows that low levels are linked to reduced brain function and an increased risk of dementia. Ongoing research is looking at using folate as both a prevention and treatment of mental health conditions.

Potassium is an essential mineral for brain health, ensuring that the brain has sufficient oxygen to function effectively. It also helps to activate the neurons involved in positive thoughts and feelings.

Manganese is closely involved with how neurons communicate with each other. It is a "cofactor" for many enzymes that work as antioxidants, ensuring the enzymes work effectively to lower oxidative stress in the body. A deficiency has been linked to reduced mental health.

SUGGESTED SERVING

Include endive in your 7–10 portions a week of green leaves. A serving is 3½–5½oz (100–150g).

HOW TO ENJOY

Belgian endive is often baked or braised, creating a mellow, sweet flavor, but it is also delicious eaten raw, which ensures maximum nutritional benefits.

Combine with sweet, nutty flavors for a brain-supporting salad.
➤ *Toss the sliced leaves with apples, vitamin B-rich chestnuts, and a store-bought or homemade blackberry vinegar dressing for a vitamin C boost. Or mix them with mineral-rich pears and walnuts, to up your antioxidant quota, and add a blue cheese dressing.*

The boatlike leaves are perfect for filling or dipping.
➤ *Separate the leaves and use them as a scoop for your favorite dips.*

PURSLANE

Purslane, a small family of sprawling plants, mainly grow wild, though common purslane is also cultivated. Both the leaves and stems can be eaten. The succulent, slightly sour and salty leaves add a crunchy texture to dishes.

BENEFITS

Purslane boasts significant amounts of antioxidants, B vitamins, magnesium, iron, calcium, and potassium, all of which support mental wellness. Purslane also contains pectin, a water-soluble fiber that supports gut health, and the fresh leaves contain more alpha-linolenic acid—an omega-3 fatty acid—than any other leaf.

Alpha-linolenic acid (ALA), an essential polyunsaturated fatty acid, is needed for growth and development. Our bodies are unable to make ALA, so we have to get it from our diets. ALA reduces the risk of hypertension, which is associated with feelings of negativity that can lead to stress and depression. ALA can also be converted into longer-chain fatty acids, which exert a powerful anti-inflammatory effect, to combat the inflammation that can be caused by chronic stress.

➤ CONTINUED...

Pectin, a soluble fiber found in plant cell walls, helps maintain good gut health. Research suggests that pectin has a prebiotic effect, which means it feeds beneficial bacteria in the gut and supports a healthy microbial balance. A healthy gut in turn supports our mental health via the gut–brain axis. Pectin also helps stabilize blood sugar levels, low levels of which can exacerbate irritability and a low mood.

SUGGESTED SERVING

Add a handful of about 3½– 5½oz (100–150g) to salads once or twice a week.

HOW TO ENJOY

The mucilaginous nature of the leaves can help to thicken sauces and soups.

Add texture to soups.
➡*Thicken a tomato soup with a handful of chopped leaves for a powerful antioxidant blend.*
Make a gut-supporting pickle to liven up rice or potato dishes.
➡*Cut the stems into 1½in (4cm) pieces. Submerge in brine (2 tbsp salt to 1¾ pints/1l water) for 7–10 days at room temperature. Store in a lidded jar in the fridge for up to 1 month.*
Toss the young leaves into salads.
➡*Try nitrate-rich shaved beets with purslane and drizzle over a mustard seed dressing.*

" Refreshing spinach is full of rejuvenating chlorophyll."

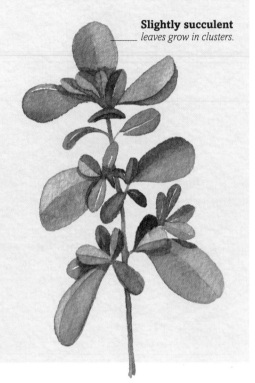

FOCUS ON

Purslane

PROFILE
This hardy plant grows widely in Europe and Asia. With small, succulent leaves, it thrives in temperate climes with a minimum of water.

PROPERTIES
Purslane is a rich source of antioxidant vitamins and essential minerals. It also has one of the highest levels of omega-3 fatty acids in leafy plants, providing anti-inflammatory and brain-building properties.

Slightly succulent *leaves grow in clusters.*

SPINACH

Light and refreshing, spinach contains a wealth of nutrients, such as vitamin B6 and folate, that support brain health. The bright green leaves are also full of cleansing and rejuvenating chlorophyll. Easy to source and versatile, it is effortless to include spinach in your diet.

BENEFITS

The nutritional benefits of spinach are far-reaching, helping to boost immunity, stabilize blood sugar, and detoxify, all of which support a healthy brain. Nutrients specific to brain functions include iron, beta-carotene, magnesium, folate, and vitamins C, K, E, and, in particular, B6. It also provides alpha-linolenic acid, an omega-3 fatty acid with anti-inflammatory properties that support brain health.

Vitamin B6 works in synergy with other B vitamins to extract energy from food. Since the brain needs a lot of energy to function properly, a deficiency in any of this important group of vitamins can negatively impact how the brain performs. Vitamin B6 is essential for the synthesis of numerous neurotransmitters, including the feel-good chemical serotonin. Insufficient vitamin B6 in the diet can lead to poor concentration and contribute to feelings of depression.

Folate is part of the B complex of vitamins. A deficiency in any of the B vitamins can disrupt normal brain function. Folate is important for brain function because it helps to support neuron messaging in the nervous system. Low levels of folate have been associated with an increased risk of depression, in particular postnatal depression, which folate deficiency is thought to contribute to significantly.

SUGGESTED SERVING

Enjoy 3½–5½oz (100–150g) per serving of spinach as part of your 7–10 weekly portions of leafy greens.

HOW TO ENJOY

Spinach is easy to combine with a variety of foods, ensuring that you gain the maximum nutritional benefits to support mental and physical wellness.

Whizz up a brain-supporting smoothie.
➡ *Blitz a handful of spinach with flavonoid-rich, mood-boosting blueberries, a dollop of gut-supporting yogurt, and zingy fresh ginger.*
Enjoy a chlorophyll "energy" burst drink to kickstart the day.
➡ *See box, below.*
Eat with eggs, which provide the amino acid tryptophan, needed to produce the feel-good hormone serotonin, as well as protein, which helps to stabilize blood sugar levels.
➡ *Gently wilt then add to an omelette.*

WHEN TO AVOID
Spinach may be best avoided if you are susceptible to kidney stones, due to the high content of the compound oxalate.

BENEFITS

Romaine is the most nutrient-rich variety of lettuce. It is a good source of vitamin K, beta-carotene, vitamin C, folate, and molybdenum. The lettuce also contains lactucarium, a phytonutrient that eases tension and promotes relaxation. A good source of fiber, romaine promotes a healthy gut environment and its high water content helps to keep the body hydrated, both benefits essential for the health of the brain.

Vitamin K supports proteins that play a key role in the nervous system. It is thought to support Alzheimer's patients by limiting neuron damage in the brain.
Beta-carotene, an important antioxidant, has been shown to improve symptoms associated with anxiety and depression. Studies show that lower levels of beta-carotene are connected to a low mood.
Vitamin C is a vitally important antioxidant. The highest concentration of vitamin C in the body is found in the brain, where one of its tasks is to neutralize damaging free radicals.
Folate supports the nervous system because it is involved in the production of messaging molecules that are used by nerves to transmit messages throughout the body. Low levels of folate have been associated with depression.
Molybdenum, an essential nutrient, helps metabolize iron, a vital mineral that plays a part in moving oxygen around the body to keep us energized.

SUGGESTED SERVING

Include 3½–5½oz (100–150g) per portion of romaine as a varied part of your 7–10 servings weekly of green leaves.

HOW TO ENJOY

Romaine is best eaten as soon as possible after it is picked. To store, wash and dry the leaves, wrap in a damp cloth, and refrigerate in the vegetable drawer.

Use sturdy romaine leaves as wraps.
➡ *Fill with chopped avocado, diced red pepper, and basil to ease anxiety and lift the spirits.*
Add older leaves to a brain-hydrating pea and lettuce soup.
➡ *Soften shallots and garlic in a pan with a little olive oil and water. Add romaine and wilt. Add peas, stock, and a few mint leaves. Simmer gently for 10 minutes then process to a puree.*

ROMAINE

Romaine (sometimes called cos lettuce) is a head-forming variety of lettuce that has flavorful, long green leaves with a crisp texture. Lettuce is often overlooked as a nutritious leaf, and it is true that it has fewer nutrients than many other leafy greens, but this hydrating food boasts a range of nutrients that support mental health and well-being. Moreover, it is available all year and is an easy addition to salads, snacks, and sandwiches.

RECIPE

Energizing spinach juice

Roughly chop a fennel bulb. Place in a food processor or blender with 2 large handfuls of spinach and a lemon, halved, peel included. Process to the desired consistency.

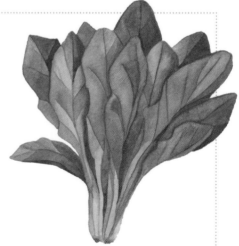

BRASSICAS

This vegetable group comes in a variety of forms. Each key brassica here is rich in vitamins, minerals, and brain-supporting phytonutrients. They also contain glucosinolates, unique compounds found almost exclusively in brassicas. When activated by chopping, chewing, or gut bacteria, they transform into molecules with potent antioxidant and anti-inflammatory effects to support mental wellness.

CABBAGE

Cabbages have a long history of use as both food and medicine. White and green cabbage, when raw, is peppery and slightly bitter, becoming sweeter when cooked. Red cabbage has an earthier, more robust flavor. The color of red cabbage reflects a potent concentration of antioxidant and anti-inflammatory compounds, just tipping the scale in its favor as the healthiest choice of cabbage.

BENEFITS

White, green, or red, all cabbages are brimming with vitamin K, vitamin C, vitamin B6, manganese, and potassium. Cabbage is also a good source of fiber that, along with the compounds made from cabbage's glucosinolates, supports a healthy gut and, in turn, a healthy brain.

Cabbage is high in antioxidants such as indole-3-carbinol, helping to maintain a healthy brain by combatting the cellular damage—or oxidative stress—caused by toxins known as free radicals that can lead to harmful inflammation.

Vitamin C is a powerful antioxidant that is essential for the production of the myelin sheath that encloses neurons in the brain and is needed to synthesize neurotransmitters, the chemicals that transmit messages between brain cells, ensuring a healthy brain function. The body is unable to make or store vitamin C so we need to include good sources in our daily diet.

SUGGESTED SERVING

Ideally, you should aim to eat 7–10 servings of brassica vegetables each week, of which cabbage could be at least a couple of servings. A serving of cabbage is 2½–3½oz (75–100g).

HOW TO ENJOY

To make the most of the many benefits of cabbage, it is best to eat it both cooked and raw. When eaten raw, cabbage has much higher levels of vitamin C, while cooked cabbage can provide more of the powerful antioxidant, indole-3-carbinol. Some find cooked cabbage easier to chew and digest, while others enjoy eating it raw, so this may influence how you eat it.

To preserve the most nutrients when cooking cabbage, steam or sauté it, using a little olive oil and water.
➡*Steam cabbage with caraway, garlic, ginger, or chili.*

RECIPE

Sauerkraut

Add 2 tsp salt to every 1lb (450g) shredded cabbage. Gently massage until juices flow. Pack in a jar, weighted, to submerge in the juice. Cover. Ferment at room temperature for up to 3 weeks, keeping it submerged. Store, lidded, in a cool dry place.

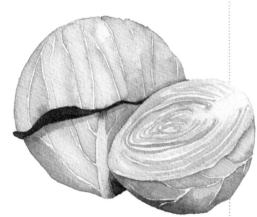

Make a jar of sauerkraut—naturally fermented cabbage is one of the most beneficial ways to eat cabbage. The fermentation process enhances antioxidant activity, increases vitamin C, and supports gut health by promoting the growth of beneficial bacteria, in turn supporting mental well-being via the gut–brain axis.
➤*See recipe, opposite.*

Juiced cabbage is loaded with nutrients to support gut health and is easier to digest for people who struggle with the high fiber content.
➤*Juice with pears, lemon, and ginger.*

WHEN TO AVOID

If you have histamine intolerance, you might have to limit or avoid fermented foods such as sauerkraut. If you take blood thinners or have hypothyroidism, while the brassica family is generally considered fine in moderation, it is best to limit your intake. Seek professional advice if in doubt.

CAULIFLOWER

This incredibly versatile brassica is available all year round. The creamy white-headed variety is most familiar, but there are also yellow, green, and purple varieties. Lime green Romanesco cauliflower, sometimes called broccoli, has a delicious sweet, nutty flavor. All varieties have beneficial nutrients.

BENEFITS

Cauliflower is rich in antioxidants, including the brain-supporting vitamins C and K, and has anti-inflammatory properties, which promote all-around health. It also contains soluble and insoluble fiber, to support the gut and, in turn, mental health via the gut–brain axis.

"Cauliflower has anti-inflammatory properties that help to support the healthy functioning of the brain."

Vitamin C, a vital antioxidant for brain health, is needed to synthesize the brain chemicals, or neurotransmitters, that help to regulate our moods.

Vitamin K deficiency might be related to the onset of cognitive impairment. There is also some evidence that suggests vitamin K can help prevent the onset of Alzheimer's disease.

Fiber is key to a healthy gut microbiome. The gut's connection to the brain via the vagus nerve means that a healthy gut supports our mental well-being. Cabbage contains both insoluble fiber, which supports the movement of stools through the colon, and soluble fiber, which provides food for the trillions of bacteria that live in our gut.

SUGGESTED SERVING

Include a 3½oz (100g) portion as part of the 7–10 servings of brassicas per week.

HOW TO ENJOY

Cauliflower is delicious raw or cooked. Raw is thought to preserve more key antioxidants, though some studies suggest that light cooking increases the bioavailability of some of its nutrients.

Steam and mash with herbs as a nutritious alternative to potatoes.
➤*Try with chopped rosemary, which is anti-inflammatory and supports memory and cognitive function.*

Enjoy light cauliflower rice.
➤*Chop and grate the cauliflower and add herbs for a raw rice dish, or lightly cook with oil and spring onions.*

Cook with spices for a flavorful boost.
➤*Sauté in a little oil with turmeric and ginger, both anti-inflammatories and soothing for digestive disorders.*

Eat raw as crudités.
➤*Enjoy the florets in a dipping sauce.*

WHEN TO AVOID

If you take blood thinners or have hypothyroidism, while the brassica family is thought fine in moderation, it is best to limit your intake. Seek professional advice if in doubt.

BROCCOLI

One of the best-known brassicas, broccoli is packed full of vitamins, minerals, and phytonutrients with antioxidant benefits. Its compounds help with detoxification in the body, helping to reduce stress from toxins.
Purple sprouting broccoli is a delicious alternative to the green-headed broccoli and has even more antioxidants than its green cousin.

BENEFITS

Broccoli contains high levels of beta-carotene and antioxidant vitamin C. Many of the B complex family of vitamins, including folate, are present in broccoli, all of which play an important role in brain chemistry. Broccoli is a good source of calcium and magnesium, both of which are essential for healthy brain function. Broccoli is also a rich source of plant-based choline.

➤ CONTINUED...

Folate is part of the vitamin B complex. Deficiency in any B vitamin can affect brain health, as they work in synergy to extract energy from food to provide the brain with a constant supply. Evidence suggests that folate supports a positive mental attitude and healthy cognition. Depression is linked to low levels.

Choline is produced in our livers, but in insufficient amounts to meet our needs, so a dietary source is key. It is required to produce acetylcholine, a neurotransmitter that passes signals between brain cells and is involved in regulating memory and mood.

SUGGESTED SERVING

Enjoy broccoli often in season, as part of your weekly 7–10 servings of brassicas. One portion is 3½oz (100g).

HOW TO ENJOY

Eat raw or steam, sauté (see recipe, opposite), or roast. To save nutrients, keep cooking times short and sauté and roast at low temperatures.

Lightly steam for a warm broccoli salad.
➡️ *Toss with olives and feta for beneficial oleic acid and protein.*
Eat raw for extra crunch and nutrients.
➡️ *Mix raw florets with yogurt and chopped walnuts for healthy fats. Add anti-inflammatory chili.*

A DECORATIVE TOUCH

As well as the leaves, arugula flowers are also edible. Try adding the delicate, subtly peppery petals to salads.

RECIPE

Sautéed broccoli

Lightly sauté broccoli in equal amounts of olive oil and water with garlic, chili, and slivered almonds.

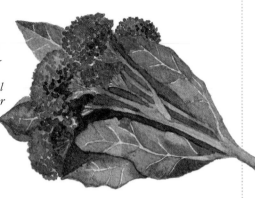

WHEN TO AVOID

If you take blood thinners or have hypothyroidism, while the brassica family is considered fine to eat in moderation, it is best to limit your intake. Seek professional advice if you are in doubt.

WATERCRESS AND ARUGULA

Flavorful watercress and arugula pack a peppery, nutrient-rich punch. The leaves of both plants are bursting with cleansing and rejuvenating chlorophyll and are good sources of sulphur compounds, which boost the production of glutathione, a potent antioxidant. Being very delicate, the leaves are best eaten soon after picking. When freshly harvested, they contain a range of beneficial phytochemicals.

BENEFITS

Arugula and watercress are rich in antioxidants that help protect against oxidative damage from free radicals. They contain many nutrients necessary for brain health, including iron, zinc, beta-carotene, calcium, and vitamin K.

Both are good sources of magnesium and potassium, whose actions are thought to help ease depression and support positive thoughts and feelings.

Magnesium supports electrical activity in the brain, aiding cognitive function. It calms nerves and relaxes muscles and is used to relieve anxiety and depression. Stress increases the rate at which we lose magnesium in our body, which can cause a deficiency. A magnesium-rich diet helps to avoid a downward spiral, as a deficiency places the body under extra stress.

Potassium is one of the major minerals in the body and plays an essential role in mental wellness. Potassium ensures the brain has sufficient oxygen to function well, and low levels have been linked to depression. Research also suggests that potassium helps the brain properly utilize the feel-good chemical serotonin, which helps regulate our mood and feelings.

SUGGESTED SERVING

Eat a 3–3½oz (80–100g) serving two or three times a week, in season, as part of your 7–10 weekly servings of brassicas.

HOW TO ENJOY

Neither watercress nor arugula keeps well, so eat them as fresh as possible.

Add flavor to a sustaining salad.
➥*Partner with tomatoes, eggplant, walnuts, and goat cheese.*
Make a delicious zesty pesto with either watercress or arugula.
➥*Combine 1¾oz (50g) of watercress or arugula, 1oz (30g) chopped walnuts, 1 crushed garlic clove, the zest of 1 lemon and 1 tablespoon of lemon juice in a food processor. Add a little olive oil while blending. Season with salt and pepper.*
Serve both with cooked dishes.
➥*Wilt older leaves of either in a little olive oil and toss through pasta or steamed vegetables, or enjoy the raw, fresh leaves as a garnish for risotto.*
Add to potato soup.
➥*Blanch the watercress and add to the soup just before blending, to ensure the chlorophyll is not lost.*

WHEN TO AVOID

If you are taking blood thinners or have hypothyroidism, watercress and arugula are fine in moderation, but it is advisable to seek professional advice.

KALE

There are several varieties of kale and each one is an excellent source of essential nutrients for mental health and well-being. Kale is one of the most nutrient-dense vegetables you can eat.

BENEFITS

Kale is packed full of brain-healthy nutrients. It is a spectacular source of vitamin K and contains high levels of beta-carotene and vitamin C, all antioxidants that protect the brain from oxidative damage by toxins. Kale is also an excellent source of iron, magnesium, omega-3 fats, protein, and fiber, all of which are beneficial for brain health. It is also bursting with cleansing chlorophyll.

Chlorophyll improves liver function, helping ensure the removal of toxins from the bloodstream, and supports a healthy gut microbiome. A sluggish liver is associated with mood swings, irritability, and irascibility.
There are two forms of vitamin K: K1 and K2. K1 is found in plants, and kale is one of the best plant sources of this vitamin. Both vitamins K1 and K2 act as antioxidants that are vital for keeping the brain healthy.
Beta-carotene is an important antioxidant that is found in plants. Like other antioxidants, it helps counteract oxidative stress in the brain, which is thought to be a key factor in cognitive decline. Beta-carotene is converted in the body to vitamin A, which is essential for healthy immune function.

SUGGESTED SERVING

Enjoy kale as a part of your 7–10 weekly portions of brassicas. A daily portion is about 3½oz (100g).

HOW TO ENJOY

This versatile vegetable can be juiced, massaged to break down the cell structure, sautéed, steamed, or crisped.

Eat with a healthy source of fat to improve the absorption of vitamin K1 and beta-carotene.
➥*Wilt in a little olive oil and water and top with a poached egg. Or toss together with avocado and shelled hemp seeds in a nutritious salad.*

WHEN TO AVOID

If you take blood thinners or have hypothyroidism, eating kale in moderation is fine, but seek professional advice if in doubt.

FOCUS ON

PROFILE
This distinctive member of the cabbage family is a hardy plant that grows successfully in cooler climes.

PROPERTIES
Kale is abundant in antioxidant nutrients, most of which are stored in its leaves and which reduce the risk of chronic inflammation in the body.

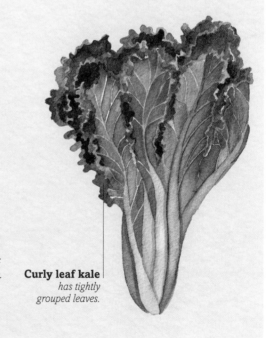

Curly leaf kale
has tightly grouped leaves.

RECIPES FOR MENTAL WELLNESS

SMOOTHIES

Rustled up in minutes, delicious smoothies are an effortless way to enjoy a nutrient-dense snack or start to the day. These sustaining drinks are packed with antioxidant-rich and energizing ingredients that deliver an impressive range of nutrients for the brain and gut, protecting both from harmful inflammation and supporting a healthy gut–brain axis for mental health and well-being.

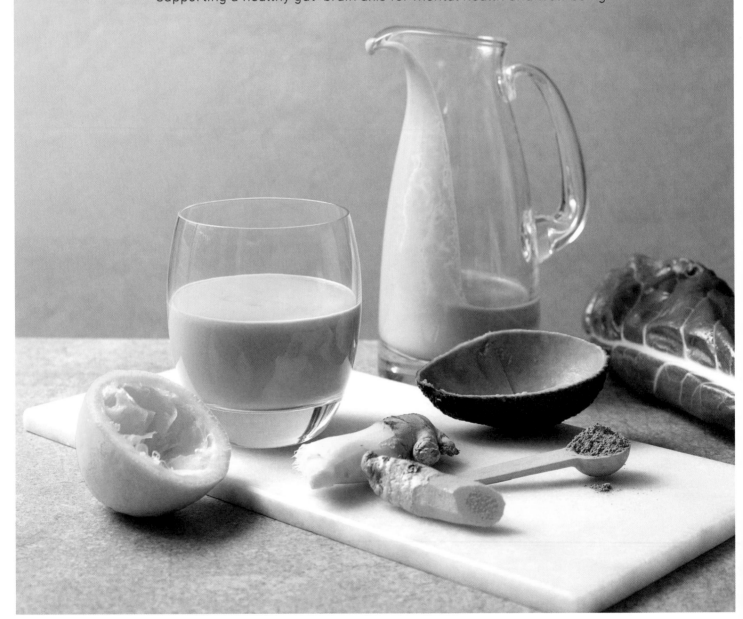

1

Mood-lifting smoothie

Lift your spirits with this zesty and comforting smoothie. Chard provides positivity-boosting magnesium, while anti-inflammatory ginger and turmeric support brain health, helping ward off inflammation linked to anxiety and depression. Avocado is full of brain-beneficial omega-3 fats, while matcha calms and energizes.

SERVES **1–2** | PREP TIME **5 MINS**

Peel and chop **½ avocado** and grate a **¾in (2cm) piece** each of **turmeric** and **ginger**. Place in a food processor, together with a **handful of chard**, the **juice of ½ lemon**, **1 tsp matcha powder**, and **7½fl oz (225ml) kefir** or **almond milk**. Blend all the ingredients together until smooth and creamy.

2

Brain-protecting winter refresher

Boost immunity and brainpower in the winter months with this nourishing smoothie. Fiber-rich pears and probiotic yogurt promote a healthy gut, in turn supporting brain health via the gut–brain axis. Vitamin K-rich kale, polyphenols in cacao, and memory-boosting cinnamon aid cognition, and antioxidants protect mind and body.

SERVES **1–2** | PREP TIME **5 MINS**

Core and chop a **pear**. Remove the stems from a **handful of kale** and roughly tear the leaves. Place the pear and kale in a food processor, along with a **handful of frozen blueberries**, **1 tbsp shelled hemp seeds**, **2 tbsp live yogurt**, **1 tsp raw cacao powder**, a **good pinch of cinnamon powder** and, if you wish, **1 tsp raw honey**. Blend all the ingredients together, adding a little **water** to reach the desired consistency.

3

Start-the-day energizer

This summery smoothie with antioxidant-rich raspberries delivers a sustaining and uplifting start to the day. Hemp provides essential fatty acids and protein, and vitamin B6 in spinach helps extract energy from food. In addition, mood-boosting folate in hazelnuts and refreshing mint lift stress and anxiety.

SERVES **1–2** | PREP TIME **5 MINS**

Place **1 large handful** each of **raspberries** and **spinach**, **1 tbsp** each of **hazelnut butter** and **shelled hemp seeds**, **3 frozen banana chunks** (about 1in/2.5cm) and **3 mint leaves** in a food processor. Blitz them all together, adding enough **water** to make a smooth and creamy consistency.

ROOTS AND TUBERS

Versatile and easy to store, roots and tubers have been a staple crop for thousands of years. Roots, such as carrots and parsnips, feed nutrients to the plant, while tubers, such as Jerusalem artichokes and potatoes, are storage vessels that propagate new plants. Root crops generally contain simple carbohydrates while tubers have more complex starches. Both are rich in fiber and highly nutritious.

CARROT

The orange carrot is one of our best-known vegetables and some of the original white, purple, red, and yellow varieties are also regaining popularity. All contain beneficial phytonutrients. Orange carrots provide an abundance of carotenoids, with beta-carotene the most plentiful. Research suggests that people who eat a diet high in brightly colored fruit and vegetables are less likely to suffer from depression.

BENEFITS

The antioxidants in carrots, including vitamin C, vitamin K, and phytonutrients, help prevent oxidative damage in the brain. Carrots also contain a number of the vitamin B complex, all of which support a healthy nervous system. They are a good source of fiber and an excellent source of beta-carotene.

Biotin, or B7, is part of the B complex of vitamins. With other B vitamins, it helps convert food into energy. It is particularly useful for regulating blood glucose, helping to avoid fatigue and mood swings. The brain uses biotin more than any other organ.

Beta-carotene is a carotenoid with potent antioxidant properties, which have been found to improve anxiety and depression by reducing oxidative damage. There are more than 600 carotenoids, but the body only converts three to vitamin A, with beta-carotene the most efficient. Beta-carotene in itself is not an essential nutrient, but vitamin A is vital for a healthy immune system.

SUGGESTED SERVING

Include 2 carrots (about 4½oz/125g, raw weight) as one of your daily portions of brightly colored vegetables.

HOW TO ENJOY

Raw, cooked, or juiced, carrots give a bumper dose of vitamins and minerals for radiant health and well-being.

Bake some carrot muffins. Adding cinnamon and ginger sharpens focus and helps ease anxiety. The aroma will lift your mood, too.
➥ *Use whole wheat spelt and spice with cinnamon and ginger.*
Rustle up an uplifting salad.
➥ *Mix grated carrots with lemon, mint, black pepper, olives, and olive oil. The fat enables the conversion of beta-carotene into vitamin A.*

RECIPE

Beet relish

Shred 3 medium beets and 2in (5cm) root of fresh horseradish. Add 1 tbsp salt and ¼ tsp each ground cloves and grated star anise. Firmly press into a jar to release the juices, weighing down the beets so they stay submerged. Cover and ferment at room temperature for a week. Close with a lid, and store.

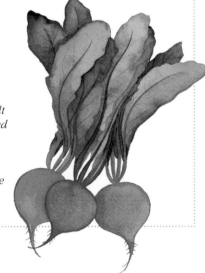

" Beet leaves are a good source of phytonutrients to help optimize brain health."

BEET

Typically thought of as red, beets can also be found in white, golden, and striped varieties. They have a sweet, earthy taste, with the red varieties tending to have the most vibrant flavor. Beets are packed full of beneficial plant compounds, including nitrates that convert in the body to nitric oxide, which dilates blood vessels to support a healthy blood flow to the brain.

BENEFITS

Beets are a great source of nutrients for brain health, including folate, vitamin C, manganese, potassium, and iron. They contain the phytochemical betaine, which aids liver function and provides anti-inflammatory benefits. The beneficial compounds called betalains in beets are responsible for their bright colors.

Betalains are a family of water-soluble pigments found in only a few plants. With potent antioxidant properties, betalains are able to neutralize toxins and help to protect brain cells from inflammation.

Folate is needed to produce mood-regulating neurotransmitters such as dopamine and serotonin. Low levels are associated with depression.

Manganese is a component of the powerful antioxidant enzyme superoxide dismutase (SOD). This helps protect the brain from free radicals, the toxins that can cause oxidative damage, which lead to disease.

SUGGESTED SERVING

Consume daily in a juice. Or include 1 medium or 2 small beets in your meals 2–3 times a week.

HOW TO ENJOY

Prepare beets in a variety of ways to maximize the nutritional benefits. To benefit most from the betalains in beets, the vegetable is best consumed raw, in a juice, though this does lose fiber. Beet leaves can also be eaten; these are a rich source of phytonutrients such as the carotenoids zeaxanthin and lutein, which help improve brain health.

Juice beets. Scrub but don't peel the beets before juicing to preserve the most nutrients.
➡ *Juice alone or with other ingredients.*

Make a beet relish for gut health.
➡ *See recipe, opposite.*

Enjoy grated as a side dish, leaving skin on for extra fiber, if you want. Adding pumpkin seed oil boosts serotonin levels to lift mood.
➡ *Dress grated beets with a little soy sauce and pumpkin seed oil.*

Try a warm salad if you prefer cooked beets. Slow-roasting retains the most nutrients when cooking.
➡ *Toss slow-roasted beets with peppery arugula and feta cheese.*

WHEN TO AVOID

Beets contain oxalates, which, for a few susceptible people, may lead to kidney stones. If taking high blood pressure medication, seek advice before drinking beet juice.

SWEET POTATO

Evidence from Peruvian caves shows sweet potatoes have been consumed since ancient times. Sweet potatoes range in color from white to vibrant orange and purple. The orange-fleshed variety is one of the best-known sources of beta-carotene, converted in the body to vitamin A. The purple variety is an excellent source of anthocyanins, part of the group of compounds known as flavonoids with well-documented antioxidant properties.

BENEFITS

Sweet potatoes are an excellent source of fiber and very high in beta-carotene. They also contain choline, essential for brain growth and development; manganese, which supports neurotransmitters and helps protect the brain from oxidation; magnesium, which calms the brain, promoting relaxation; and potassium, which ensures the brain properly utilizes the feel-good chemical serotonin.

The fiber in sweet potatoes is both soluble and insoluble. Soluble fiber provides food for beneficial gut bacteria, while insoluble fiber speeds up the movement and processing of waste. In addition, sweet potatoes contain "resistant" starch. This is starch that passes through the digestive tract unchanged so that when it arrives in the colon, it provides food for friendly gut bacteria. This in turn increases the production of short-chain essential fatty acids, which keep the cells of the colon wall healthy. Fiber and resistant starch in sweet potato both play a role in keeping the body's blood sugar levels stable, which helps to avoid sudden mood swings and promote a sense of calm and well-being.

➤ CONTINUED...

Beta-carotene in one medium-sized sweet potato provides more than 400 percent of our average daily needs; the excess is harmless to the body. The ability of beta-carotene to reduce free radicals helps improve cognitive function, reducing symptoms of anxiety and depression.

SUGGESTED SERVING

Eat 1 medium sweet potato, about 5½oz (150g) raw weight, as often as you like. Bear in mind, it is best to eat a variety of colorful vegetables.

HOW TO ENJOY

Steam, roast, bake, grill, or stir-fry, there are plenty of ways to enjoy sweet potatoes. You will significantly increase the amount of beta-carotene the body absorbs if you include a little fat when you eat sweet potatoes. Most of the fiber and many of the antioxidants in sweet potatoes are found in the skin.

Bake whole sweet potatoes and fill with your favorite flavors. This sustaining lunch will keep blood sugar steady to maximize focus through the day.
➡ *Bake in the oven until the skin is crispy and the insides soft. Add a little seasoning, a small amount of butter, and fillings of your choice.*

Make a comforting, warming sweet potato soup. Adding garlic promotes healthy blood flow to the brain, while hemp oil aids the absorption of beta-carotene and provides omega-3 fat, essential for brain health.
➡ *Add plenty of crushed garlic and finish with a swirl of hemp oil.*

Enjoy a sustaining, mood-enhancing sweet potato bowl.
➡ *Combine roasted sweet potato with steamed kale, top with a black bean and avocado salsa, and add a splash of olive oil.*

RECIPE

Crunchy celeriac slaw

Make a celeriac slaw with the four fat-soluble vitamins—A, D, K, and E—which work in synergy and are key for healthy brain function. Combine fine shreds of celeriac and carrot in a mayonnaise made from eggs and olive oil.

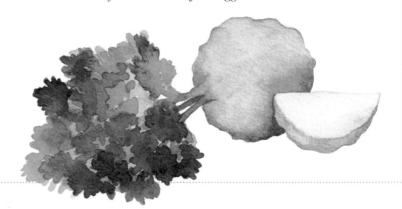

JERUSALEM ARTICHOKE

The Jerusalem artichoke is a perennial sunflower producing a grey-, purple-, or pink-skin tuber with a sweet, delicate-textured white flesh inside. Jerusalem artichokes contain inulin, a prebiotic that supports a healthy gut, and their starchy fiber prevents spikes in blood sugar levels.

BENEFITS

Jerusalem artichokes contain a number of antioxidants, including vitamin C and carotenoids, both of which offer the body protection from inflammation. The tubers are an excellent source of minerals, especially potassium, iron, and copper— all important for mental health and brain function. Jerusalem artichokes are also one of the richest sources of inulin, a prebiotic fiber with many health benefits, especially for the gut.

Inulin is found in many plants and belongs to a type of dietary fiber known as a fructo-oligosaccharide (FOS). It is a prebiotic because it is not absorbed in the small intestine, so moves into the large intestine where it feeds beneficial gut bacteria. Inulin selectively promotes the growth of *Bifidobacteria* and *Lactobacilli*. These help maintain a healthy gut, which in turn plays a crucial role in regulating brain function via the brain–gut axis, helping to moderate processes such as the stress response.

Iron is needed to form the red blood cells that carry oxygen around the body. A deficiency in the diet limits the amount of oxygen reaching cells, resulting in tiredness and a reduced ability to cope with stress and feelings of anxiety.

Potassium is also essential in ensuring the brain has enough oxygen to function at its best. Potassium helps to maintain a healthy blood pressure, which, in turn, helps to reduce stress and anxiety.

SUGGESTED SERVING

The production of gas as gut bacteria break down inulin is a side effect of eating Jerusalem artichokes. Large quantities can cause discomfort so you may wish to limit Jerusalem artichoke servings to about 2½oz (75g) raw weight once or twice a week.

HOW TO ENJOY

Some varieties of Jerusalem artichokes are very knobbly and can be hard to peel; in this case it is best to roast them, skin on, with a selection of other vegetables, for a side dish packed with a variety of nutrients. You can turn smoother varieties that are easy to peel into soups and dips.

Eat with other antioxidant-rich vegetables to help soothe anxiety. Combining with carrots helps to reduce the gas effects of artichokes considerably.
➡ *Whizz up a soup with carrots and artichokes.*
Make a gut-supporting pickle. Crunchy, full of flavor, and brimming with lactic bacteria, pickling also reduces the inulin content, which in turn helps limit digestive gas.
➡ *Ferment Jerusalem artichokes with garlic and chili for a week. Serve with wilted greens, add to a wrap, or spice up a rice dish.*
Enjoy roasted artichokes, leaving skin on, if desired, to help them keep their shape.
➡ *Combine with shiitake mushrooms, kale, and walnuts for a delicious combination loaded with brain-boosting nutrition.*

WHEN TO AVOID
Those suffering with irritable bowel syndrome (IBS) may want to avoid eating Jerusalem artichokes if these cause additional discomfort from gas and bloating.

" Prebiotic nutrients in Jerusalem artichokes feed healthy gut bacteria."

CELERIAC

Celeriac, also known as celery root, is a large knobbly root vegetable closely related to celery and parsley, with a nutty flavor and a crunchy texture. If you can source it freshly harvested, the stalks and leaves are also edible. Celeriac is an excellent source of fiber for gut health.

BENEFITS

Celeriac is rich in antioxidants, which disarm free radicals, protecting our cells from damage. It is a particularly good source of vitamins K and C.

Vitamin K is the name given to a group of fat-soluble vitamins. Of the two forms, vitamin K1 is produced by plants, and K2 is found in animal and fermented foods. Though the two types have different roles, K1 can be converted in the body to K2. Vitamin K is involved in the synthesis of sphingolipids, a major component of the myelin sheath around nerves.
Vitamin C is a vitally important molecule for brain health. The highest concentrations of vitamin C are found in the brain. In addition to its well-known role as an antioxidant, vitamin C is needed to convert dopamine to serotonin, the hormone that stabilizes our mood, helping promote well-being.

SUGGESTED SERVING

Eat as often as desired as part of your weekly servings of varied vegetables.

One portion is ¼ of a medium celeriac, about 4½oz (125g) raw weight.

HOW TO ENJOY

Raw or cooked, celeriac is highly versatile. Use as a base for coleslaws or salads, or mash, bake, roast, or boil. Eating raw maximizes the vitamin C content.

Make celeriac rice as a nutritious alternative for rice-based dishes. Using miso adds beneficial bacteria.
➡ *Process to a ricelike texture and moisten with unpasteurized white miso.*
Enjoy a warming soup with an antioxidant boost.
➡ *Add turmeric to celeriac soup to make a potent blend for brain health.*
Make crunchy celeriac slaw.
➡ *See recipe, opposite.*

WHEN TO AVOID
People can be allergic to celeriac. Symptoms may be mild, but celeriac has also been known to cause anaphylactic reactions.

MYELIN SHEATHS

Myelin is an insulating layer around nerves and is vital for the proper conduction of nerve cells and high levels of brain function.

STEMS AND BULBS

Eating stems and bulbs provides a range of potent phytonutrients, essentially the plants' immune systems, which we harness the benefits of when we consume them. The following foods are all excellent sources of antioxidant and anti-inflammatory flavonoids, which support our overall health by preventing damaging inflammation in the body and brain.

ASPARAGUS

Fresh, fragrant-tasting asparagus is a seasonal treat. There are three main types of asparagus: green, grown mostly in America and the UK, purple, grown in France, and the Dutch white variety. Purple asparagus is a source of anthocyanins, phytonutrients that help to slow down the age-related decline in brain function; while the green variety has a higher antioxidant activity than white.

BENEFITS

Asparagus contains a range of B vitamins and is an excellent source of the fiber inulin. It also contains an abundance of phytonutrients, rich in antioxidant activity. It is one of a handful of plant foods that contain preformed—bioavailable—glutathione, a vital antioxidant that is particularly efficient at breaking down free radicals. It is also an excellent source of vitamin K and provides selenium and vitamins C and E.

Inulin is a type of fiber that acts as a prebiotic—providing food for beneficial bacteria as it passes through the gut. As good bacteria thrive and multiply, they keep the number of harmful bacteria in check. Inulin helps waste to move efficiently through the body keeping the digestive tract in good working order.

Each B vitamin has its own independent role in the body while also working together with the other B vitamins. The B vitamin family plays a critical role in health and vitality and has a direct effect on brain function. B vitamins extract energy from our food, crucial for the brain, which uses more energy than any other organ. They are also involved in DNA and RNA synthesis, help build vital molecules, and regulate the metabolism of neurotransmitters. A deficiency can disrupt normal brain function.

SUGGESTED SERVING

Enjoy 8 spears 2 to 3 times a week when in season.

HOW TO ENJOY

All types of asparagus can be enjoyed raw as well as lightly steamed or baked. Snap off woody ends before eating, and if you need to store asparagus, keep it fresh by placing it upright in a jar of water.

Eat with eggs for an energizing start to the day. Eggs provide vitamin B12, so combining these two ingredients provides the whole B vitamin family.
➡ *Top lightly cooked asparagus spears with a poached egg for a weekend breakfast or brunch.*

Pair with fish for a great flavor combo. Try with salmon for brain-supporting omega-3 fatty acids.
➡ *Serve with lightly poached salmon.*

Enjoy an asparagus and avocado salad. Healthy fats in avocado and olive oil significantly boost the bioavailability of vitamins A and K in asparagus.
➡ *See recipe, opposite.*

"With its high water content, regularly snacking on celery is a great way to help keep the brain hydrated."

RECIPE

Asparagus and avocado salad

Using a vegetable peeler, shave a handful of raw asparagus spears. Combine with chopped avocado and spring onions and a squeeze of lemon juice, and drizzle with some extra virgin olive oil.

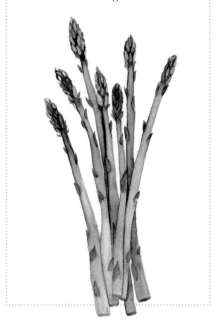

CELERY

Celery has thick, juicy stalks and parsleylike green leaves that are also edible. The stalks are crunchy with a slightly bitter, very mild, salty flavor. Pectin-based polysaccharides in celery are soluble fibers that provide food for beneficial bacteria, promoting a healthy gut microbiome. This, in turn, supports mental well-being via the gut–brain axis—the vagus nerve, which links the gut and brain.

BENEFITS

With a high water content, celery provides essential hydration. It also provides a variety of beneficial phytonutrients, including the flavonoid luteolin, as well as vitamin K, molybdenum, and folate.

Luteolin in animal and cell studies has demonstrated its ability to protect the brain from inflammation and oxidative stress. It is also thought to help reduce the "brain fog" associated with inflammatory brain conditions.

Molybdenum, an essential mineral, maintains a proper balance of sulphur in the body. Sulphur helps our bodies produce their own natural antioxidants and builds healthy connective tissues.

Hydration is critical for every cell in our body. Vegetables that have a high water content, such as celery, play a significant part in keeping the body hydrated. When the brain is fully hydrated, it can receive nutrients and eliminate toxins efficiently. If water levels are not maintained, our brains cannot function properly, leading to cognitive problems. By the time you feel thirsty, the body is already dehydrated.

SUGGESTED SERVING

Eat a couple of stalks regularly.

HOW TO ENJOY

Celery is one of the classic "mirepoix" ingredients, together with carrots and onions, that is used in the West as a flavor base for soups, stews, and casseroles. It is also easy to incorporate raw celery into your diet.

Enjoy a "pick-me-up" juice to help combat stress. As well as being hydrating, celery juice is a speedy way to deliver nutrients around the body.

➡*If the taste of celery juice on its own is too strong, mix with carrots, green leaves, red pepper, and lemon.*

Make an uplifting salad with this medley of mood-boosting ingredients.

➡*Chop a couple of celery stalks, an apple, and a beet. Add some carrot sticks and serve with a tamari and walnut oil dressing.*

WHEN TO AVOID

Celery is one of the 14 major food allergens. While symptoms may be mild, celery can also cause anaphylactic reactions.

FENNEL

Fennel has a unique, aromatic, aniseed taste and a crunchy texture. All parts of the fennel plant are edible. The stalk tends to be a bit fibrous with a stronger flavor, while the fronds are tender and fragrant. The thick white leaves at the base of the fennel form the bulb, which is packed full of powerful antioxidants that help reduce inflammation in the body and brain.

BENEFITS

Fennel contains a good amount of vitamin C as well as folate and the phytonutrient rutin. It also contains manganese, which helps protect the brain from damaging free radicals; potassium, an electrolyte that supports brain signaling, in turn promoting positive thoughts and feelings; and magnesium, which has a calming effect on the body.

Folate is needed to break down homocysteine, an amino acid made in the body as part of the biochemical process. A buildup of homocysteine can cause symptoms such as dizziness, fatigue, and mood changes.

➤ CONTINUED…

Vitamin C is a vital antioxidant molecule and a cofactor in the synthesis of brain neurotransmitters that regulate anxiety, happiness, and balance mood. This stress-busting nutrient is known to reduce both the physical and psychological effects of stress, and people with high levels of vitamin C seem to cope better. Our bodies cannot synthesize or store vitamin C, so daily sources are needed.

Rutin strengthens blood vessels and improves circulation. It is a powerful antioxidant that helps prevent inflammation and protects the brain.

SUGGESTED SERVING

Include 1 fennel bulb as part of your daily serving of vegetables.

HOW TO ENJOY

Fennel is easy and versatile to use. If you find the aniseed flavor too strong to eat raw, try braising fennel, which makes it much milder, with a soft, melt-in-your-mouth texture.

Ferment fennel to provide probiotic gut bacteria for healthy body and brain. Ferment with cabbage for a delicious aniseed-flavored sauerkraut.
➨*Combine chopped fennel and shredded cabbage with salt and spices. Pack into a jar, pressing down to release juices. Weight the ingredients to keep them submerged. Cover and ferment for 1 week at room temperature, then lid and store.*

Combine fennel with walnuts to provide alpha-linolenic acid (ALA)—an essential fatty acid needed for a healthy brain.
➨*Blend up a fennel soup, with chopped walnuts adding texture as well as nutrients.*

Enjoy a warming fennel dish with mood-lifting ingredients.
➨*Slowly braise with carrots and shallots.*

Add to a stir-fry for a meal brimming with antioxidant and anti-inflammatory phytonutrients.
➨*Stir-fry chopped fennel with red onions, peppers, and tomatoes.*

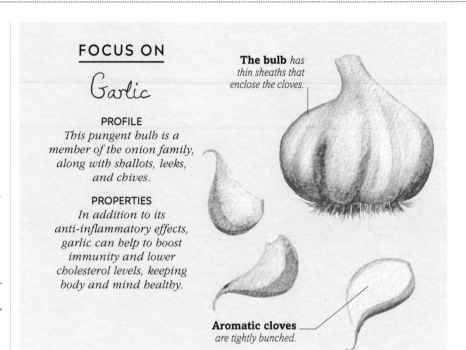

FOCUS ON

Garlic

PROFILE
This pungent bulb is a member of the onion family, along with shallots, leeks, and chives.

PROPERTIES
In addition to its anti-inflammatory effects, garlic can help to boost immunity and lower cholesterol levels, keeping body and mind healthy.

The bulb *has thin sheaths that enclose the cloves.*

Aromatic cloves *are tightly bunched.*

GARLIC

Garlic has been an integral part of many food cultures for centuries. The abundant sulphur compounds in garlic are responsible for its pungent, aromatic flavor. Eating garlic regularly has been shown to provide significant physical health benefits, including helping to regulate blood pressure, strengthen immunity, and lower the risk of heart disease. Poor physical health can exacerbate anxiety and stress, leading to an increased risk of mental health problems.

BENEFITS

Garlic is a good source of a variety of beneficial nutrients, including manganese, selenium, and antioxidant vitamin C. However, it is the sulphur-rich compounds found in garlic that are so immensely beneficial to our health and well-being.

"Eating immunity-boosting garlic raw provides the most therapeutic effects for body and mind."

Sulphur plays a critical role in health, and garlic is abundant in sulphur compounds, often in unique forms. Allicin in raw, crushed garlic is a well-studied therapeutic sulphur compound. The action of crushing or chewing raw garlic cloves releases the enzyme alliinase, which converts the compound alliin in garlic to allicin. Allicin reduces inflammation and protects the body from damaging free radicals. Garlic also contains several sulphur-containing amino acids, including cysteine and methionine. In addition, sulphur is required for glutathione synthesis, a potent antioxidant for the brain.

SUGGESTED SERVING

Try eating a raw garlic clove daily and add garlic regularly to cooked dishes, too.

HOW TO ENJOY

Eating garlic raw is the best way to benefit from its therapeutic effects. If you cook with garlic, crush the garlic first, then allow it to rest for 10 minutes before adding it to your dish. This is because heat destroys the enzyme alliinase, so resting chopped or crushed garlic gives allicin time to form before cooking. Resting crushed garlic also allows numerous other beneficial sulphur compounds to form. Allicin is reasonably tolerant of heat for a short time. A good way to preserve allicin is to add garlic toward the end of cooking. Cooking does not destroy all the compounds in garlic, so this pungent bulb can be included in your diet in a variety of ways.

Add a garlic clove to your morning juice. Blend with antioxidant-rich ingredients for flavor and sweetness. The combination here helps to lift spirits if you are feeling down.
  ➡*Try a blend of red pepper, tomato, chili, garlic, and basil.*

Make a pesto with garlic, basil, and walnuts. Basil is mentally stimulating and walnuts contain alpha-linolenic acid (ALA), vital for brain health.
  ➡*Add raw garlic to your pesto ingredients and process until smooth.*

ONION

Onions are one of the world's oldest cultivated plants, used as food and medicine for thousands of years. An excellent source of antioxidant and anti-inflammatory phytonutrients, onions are found in a variety of sizes and flavors, ranging from jumbo onions to shallots, and from sweet to pungent. The distinctive flavor of onions comes from the beneficial sulphur compounds.

BENEFITS

Many of the health benefits of onions come from their antioxidant content, including vitamin C and the phytonutrient quercetin; red onions also contain anthocyanins. Other onion nutrients include vitamin B6, biotin, and copper.

Quercetin is a flavonoid and a very important phytonutrient in our diets. Research shows quercetin plays a role in protecting the brain against oxidative stress and inflammation. Dietary flavonoids have also been found to lessen the effects of Alzheimer's disease.

All B vitamins play an essential role in the central nervous system, helping to maintain emotional balance. Vitamin B6 is involved in hemoglobin production, the blood protein that carries oxygen to the brain and around the body. Biotin is a B vitamin that is especially useful for maintaining blood sugar levels, helping to avoid fatigue and mood swings.

IDEAL STORAGE

Store onions and garlic in a cool, dark, dry place. Putting them in a paper bag with ventilation holes can help them last even longer.

Copper is necessary for activating certain enzymes in the brain, including dopamine. Dopamine plays many essential roles in the body and low levels of this enzyme can negatively affect mood.

SUGGESTED SERVING

Try to include an onion in your cooking every day.

HOW TO ENJOY

Onions are integral to a vast number of dishes as a flavor base. Enjoy onions in a variety of ways. Raw, they are crisp and pungent; cooked, they are soft and silky; caramelized, they are sweet and utterly delectable.

Add to a chunky guacamole for a perfect summery dish that is loaded with healthy ingredients to boost brain function.
  ➡*Make a guacamole with red onions, tomatoes, avocado, and jalapeno.*
Slow-roast whole onions. Many onion nutrients are found in, or lie just under, the skin so softening the skin during cooking provides nutrients to help keep the heart healthy, immunity strong, and moods balanced.
  ➡*Just remove the top, leave the onion unpeeled, and cook slowly until soft and sweet.*

VEGETABLE FRUITS AND FLOWERS

Some of our favorite foods that we think of as vegetables are, botanically, seed-producing fruits. Flowering vegetables are plants where the flower is eaten as a vegetable, the best-known and the most nutritious being the globe artichoke.

RED PEPPER

All peppers, from the sweet red bell pepper to the mellow warmth of jalapeño and the fiery habanero, are known as capsicums. Bell peppers come in a rainbow of colors, from the slightly bitter green, chocolate brown, and purple to the sweet and succulent yellow, orange, and red. Red peppers ripen on the vine the longest and have the most nutrients.

BENEFITS

Red peppers are a dense source of vitamin C and carotenoids, many of which are potent antioxidants. They are also a good source of vitamin B6 and folate, which play an important role in brain health—a deficiency in any of the B vitamins can be detrimental to the health of the brain.

Vitamin C is an extremely powerful antioxidant that we need to include in our diet each day. One red pepper contains more than 200 percent of our daily vitamin C needs. Vitamin C protects against the harmful effects of toxins known as free radicals and is a vital antioxidant molecule in the brain, which has the highest concentration of vitamin C in the body. This stress-busting nutrient helps our bodies to cope better with the effects of stress. Vitamin C also increases the amount of iron from plant sources that the body absorbs, so combining sources of plant iron with vitamin C is extremely beneficial. Studies suggest that those with an iron deficiency are more prone to depression.

Carotenoids—the pigments in plants that produce bright orange, red, and yellow colors—are found abundantly in red peppers. The powerful antioxidant action of these compounds is thought to help prevent cognitive decline.

SUGGESTED SERVING

Eat ½ of a large or 1 small red pepper daily in season if you wish. Make sure, though, that you eat a variety of colorful vegetables for a range of nutrients.

HOW TO ENJOY

Red peppers are delicious eaten raw as a snack or in salads and juices. You can also intensify their natural sweetness and flavor by grilling or roasting. Eating peppers raw preserves the most vitamin C, which can be destroyed with heat, although cooking red peppers can increase the availability of carotenoids.

RECIPE

Squash salad

Peel, dice, and seed a butternut squash and roast for 25–30 minutes at 400°F (200°C). Toss the roasted squash with steamed broccoli, quinoa, avocado, and olives and top with a garlic dressing.

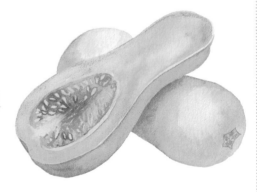

"Red peppers are densely packed with vitamin C, an essential vitamin for brain function."

Make a rainbow super-juice packed full of essential nutrients.
➡ *Blend 1 seeded red pepper, 1 beet, 2 carrots (scrubbed but not peeled), a handful of spinach, and 2 thick lemon slices with pith and rind.*

Whizz up an antioxidant-rich soup.
➡ *Puree red peppers, tomatoes, onion, and garlic together. Add a little water if needed. Serve cold with basil leaves, or gently warm through if you prefer.*

Mix peppers with greens to help iron absorption.
➡ *Top roasted peppers with wilted greens and scatter over some shelled hemp seeds to add brain-supporting essential fatty acids.*

WHEN TO AVOID

Peppers, along with tomatoes, potatoes, and eggplant, belong to the nightshade family. Some believe these contribute to inflammatory conditions such as rheumatoid arthritis and are best avoided if this is a concern.

MOISTURE TRAP

Peppers lose moisture via their green stems and quickly dry out if these are removed. Prepare and chop just before use.

BUTTERNUT SQUASH

The distinctive butternut squash grows on a trailing vine and is valued for its compact size, thin edible skin, and sweet, rich flavor. The seeds of butternut squash are also edible and are a good source of vitamin E. Butternut squash's bright orange flesh signifies that this vegetable fruit is high in antioxidant and anti-inflammatory carotenoids, with their benefits for brain health.

BENEFITS

Butternut squash contains plenty of beneficial fiber that helps to support a healthy gut and, in turn, healthy brain function via the gut–brain axis. It is also an excellent source of vitamin B6 as well as vitamin B2, vitamin B3, folate, and pantothenic acid, which can help reduce fatigue and lift a low mood. Butternut squash is an especially rich source of antioxidant carotenoids.

The four carotenoids that are particularly high in butternut squash are alpha-carotene, beta-carotene, lutein, and zeaxanthin. Beta-carotene, and to a much lesser extent alpha-carotene, are converted in the body to vitamin A, vital for our vision as well as cellular communication and our immune function, which can be impacted by chronic stress over time. Lutein and zeaxanthin are essential for eye health, but recent research also suggests they are important for our brain health, too. Lutein, in particular, is associated with better learning and memory. Lutein has anti-inflammatory properties and it is thought that inflammation in the body is detrimental to the function of the hippocampus, involved in memory.

Vitamin B6, along with the entire complex of B vitamins, is incredibly important for our mental well-being. Vitamin B6 is required to synthesize numerous neurotransmitters, such as serotonin, which helps us cope with frustration and stress, and dopamine, which creates a sense of vitality, making you feel uplifted.

SUGGESTED SERVING

You can eat 5½oz (150g) of butternut squash daily if you wish. Make sure you eat a variety of colorful vegetables to maximize your nutrient intake.

HOW TO ENJOY

The dense-fleshed butternut squash is extremely versatile and can be mashed, steamed, or roasted with or without its skin. The flesh holds its shape well in a stew and makes a delicious curry.

Try combining squash with hazelnut butter—the oil from the butter helps the absorption of carotenoids.
➡ *Mix baked butternut flesh with the hazelnut butter for a brain-boosting dip.*

Create an immune-boosting, mood-lifting squash salad.
➡ *See recipe, opposite.*

Enjoy butternut squash with calming and revitalizing foods to help ease persistent anxiety.
➡ *Steam cubes of butternut squash and toss gently in olive oil with ginger, chili, and basil.*

TOMATO

We tend to think of tomatoes as red, but they come in a diverse range of colors and shapes, from huge purple beefsteak to small, red, plum tomatoes. Nutritional content varies according to the type, how the tomato was grown, and how ripe it was when picked from the vine. Picked fresh from the vine, tomatoes are succulent, flavorful, and densely packed with nutrients.

BENEFITS

Tomatoes have a high water content and are most hydrating when fresh; staying adequately hydrated is essential for our mental health, helping to support brain function and keeping us energized and alert. Tomatoes are also a good source of vitamins and minerals, including vitamins C and K, biotin, and potassium; they are rich in carotenoids, and are especially high in the antioxidant lycopene.

Biotin, also known as vitamin B7, is one of the vitamin B complex, which together protect our brains, improve memory, and generally help us to

> " Fresh tomatoes have a high water content, which helps to support brain function."

FOCUS ON

Globe artichoke

PROFILE
This handsome vegetable was popular with the Greeks and Romans, and most artichokes today are grown in the Mediterranean region.

PROPERTIES
As well as being high in antioxidants, artichokes are often used to help soothe digestive problems, which may be linked to stress.

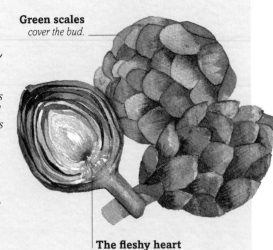

Green scales *cover the bud.*

The fleshy heart *is the most succulent part of the bud.*

maintain a positive outlook. A deficiency in biotin has been linked to lethargy and depression.

Lycopene is an important carotenoid for brain health. This powerful antioxidant prevents oxidation of the high density of healthy polyunsaturated brain fats and also protects the brain from inflammation. Consuming lycopene with a source of fat increases its absorption. Lycopene is made more available in cooked tomato products such as tomato paste and sauce.

The electrolyte potassium fires up our brain neurons. Low levels slow the brain down, causing brain "fog," and have been linked to depression. Concentrated tomato products such as tomato puree provide the highest amount of potassium.

SUGGESTED SERVING

Eat 1 large or 8 cherry tomatoes daily if you wish, but be sure you eat a variety of vegetables to maximize nutrients. When out of season, processed tomato products are a good alternative.

HOW TO ENJOY

Tomatoes form the basis of many dishes. Make and store the sauce when fresh tomatoes are not in season.

Enjoy tomatoes with their skin on as this contains essential phytonutrients.
➡ *Make a salsa from diced fresh tomatoes, red onions, garlic, chili, cilantro, and lime.*

The absorption of carotenoids in tomatoes is significantly increased with the addition of olive oil.
➡ *Toss sliced tomatoes with olive oil, basil, and some salt and black pepper.*

Cooking tomatoes increases the bioavailability of lycopene.
➡ *Roast tomatoes with oil and herbs.*

WHEN TO AVOID

Tomatoes belong to the nightshade family, which some believe contribute to inflammatory conditions such as rheumatoid arthritis, so are best avoided if a concern. Allergies are rare, but those allergic to grass pollen are most likely to be affected by tomatoes.

AVOCADO

Avocados grow in tropical and Mediterranean climates; the most commonly cultivated one is Hass. Their creamy, rich flesh is due to their fat content—avocados are one of the fattiest plant foods you can eat. Oleic acid, a healthy monounsaturated fat, is the primary fatty acid found in avocados.

BENEFITS

Avocados contain an abundance of minerals and vitamins. They are a good source of potassium and copper, both needed for a healthy brain. They are also high in vitamin K, stress-busting B vitamins, especially folate, are an excellent source of vitamin E, and are packed full of fiber.

Fiber—essential for gut health—is either soluble, which helps beneficial bacteria to thrive, or insoluble, which speeds up the movement of waste through the colon. The fiber in avocado is mostly insoluble. Both fibers help keep the gut healthy, which, as the gut communicates with the brain via the gut–brain axis, is essential for a healthy brain.

Vitamin E is a potent antioxidant and a fat-soluble vitamin that helps protect the fats in the brain and prevents inflammation.

Folate, involved in neuron messaging, is needed to break down homocysteine, an amino acid made by the body as part of biochemical processes. A buildup of homocysteine is thought to slow down the flow of nutrients to the brain. Research shows a link between depression and low levels of folate.

SUGGESTED SERVING

Enjoy 1 or 2 avocados a week.

HOW TO ENJOY

Ripen avocados in a paper bag with an apple or banana. Refrigerate once ripe.

Make a sustaining smoothie.
➥*Blend ½ avocado with ½in (1cm) piece each turmeric and ginger, grated, 2 tbsp hemp seeds, 9fl oz (250ml) coconut water, and black pepper.*
Make a fiber-boosting spread.
➥*Chop and dress with a squeeze of lime and chili sauce. Pile on sourdough rye toast or use to top black bean soup.*
The fat in avocado increases the absorption of antioxidants.
➥*Eat with brightly colored vegetables.*

WHEN TO AVOID

If you have a latex allergy, you may have a similar reaction to avocados.

GLOBE ARTICHOKE

Originating in the Mediterranean, these have been cultivated for centuries for both food and medicine. They belong to the thistle family, and the part that you eat is the immature flower. Both the leaves and the heart contain health-supporting nutrients.

BENEFITS

Globe artichokes are a good source of mood-regulating folate and magnesium as well as the powerful antioxidant vitamin C. They also contain a high concentration of the polyphenol cynarin and are rich in the soluble fiber inulin.

Polyphenols are beneficial plant compounds. Eating a diet rich in polyphenols helps prevent disease and supports brain health. Cynarin, a polyphenol found in globe artichokes, has a long history of use to stimulate bile flow and support the liver. A vital function of the liver is to disarm toxins. When liver function is impaired, toxins can build up, affecting the nervous system's role and brain health. Polyphenols quercetin and rutin, also found in globe artichokes, fight inflammation and protect the brain.

Inulin is a soluble fiber and acts as a prebiotic, feeding beneficial gut bacteria. In turn, the bacteria produce nutrients that support the health of colon cells and short-chain fatty acids, lowering inflammation. The intimate connection between the gut and brain makes eating foods that support gut health vital for our mental well-being.

SUGGESTED SERVING

In season, eat 1 artichoke up to 3 times a week. Out of season, enjoy the hearts preserved in brine or oil once a week.

HOW TO ENJOY

Artichokes can be eaten hot or cold.

Eat tender artichokes by hand.
➥*Boil or steam for 20 minutes, then pull the leaves off one by one. Dip the leaves into a sauce such as olive oil with balsamic vinegar, chopped garlic, and black pepper, or a lemony mayonnaise, then scrape off the fleshy leaf base between your teeth. Discard the hairy central piece then eat the fleshy heart.*
Enjoy the bottled hearts in a salad.
➥*Add to a potato salad with lemon zest and parsley, or make a salad from arugula, olives, artichoke hearts, and goat's cheese.*

WHEN TO AVOID

Globe artichokes may trigger a reaction in people who are allergic to ragweed pollen or are sensitive to members of the *Asteraceae/Compositae* plant family.

FUNGI AND SEAWEEDS

Traditionally foraged for, fungi—or mushrooms—and seaweeds are rich in nutrients. Mushrooms are the fruiting body of certain fungus. Many edible ones are cultivated, including button, crimini, oyster, portobello, and shiitake. There is a vast variety of edible seaweeds, including wakame, kombu, arame, nori, and dulse. Iodine, an essential mineral for mental wellness, is present in seaweed.

SHIITAKE

Mushrooms are high in protein, complex carbohydrates, and a range of other compounds that promote mental wellness. Shiitake is one of the most studied mushrooms, both for its food and medicinal benefits. They are a rich source of B vitamins, which help to convert our food into energy, and are abundant in antioxidants. Readily available, they have a delicious earthy flavor.

BENEFITS

Shiitake mushrooms are excellent sources of the antioxidants ergothioneine and selenium, as well as copper, zinc, and lentinan, a polysaccharide. Shiitake can also be a good plant source of vitamin D. Research shows that exposing the gills of fresh shiitake to the sunlight produces vitamin D2, which has anti-inflammatory and immune-boosting properties that help to protect the brain. A deficiency in vitamin D has been shown to increase the risk of suffering with depression.

Ergothioneine is a potent antioxidant and anti-inflammatory, and some of the highest levels are found in mushrooms. Recent research has found that people who eat mushrooms have a lower risk of a decline in memory and thinking skills, which has been attributed, in part, to ergothioneine. In addition, ergothioneine can help to prevent stress-induced sleep disturbances.

Selenium, an essential mineral, is involved in many brain functions. Adequate levels in the diet are thought to be crucial for helping to prevent anxiety and symptoms of depression. Selenium, an antioxidant, plays an essential role in the immune system. It helps to lower oxidative stress caused by toxins in the body, which in turn reduces inflammation and enhances our immunity. Maintaining a healthy immune system promotes the long-term health of the brain.

SUGGESTED SERVING

Aim to eat a portion (3½oz/100g) of mushrooms 3–4 times a week.

HOW TO ENJOY

Shiitake mushrooms can be cooked in a little olive oil. Their flavor goes well with eggs, pasta, rice, fish, and many vegetables, including potatoes, eggplant, kale, and cauliflower. Or add a teaspoon of powdered shiitake to a smoothie.

RECIPE

Shiitake broth

Gently simmer 9oz (250g) sliced shiitake, 1 red onion, 2 cloves of garlic, 2 celery sticks, and 2 carrots, all chopped, in 1¾ pints (1 liter) well-flavored vegetable stock for 45 minutes, for a rich, earthy broth.

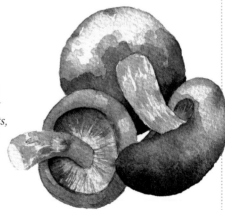

Make a soothing and calming
shiitake broth.
➠*See recipe, opposite.*
Cook with herbs for a toast topping.
➠*Gently soften sliced shiitake in
ghee, add sage and serve on rye toast.
The fiber in rye helps with digestion
and sage helps with memory.*

WHEN TO AVOID
Never pick or eat wild mushrooms
unless correctly identified by an expert.

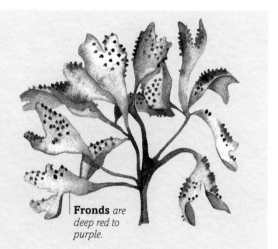

FOCUS ON

Dulse

PROFILE
*This red edible seaweed
grows wild in the north
Atlantic and Pacific.*

PROPERTIES
*High in micronutrients,
dulse also provides fiber,
promoting a healthy gut.*

Fronds *are
deep red to
purple.*

DULSE

**Seaweeds offer one of the broadest
range of minerals of all foods, and
dulse has one of the highest iron and
vitamin C contents of any seaweed.
This medium-sized red seaweed
grows along the low waterline on
rocky coastlines. It is possible to buy
fresh dulse, and it is one of the
seaweeds you can eat raw. More
often than not, though, it is sold
dried. It is easy to incorporate in a
variety of dishes, and you can also
eat it straight from the bag.**

BENEFITS

Dulse is an excellent source of iodine
(see right). It also contains vitamin B6,
which aids in the production of
neurotransmitters; iron, vital for memory;
potassium, which helps our nerves to
work; and the antioxidant beta-carotene.
The iron, zinc, and iodine found in dulse
are key nutrients that make an important
contribution to maintaining healthy
cognitive function.

Iodine is critical for a healthy thyroid,
the gland positioned in the neck
that helps produce and regulate
hormones. Iodine is needed to make
the thyroid hormones thyroxine (T4)
and triiodothyronine (T3). In the

brain, T4 and T3 activate dopamine,
serotonin, and the amino acid
gamma aminobutyric acid (GABA),
all key neurotransmitters that
affect our moods. Low levels of
T4 and T3 in the body can increase
the risk of experiencing depression
and can also affect our ability to
concentrate. During pregnancy,
iodine is essential for the correct
development of the brain.
Worldwide, iodine deficiency
has been found to contribute
to preventable brain damage.

SUGGESTED SERVING

Dulse contains between 150 and
300mcg per gram of iodine.
The adult recommended daily
amount is 150mcg, rising to
200mcg during pregnancy and
lactation. Include no more than
10g of dulse weekly in your diet.

HOW TO ENJOY

All seaweeds have flavor-enhancing
properties thanks to the polysaccharide
alginates and glutamate flavor
compounds that provide the "umami"
taste. There are few savory dishes
that dulse does not improve.

Add as an iron-rich topping to
dishes of all kinds.
➠*Crisp the dulse in a pan before
topping soups, salads, and baked
potatoes, or mixing into risottos
and paella.*

WHEN TO AVOID
If you have thyroid issues, consult
your health practitioner before
eating a lot of seaweed. Seaweeds
can accumulate heavy metals, so
always source sustainably harvested
seaweeds from clean ocean or
aquaculture waters.

"*Dulse has one of the highest
levels of iron and vitamin C
of any of the seaweed family.*"

BERRIES

Juicy, brightly colored berries are some of the healthiest foods you can eat. Blackberries, raspberries, blueberries, strawberries, and other berries are brimming with phytonutrients that play a significant role in easing anxiety and symptoms of depression to support mental well-being. Eating a variety of berries delivers the most extensive range of phytonutrients.

RASPBERRY

A member of the rose (*Rosaceae*) family, these have a vibrant, sweet taste with a hint of sourness and are at their flavor-best when freshly picked. A top brain-supporting food, raspberries boast an impressive list of health-protecting phytonutrients, including anthocyanins, compounds that give fruits their color.

BENEFITS

An excellent source of the powerful antioxidants vitamin C, vitamin K, and ellagic acid, raspberries also provide folic acid, crucial for brain and nerve function. Full of fiber, they promote digestive harmony, in turn supporting brain health. They also contain manganese and copper, both of which support healthy cognition.

Stress-busting vitamin C helps us to cope better with everyday pressures. Vitamin C is also needed to convert dopamine to serotonin, which regulates anxiety and balances mood.

Vitamin K is involved in maintaining and promoting healthy nerves. Eating vitamin K-rich foods helps sharpen memory and stave off dementia in older adults.

Ellagic acid belongs to the polyphenol group of phytonutrients; it is found in many fruits, but is exceptionally high in raspberries. This compound is a powerful antioxidant, helping to neutralize free radicals, the unstable molecules that damage healthy cells. In fact, ellagic acid is one of the most potent antioxidants you can include in your diet.

SUGGESTED SERVING

Eat about 5½oz (150g) of any kind, or mix, of berries daily, when in season. The maximum nutrition comes from fresh, seasonal berries.

HOW TO ENJOY

Very perishable, raspberries are best on the day of purchase. Enjoy on their own or with other foods for a synergy of benefits.

Eat with probiotic-rich yogurt.
➡ *Serve with a dollop of live yogurt.*
Make a raspberry sauce. Don't sieve out the seeds as these contain fiber, antioxidants, and essential fatty acids.
➡ *Lightly mash raspberries into a sauce and enjoy with a wide range of foods.*
Make an antioxidant-rich summer salad.
➡ *Toss with green leaves, avocado, fennel, basil, parsley, and dulse. Dress with lemon juice and hemp oil.*

RECIPE

Strawberry salsa

Make a refreshing salsa. Dice 14oz (400g) strawberries, 1 red onion, and a small, seeded red pepper. Mix with 1 tbsp lime juice and a handful of chopped cilantro.

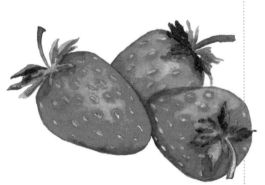

BLUEBERRY

The deep purple–blue color and complex, sweet flavor of blueberries come from various phytonutrients, the best-known being the flavonoid, anthocyanin. Blueberries contain many different antioxidants; in fact, they have one of the highest antioxidant levels of all common fruits and vegetables. This antioxidant content helps to support the heart and circulatory system, which is critical to support the health of the brain.

BENEFITS

Numerous studies demonstrate the impressive benefits of blueberries and how they can enhance brain health. One study showed that people who eat blueberries have slower cognitive decline rates, meaning that their brains remained healthier as they age. Blueberries contain good amounts of fiber, vitamin K, vitamin C, manganese, copper, and anthocyanins.

Manganese is needed by the body for the health of the nervous system and brain. Studies suggest it has a role to play in preventing neurological disorders such as Parkinson's disease.

Copper is essential in the production of hemoglobin, which carries oxygen to the brain and around the body. A shortage of copper impacts the neurotransmitter dopamine, which helps to maintain a happy mood and positive outlook.

Anthocyanins are powerful antioxidant compounds that fight oxidative stress. They are found in red, purple, and blue foods, and they are particularly high in blueberries. Eating foods rich in anthocyanins is hugely beneficial, as studies indicate a link between free radicals and mood disorders such as anxiety and depression.

SUGGESTED SERVING

Eat about 5½oz (150g) of any kind, or mix, of berries daily, when in season. The maximum nutrition comes from fresh, seasonal berries.

HOW TO ENJOY

Blueberries will last for up to a week in the fridge and also freeze well, so pop a few bags in the freezer for winter smoothies. These versatile berries can be easily added to muffins, turned into sorbets, and tossed into salads.

Enjoy a nourishing pudding. Adding chia seeds to this creamy pudding provides magnesium, the "relaxing mineral," to ease stress and anxiety.
➥*Combine blueberries with coconut milk and scatter with some chia seeds.*

Make an antioxidant-rich rice dish.
➥*Add red onions, blueberries, and walnuts to pilaf rice.*

Enjoy as an afternoon pick-me-up.
➥*Skip sugary snacks and eat a handful of blueberries instead.*

STRAWBERRY

This luscious, ever-popular scarlet red summer fruit is juicy and sweet. Many different compounds make up the unmistakable irresistible aroma of strawberries. Foraged wild strawberries provide a sharp, sweet, and juicy burst of flavor. Both wild and cultivated strawberries have excellent health benefits.

BENEFITS

Strawberries contain numerous nutrients beneficial for mental well-being. As well as vitamin C, folate, and iodine, they provide copper, potassium, and manganese, all key to cognitive function.

Vitamin C is a key brain antioxidant that helps combat inflammation. It has been found to help improve anxiety and depression symptoms.

Folate is part of the vitamin B complex and a deficiency in any of this group can disrupt brain function. Folate helps the body produce mood-regulating neurotransmitters such as dopamine and serotonin. Clinical trials found that folate can have a therapeutic effect on depression.

Iodine is essential to make thyroid hormones, which control metabolism. Low levels of iodine lead to "brain fog," fatigue, anxiety, and depression. Our bodies are unable to make iodine so we must obtain it from our food.

SUGGESTED SERVING

Eat about 5½oz (150g) of any kind, or mix, of berries daily, in season. Maximum nutrition is in fresh, seasonal strawberries.

HOW TO ENJOY

Enjoy in season or dehydrate for winter use. If you do not have a dehydrator, you can dry on the lowest oven heat, cutting large strawberries into thick slices.

Make a nerve-calming fruit salad.
➥*Combine with flavorful lemon balm.*

Enjoy healthy strawberries and cream with essential fatty acids in hemp.
➥*Top a bowl of strawberries with hemp cream (see p.167).*

Enjoy on a buckwheat pancake. Buckwheat provides excellent protein for the brain, and yogurt adds probiotics for a healthy gut.
➥*Top a buckwheat pancake with strawberries, yogurt, and mint.*

Make a revitalizing salsa.
➥*See recipe, opposite.*

WHEN TO AVOID

Though uncommon, strawberry allergies and intolerances exist.

RECIPES FOR MENTAL WELLNESS

SAUCES AND TOPPINGS

These delicious accompaniments not only lend flavor complexity and depth to dishes and snacks, but are also an excellent way to add a whole range of essential micronutrients to our food. As well as being nutrient-dense, compounds in spices, herbs, and garlic aid the digestive process, helping to optimize the absorption of essential nutrients in the gut that are needed for brain health, cognition, and overall well-being.

1

Salsa verde

This tangy salsa, a delicious accompaniment to fish and chicken, contains a medley of antioxidant herbs to combat the effects of stress. Parsley is a source of vitamin C, the immune-boosting vitamin needed to synthesize the neurotransmitters in the brain that help to regulate mood. Garlic and shallots provide sulphur compounds, which convert to anti-inflammatory alliin, protecting against oxidative stress.

MAKES **10FL OZ (300ML)** | PREP TIME **10 MINS**

Finely chop the leaves of a **bunch** each of **parsley** and **basil**. Snip a **small bunch** of **chives**, and rinse, dry, and roughly chop **2 tbsp salted capers**. Place the herbs in a bowl with the capers, **1 finely chopped shallot** and **2 finely chopped garlic cloves**. Stir in **1 tbsp apple cider vinegar** and **1 tsp Dijon mustard**. Beat in **5fl oz (150ml) olive oil** until you reach the desired consistency. Season with **sea salt flakes**. Taste, adding more vinegar and salt as needed.

2

Toasted spice condiment

Enjoy this nutty condiment sprinkled over soups, baked dishes, and salads. Hazelnuts provide folate, which has a protective action against depression, while sesame is a source of protein, crucial for brain health. Coriander and cumin act as digestive aids, helping the absorption of essential brain-supporting nutrients.

MAKES **3OZ (85G)** | PREP TIME **10 MINS**

Put **2 tbsp sesame seeds**, **1 tbsp coriander seeds**, and **1 tsp cumin seeds** in a dry frying pan over medium heat. Cook gently, shaking the pan to ensure even toasting, until the spices crack and release their strong aroma. Grind the sesame, spices, and **¼ tsp sea salt flakes** together with a mortar and pestle. Mix with **2 tbsp finely chopped hazelnuts**. Keep in an air-tight container in the fridge for up to a week.

3

Lacto-fermented chili sauce

This rich, fiery, fermented sauce can pep up a whole range of dishes. As well as providing stimulating chili, the fermentation process supplies the gut with beneficial bacteria, creating a healthy gut microbiome that in turn supports brain health. When we eat chilli peppers, our brains release endorphins, the natural feel-good chemicals.

MAKES ABOUT **1¾ PINTS (1 LITER)** | PREP TIME **5 MINS** | FERMENTATION UP TO **2 WEEKS**

Fill a Mason jar with **2¼lb (1kg) chilies**, stalks removed, seeded, and coarsely chopped, and **6 finely chopped garlic cloves**. Add **2 tbsp fine salt** to **1¾ pints (1 liter) water** for a brine. Pour over enough brine to cover the chilies and garlic. Top with a weight, cover with muslin or an airtight lid, and let ferment at room temperature, away from direct sunlight, for 2 weeks, checking that the chilies remain submerged. Once pleasantly sour, strain and reserve the brine. Process the mix in a blender with enough of the reserved brine for a thick sauce. Transfer to bottles and store in the fridge for up to 3 months.

CITRUS

Citrus fruits include oranges, grapefruits, lemons, and limes. All are good sources of vitamin C and antioxidant and anti-inflammatory plant compounds. Flavonoids, in particular, support mental well-being, protecting the nervous system, improving brain function, and aiding memory. The whole fruit also provides fiber, which supports a healthy gut and in turn mental health via the gut–brain axis.

GRAPEFRUIT

White, pink, and red varieties of grapefruit have a refreshing sweet, sour, and tangy flavor. A high water content makes the fruit an extremely hydrating one for our brains, which depend on adequate hydration to function properly. Red and pink grapefruit are excellent sources of the antioxidant lycopene, and all grapefruit contain potassium, which helps reduce symptoms of stress.

BENEFITS

Studies have shown that eating grapefruit before a meal can help with weight loss. Being overweight increases the risk of cognitive decline and can lead to Type 2 diabetes, which makes depression 2–3 times more likely. Grapefruit also provides vitamin B1, which helps maintain nerve function; vitamin B5, which improves focus; stress-busting vitamin C; and the soluble fiber pectin.

Lycopene, a caretonoid phytonutrient, is found in pink and red grapefruit. Its potent antioxidant powers eliminate free radicals, protecting the brain, which is especially vulnerable to oxidative damage.

Potassium, an electrolyte, helps ensure the brain has enough oxygen to work at its best. It fires up the brain; low levels have been shown to slow the brain, causing fatigue and "brain fog."

Pectin is a soluble fiber with numerous health benefits. It acts as a prebiotic, feeding beneficial gut bacteria that support mental health via the brain–gut axis.

SUGGESTED SERVING

If you want to lose weight, eating ½ grapefruit before a meal may help as part of a balanced diet. Otherwise, include 1 grapefruit as one of your 3 fruits a day.

HOW TO ENJOY

Eating grapefruit whole is the best way to obtain all the valuable nutrients and fiber.

Make a granita. This is an excellent way to preserve beneficial nutrients.
➡ *Process the segments, fibrous parts too, to a purée with honey. Freeze.*
Add zing to a salad. The vitamin C aids iron absorption from the green leaves.
➡ *Mix with green leaves and avocado.*

WHEN TO AVOID

Avoid if taking statins. Allergy is rare, but a citrus intolerance can lead to bloating, cramps, and diarrhoea.

RECIPE

Zingy citrus yogurt

Mix orange and grapefruit segments together, including the pith, with 4 tablespoons of natural yogurt. Add honey to sweeten and orange zest for a citrussy kick.

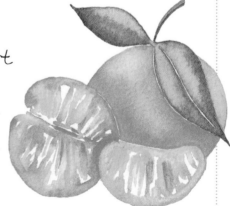

"Flavonoids in the pith and rind of oranges support healthy brain function."

ORANGE

There are a number of different types of oranges, ranging from the sour Seville orange and crimson-flushed blood orange to sweet tangerines and juicy navel and Valencia oranges. All are high in vitamin C and very good sources of fiber for a healthy gut microbiome. The navel orange is at its seasonal peak in the winter months—its color and aroma alone lift spirits.

BENEFITS

Flavonoids concentrated in the orange rind and pith strengthen blood flow, supporting brain function. As well as vitamin C, navel and Valencia oranges contain B vitamins, which play a key role in brain health, and calcium, copper, and potassium, which are all linked to better memory.

Vitamin C is in all citrus fruits and navel and Valencia oranges are excellent sources. It plays a crucial role in the central nervous system, helping the maturation of neurons and the formation of the myelin sheath that surrounds and protects nerve fibers. It also facilitates the synthesis of neurotransmitters that affect our motivation, alertness, concentration, and memory.

Folate, also known as vitamin B9, is one of the B vitamins in oranges. A deficiency is linked to an increased risk of Alzheimer's disease. It is involved in synthesizing the neurotransmitter dopamine, which aids memory, attention, and focus; and serotonin, which improves mood.

SUGGESTED SERVING

Eating oranges regularly—up to 1 a day—significantly boosts vitamin C intake.

HOW TO ENJOY

Eat the whole fruit, including the pith, rather than drink store-bought juice, which is high in sugar and low in fiber so can cause a spike in blood sugar levels.

Combine with yogurt for gut health.
➡ *See recipe, opposite.*
Enjoy a chocolate-orange mousse for an antioxidant boost.
➡ *Opt for dark chocolate for the highest cacao content.*

WHEN TO AVOID
Citrus allergy is rare but an intolerance can lead to bloating, cramps, and diarrhea.

LEMON

Lemons are available all year round. Tart and acidic in flavor, they are nevertheless incredibly refreshing. In addition to vitamin C, lemons contain other compounds with antioxidant properties, including D limonene. Research suggests that this compound, found predominantly in the lemon peel, can help to ease stress and anxiety.

BENEFITS

Lemons are an excellent source of the soluble fiber pectin, and contain folate, which reduces the risk of Alzheimer's disease; vitamin B6, which helps ease anxiety, depression, and fatigue; and potassium, which promotes positivity.

Vitamin C is a vital antioxidant that we have to obtain from our diet daily. The highest concentrations are found in the brain and central nervous system. Because of its ability to neutralize toxins, it has a crucial neuroprotective role, helping us cope with the psychological and physical effects of stress. The more stress in your life, the greater your need for vitamin C.

SUGGESTED SERVING

Liven up food and drinks daily with a good squeeze of lemon juice. Add preserved lemon pieces to grain and veggie dishes.

HOW TO ENJOY

The juice of ½ lemon in a glass of water is revitalizing, but you will miss out on fiber and compounds if you use only the juice.

Preserve a jar of lemons for a pickle. This provides the compounds and fiber found in the pith and skin.
➡ *Use organic lemons to avoid pesticide residue in the skin and the wax used to protect lemons in transit.*
Make a tangy antioxidant and probiotic-rich fermented drink.
➡ *Stir the juice of 6 lemons into 4½oz (125g) unrefined cane sugar in a Mason jar. Add 4fl oz (120ml) whey and 1¾ pints (1 liter) water. Seal. Leave in a warm place for 5 days.*

WHEN TO AVOID
It is possible to be intolerant to citrus; lemon is the most well-tolerated.

TROPICAL

Tropical fruits are packed full of luscious flavors. In addition to their delicious taste, these exotic fruits also contain a host of beneficial nutrients. Fruits such as papaya, mango, passion fruit, pineapple, and banana have plant compounds that deliver antioxidant benefits for the body and brain. They also provide plenty of fiber for digestive support, maintaining a healthy gut–brain axis.

BANANA

The tropical banana has been cultivated for thousands of years. Historically, bananas were not the sweet, creamy-fleshed, yellow variety that we eat today but the green variety that we know as plantain (see box, right). Sweet yellow bananas contain a significant amount of vitamin B6 and vitamin C, two critical nutrients for brain health; they also provide a good amount of potassium.

BENEFITS

As well as vitamins and a fair amount of fiber, including resistant starch, bananas contain manganese, which protects against oxidative cell damage; copper, essential for brain-specific enzymes; and biotin, which promotes a positive outlook.

Vitamin B6 is needed for the synthesis of several neurotransmitters, including serotonin. Low levels of this vitamin are associated with irritability, nervousness, difficulty concentrating, and depression.

Vitamin C is a vital antioxidant molecule in the brain. It helps lift a low mood and ease depression.

Potassium, a balancing electrolyte, helps to activate neurons that are involved in positive thoughts and feelings. Potassium-rich foods such as bananas may help reduce symptoms of stress and anxiety.

Fiber in bananas is mostly in the form of soluble fiber, which slows down digestion. The slow movement through the gastrointestinal tract helps prevent sugar spikes. Soluble fiber finally gets broken down by bacteria in the large intestine. Bananas also contain starches that are naturally resistant to digestion. These starches move through to the large bowel where they are fermented to make short-chain fatty acids, providing energy for gut microbes and the brain.

SUGGESTED SERVING

You can eat a banana a day, but aim to eat a variety of fruit and vegetables.

HOW TO ENJOY

Bananas are easy to include in your diet. They are the ultimate convenience food, easy to take with you when traveling and enjoyed by all ages. One banana provides a significant amount of nutrients to support mental well-being.

Make a delicious, mood-boosting iced treat. The addition of chocolate adds magnesium, and hemp seeds provide essential fatty acids.
➥*Push halved bananas on to a stick. Roll in melted raw chocolate and shelled hemp seeds, then freeze.*

FOCUS ON
Plantains

PROFILE
This green banana variety is grown as a cooking ingredient in tropical regions around the world.

PROPERTIES
Low in fat, plantains are a good source of potassium and antioxidant vitamin C.

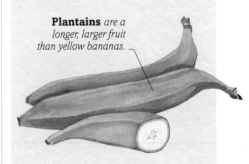

Plantains *are a longer, larger fruit than yellow bananas.*

Combine banana with oats for an effective mood-enhancing combination.
➡️*Slice up a banana and mix it in with your morning oatmeal.*
Make an energizing, gut-friendly morning smoothie.
➡️*Blend banana, yogurt, spinach, fresh turmeric and ginger, black pepper, and a squeeze of lemon.*

WHEN TO AVOID

Allergy to bananas is possible. If you have a latex allergy, you may also be allergic to bananas.

MANGO

Worldwide, the mango has proven to be one of the most popular of all the tropical fruits. In Indian Ayurvedic tradition, mangoes are called the "king of fruits" and medicinal properties are attributed to all parts of the tree, bark, flower, seed, leaves, and fruit. Mangoes are densely packed with vitamins, minerals, and antioxidants. The exotic flesh of a mango is a delicious way to boost brain health.

BENEFITS

Mangoes are an excellent source of vitamin C and a good source of the B family of vitamins. They also contain plenty of prebiotic dietary fiber, which helps to keep the digestive tract working efficiently, as well as plant compounds such as beta-carotene, and active digestive enzymes.

Vitamin C is well-known as the stress-busting vitamin. Chronic stress and anxiety can damage the brain, leading to a range of symptoms, including memory loss.

RECIPE

Mango salsa

Peel and dice a mango into small cubes. Finely dice a red onion. Seed and finely dice ½ red chili, then combine the mango, onion, and chili. Add diced avocado, chopped cilantro leaves, and a squeeze of lime.

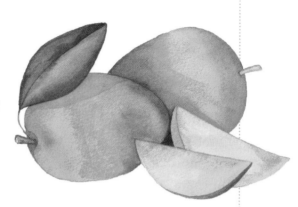

B vitamins are critical for maintaining the function of brain neurotransmitters and are also essential for a balanced mood and a good night's sleep.

Beta-carotene, a carotenoid, is the yellow-orange pigment that gives mangoes their color. Like all carotenoids, it is an antioxidant that protects the body from oxidative stress. By helping to eliminate damaging free radicals, antioxidants such as beta-carotene are thought to improve symptoms of anxiety and depression.

Highly active enzymes in mangoes aid in the breakdown and digestion of protein.

SUGGESTED SERVING

Because of its sweetness, limit mangoes to 1 a week. Aim for a variety of fruits, making the most of locally grown ones.

HOW TO ENJOY

It is hard to beat simply eating the sweet, aromatic flesh of the mango, peeled, and cut away from the stone. This is also one of the best ways to benefit from the nutrients in mango. However, this delicious fruit is also a great addition to a range of sweet and savory dishes, adding texture and sweetness.

Make a mango lassi. Combining mango with live yogurt supports gut health, providing probiotics for a healthy gut microbiome and, in turn, supporting brain health via the gut–brain axis.
➡️*Whip up a lassi with live yogurt, mango flesh, and a squeeze of lemon for a gut-boosting drink.*
Make a tasty mood-enhancing salsa.
➡️*See recipe, above.*

"Sweet, aromatic mangoes contain B vitamins that help to elevate mood and enhance sleep."

APPLES, PEARS, AND STONE FRUITS

Fruits are fiber-rich and sustaining. Hard fruits, such as apples and pears, are best eaten in season, though often store well. Soft, stone fruits such as peaches, nectarines, and cherries should be eaten fresh or dried to use in the winter months.

APPLE

Apples originated in the mountains of Kazakhstan, where the wild tree still blossoms. Today, apples are found in a wide array of varieties of various sizes and colors. They range from astringent cider apples to tart and tangy cooking apples and sweet, juicy, eating apples. All types provide large quantities of the soluble fiber pectin.

BENEFITS

Quercetin, an antioxidant, is common to all apples. Apples also contain potassium, vitamin K, B vitamins, and vitamin C. They are densely packed with beneficial phytonutrients, though the type and quantity vary depending on the variety and where an apple has grown. Many of the phytonutrients are found in the skin.

Quercetin is a powerful antioxidant phytonutrient found in many plants and is particularly abundant in apples. It protects the body from the destructive action of free radicals and also helps to reduce inflammation, protecting against degenerative brain disorders such as Alzheimer's disease. Research suggests that quercetin can help regulate blood sugar levels, helping to balance mood and avoid irritability.

Pectin in apples is a soluble fiber that acts as a prebiotic, supporting the gut by feeding beneficial bacteria. The brain and gut are in constant communication via the vagus nerve, known as the gut–brain axis; studies show that healthy gut microbes positively affect our mental well-being.

Vitamin C in the body is found in the highest concentrations in the brain, where it plays an important mood-lifting effect. Our bodies are unable to store vitamin C, so we need to obtain it from our diet every day.

SUGGESTED SERVING

Enjoy an apple daily as part of your 2–3 portions of fruit a day.

HOW TO ENJOY

Many of apples' benefits are in the skin. Enjoy in sweet and savory dishes. If you have cider apples, make raw apple cider vinegar, which is abundant in benefits.

Enjoy in an autumn salad. Walnuts provide essential fatty acids while endive has mood-lifting folate.
➥ *Toss apple slices with walnuts and Belgian endive.*

RECIPE

Sautéed pears with spinach

Sauté a diced pear in a little olive oil until softened. Toss in a small, finely diced and seeded chili and cook for 1 minute. Add a generous pat of butter and 8oz (225g) baby spinach and gently wilt.

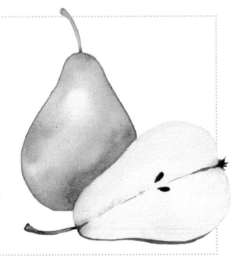

"Many of the precious phytonutrients provided by apples and pears are found within the skin."

PEAR

There are numerous varieties of pears, which come in different shades of green, brown, red, and gold. Common ones include the juicy, aromatic Williams and the earthy-flavored Comice. All pears are loaded with antioxidants and are an excellent choice to eat to help with inflammatory conditions.

BENEFITS

A good source of copper, vitamins C and K, and dietary fiber, pears also contain lots of fiber, mostly insoluble.

Copper is essential for haemoglobin production, which carries oxygen to the brain so is crucial for brain health.

Vitamin C helps soothe anxiety. People with higher levels of vitamin C in their diet have been found to cope better with stress.

Vitamin K is thought to support a sharper memory in older populations.

Insoluble fiber helps to maintain a healthy gut, which is, in turn, essential for good brain function.

SUGGESTED SERVING

When in season, include 1 pear in your daily portions of fruit.

HOW TO ENJOY

It is best not to peel pears, as much of the fiber and phytonutrients are in the skin.

Pears are generally sold before they are ripe as they bruise easily, then they soon ripen at room temperature. Pears work well in both sweet and savory dishes.

Enjoy with spinach and chili. The sweetness of the pear marries well with the slightly bitter spinach and fiery chili, while the vitamin C in the pears helps the absorption of the iron in spinach.
➨ *See recipe, opposite.*

Eat with soothing herbs to help relieve stress.
➨ *Poach pears with lemon balm.*

Pears and raw cacao are a great flavor combination. Raw cacao increases blood flow to the brain and can improve cognition, while almonds provide calming magnesium.
➨ *Blend into a smoothie with a little almond milk.*

CHERRY

There are two kinds of cherries: sweet and sour—or tart. Both contain phytonutrients that protect our brain cells from oxidative damage. The season for cherries is brief, so they can be enjoyed for only a short time. Acerola cherries, available as a powder, contain huge amounts of vitamin C; while these are called cherries and resemble cherries, technically they are "cherrylike" berries that are native to South America.

BENEFITS

Cherries are a rich source of polyphenol phytonutrients and vitamin C, both of which have antioxidant and anti-inflammatory properties. Sweet and sour cherries contain melatonin, though there are higher concentrations in sour ones.

Melatonin is a hormone produced by the pineal gland in your brain; it can also be found in foods such as walnuts, kiwi fruit, and cherries. Melatonin helps regulate the body's internal rhythms and improves sleep quality and duration. The restorative function of sleep is critical to cognitive function and well-being.

Vitamin C is a vital supportive nutrient that enables people to cope better with the physical and psychological effects that stress can cause. Chronic stress can cause the adrenal glands to become fatigued, which, in turn, affects mental health. Vitamin C helps restore healthy function to our adrenals, significantly improving mental health.

SUGGESTED SERVING

When in season, include a generous handful in your 2–3 portions of fruit a day.

HOW TO ENJOY

Sweet cherries are best eaten fresh and raw, whereas sour cherries taste much better when cooked. Dried sour cherries are available, which work well in savory dishes. You can also purchase sour cherry juice. It is hard to improve on a bowl of ripe, dark red, sweet cherries.

Combine sour cherries with saffron, which has been used for thousands of years as a natural form of antidepressant.
➨ *Toss a handful of sour cherries into saffron rice.*

PLUM

Like apples and pears, there are many plum varieties and these come in a range of colorful hues. All plums are good sources of fiber and also contain beneficial phytonutrients, although red plums tend to carry the most. Dried plums, known as prunes, can be made from most varieties and contain a similar nutritional profile. These have the added advantage of being available all year round. Despite being sweet, the high fiber content of prunes helps prevent blood sugar spikes.

BENEFITS

Plums contain beneficial polyphenol compounds; antioxidant vitamins C and K; the important brain minerals, potassium and copper; and are full of insoluble fiber for a healthy gut. Plums and prunes are often used to help "keep things moving" through the digestive system; this effect is most likely caused by the compound sorbitol found in plums, which acts as a natural laxative.

Polyphenols are plant compounds that promote and help maintain good health. There are more than 500

> " *Fiber in plums and apricots helps to ensure healthy digestion, in turn supporting well-being.* "

FOCUS ON

Plums

PROFILE
From the genus Prunus, *plums have been cultivated domestically around the world for thousands of years.*

PROPERTIES
With antioxidant and gut-promoting properties, plums are excellent for supporting overall health, including heart health, in turn increasing well-being.

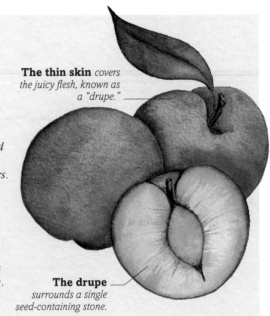

The thin skin *covers the juicy flesh, known as a "drupe."*

The drupe *surrounds a single seed-containing stone.*

polyphenols in plant-based foods, each one performing a different role. Plums contain two important polyphenol compounds that have been shown to help prevent oxidative damage to essential fats in our bodies. Our brains are made up of more than 60 percent fat, so eating plums can have a protective effect on the brain and, in turn, help to support our mental well-being.

Vitamin C is useful in preventing oxidative damage to the cholesterol in our bodies, 25 percent of which is found in our brains. Oxidized cholesterol builds up in the arteries and can lead to serious conditions such as a stroke.

Potassium helps regulate blood pressure to keep the effects of stress under control. It supports healthy nerve function, enabling clarity of thought and positive feelings.

SUGGESTED SERVING

When in season, include 3–4 plums as one of your daily 2–3 portions of fruit.

HOW TO ENJOY

Buying plums in season ensures they have the richest, sweetest-tasting flesh. If you have a dehydrator, you can dry plums for winter use. If you do not have a dehydrator, halve and stone the plums, then quarter large plums, and dry on the lowest oven heat. Keep a packet of prunes in the cupboard for an instant snack.

Enjoy with yogurt, full of friendly gut bacteria to support digestive health and the brain via the gut–brain axis.
➡ *Add a sliced plum to a bowl of live yogurt with a sprinkle of nutmeg.*

Combine with arugula, fennel, and goat cheese. Arugula and fennel support digestion, enabling nutrients to be efficiently absorbed, while goat cheese is a good source of probiotics.
➡ *Lightly caramelize plum halves and toss with arugula, fennel, and a little raw goat cheese.*

Whip up a brain-supporting smoothie.
➡ *Blend soaked prunes and the soaking water, shelled hemp seeds, fresh ginger, and cacao.*

APRICOT

The fresh, golden apricot is soft, sweet, and a little bit tart. Although the season for fresh apricots is a short one, it is possible to buy dried apricots all year round. The long lives and good health that are enjoyed by the Hunza population in the Himalayas is partly attributed to the apricots they eat. Though it may be hard to measure how true this is, apricots certainly do contain plenty of antioxidants that are key for health and vitality.

BENEFITS

As well as being an excellent source of antioxidants, including beta-carotene and vitamin C, apricots are also high in soluble fiber and are a good source of potassium, an electrolyte that is critical for regulating nerve signals.

Beta-carotene is a flavonoid that gives apricots their glorious color and is a potent antioxidant. The brain uses a large quantity of oxygen to support its immense activity, resulting in the highly unstable molecules known as free radicals. Antioxidants such as beta-carotene help to stabilize these molecules to prevent them from causing harm. By reducing free radicals that can lead to damaging inflammation, antioxidants have been found to improve anxiety and depressive symptoms.

Soluble fiber slows the movement of food through the digestive tract, making the body feel fuller for longer. It also provides food for beneficial gut bacteria, creating a healthy gut microbiome. A healthy gut helps promote good mental health and overall well-being, as the digestive system and brain are connected via the gut–brain axis.

Potassium is critical for regulating nerve signals in the brain and body. Low potassium levels can lead to difficulty thinking and "brain fog," characterized by an inability to focus and problems with memory. Potassium helps ensure the brain has enough oxygen to function well.

SUGGESTED SERVING

When in season, include 2–3 apricots as 1 of your daily 2–3 portions of fruit.

HOW TO ENJOY

Apricots are delicious eaten fresh on their own. They also add a rich, sweet taste to savory dishes and can be dried or fermented for a snack or to add to dishes when they are no longer in season.

Make apricot "leather." In the Middle East, fresh apricots are used to make a kind of fruit leather known as amardine. This is then infused in water to make a refreshing and revitalizing drink that helps to hydrate body and brain.
➡ *Stone and cook a few apricots. Add lime juice and honey to taste. Blend to a paste. Line a tray with parchment paper and spread the paste to ¼in (5mm) thickness. Dry in a dehydrator or an oven on the lowest setting. Cut into strips, roll up, and refrigerate in an airtight container. Eat or use to make an apricot-flavored drink.*

Make a lacto-fermented apricot chutney. Fermenting adds plenty of beneficial gut bacteria to antioxidant-rich apricots.
➡ *See recipe, below.*

Enjoy a fruity oat breakfast for a calming, grounding start to the day. The fiber in the apricot and oats will help to sustain the appetite, reducing the urge to snack between meals.
➡ *When in season, add chopped apricots and a pinch of cardamom to a bowl of morning oats.*

SLOW TO RIPEN

Once picked, apricots continue to ripen. Ideally, keep at room temperature away from direct sunlight and eat when softened and juicy.

RECIPE

Apricot chutney

Chop 9oz (250g) apricots, 1 red onion, 3 garlic cloves, 1 medium chili, and a 1in (2.5cm) piece of fresh ginger. Place in a Mason jar with 1 tsp salt and 1 tbsp sauerkraut juice. Weight, loosely cover, and ferment at room temperature for 5 days.

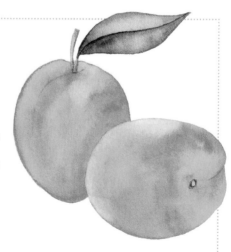

LEGUMES

Legumes are the edible seeds from the Fabacaea plant family and come in various shapes, colors, and sizes. All legumes contain plenty of healthy protein, making them an excellent addition to a plant-based diet. With a vegan diet, it is important to include a wide variety of plant foods in your diet to be sure you are getting a mix of proteins providing all nine essential amino acids.

LENTIL

Lentils are probably the oldest of the cultivated legumes. There are various types of lentils, the most common varieties being the large green and split red ones, but black beluga and French dark green lentils are also popular. All legumes are a good source of fiber, but lentils are a particularly excellent source, containing soluble and insoluble fiber, both of which are necessary for healthy digestion, supporting mental well-being via the gut–brain axis.

BENEFITS

Aside from protein and fiber, lentils are packed full of nutrients that are essential for brain health.

Molybdenum, an essential mineral, is found in all legumes, including lentils. It prevents toxins from building up and causing damaging inflammation.

Iron, another essential mineral, is used in the production of neurotransmitters and helps keep us energized and alert.

Zinc is critical for ensuring proper communication between brain cells. It also plays an essential role in supporting memory.

Folate helps support the creation of red blood cells and is critical for proper nerve function. Lentils are a particularly good source of folate.

The electrolyte mineral, potassium, is required to activate neurons involved in positive thoughts and feelings. Without the electrical charge sparked by potassium, neurotransmitters such as serotonin, which boost mood, cannot be utilized.

SUGGESTED SERVING

Enjoy a variety of nutrient-rich legumes. If you eat a plant-based diet, eat 3 rounded tablespoons of cooked legumes each day.

HOW TO ENJOY

A great source of vegetarian protein, lentils are versatile and easy to cook. If necessary, you can cook them without soaking. They add a rich, nutty flavor to soups, stews, and salads.

Make an anti-inflammatory, brain-nourishing, and aromatic soup.
➡ *Cook red lentils with onions, chili, and coconut milk for a delicious soup.*

Sprout lentils to make the beneficial nutrients in lentils more bioavailable.
➡ *Sprout whole green lentils and toss into salads. See p.170 for directions on sprouting.*

RECIPE

Lentil dahl

Cook 7oz (200g) rinsed red lentils. Heat 2 tbsp ghee. Add 1 tsp cumin seeds and cook for 1 minute. Finely dice 1 onion, 1 green chili, and 2 garlic cloves and add with the lentils. Cook for 3 minutes. Add 2 tsp grated ginger, ½ tsp each ground turmeric, cardamom, paprika, and salt. Drain.

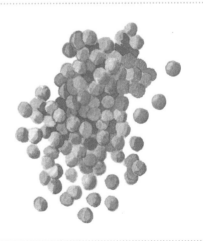

Add live yogurt to lentil dishes. Vitamin B12 in yogurt works with the vitamin B6 and folate found in lentils to control high levels of the amino acid homocysteine, a buildup of which can damage the brain.
➠*Serve spicy lentil dahl (see recipe, opposite) with full-fat live yogurt.*

PEA

Fresh peas are harvested from immature pods, whereas dried peas are produced by harvesting and drying peas from mature pods. Peas are also available whole or split— they split in half naturally when the skin is removed. The humble pea has one of the highest fiber contents of any legume.

BENEFITS

Peas contain many B complex vitamins. A deficiency in any B vitamin can disrupt normal brain function. They are also an excellent source of molybdenum, an essential mineral required by the brain, and contain a phytoestrogen isoflavone called daidzein, which is thought to help support mental health.

Vitamin B1, also known as thiamine, has a central role in brain health. The brain needs thiamine for energy; without adequate thiamine, brain cells die. The brain also needs thiamine to make acetylcholine, a neurotransmitter that serves a critical function in the brain, encoding new memories and enhancing our ability to reason and concentrate. Acetylcholine enables the growth of new synapses—the site of transmission between neurons. A lack of acetylcholine in the diet can contribute to the development of neurodegenerative diseases.

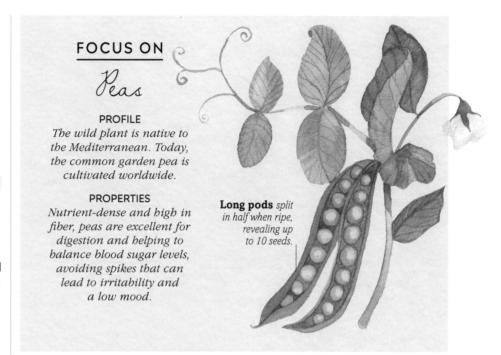

FOCUS ON
Peas

PROFILE
The wild plant is native to the Mediterranean. Today, the common garden pea is cultivated worldwide.

PROPERTIES
Nutrient-dense and high in fiber, peas are excellent for digestion and helping to balance blood sugar levels, avoiding spikes that can lead to irritability and a low mood.

Long pods *split in half when ripe, revealing up to 10 seeds.*

Vitamin B5, also known as pantothenic acid, is required for fat metabolism, energy, and normal brain function. It also boosts memory and regulates the autonomic nervous system by producing neurotransmitters such as acetylcholine.

A folate (vitamin B9) deficiency leads to an increase in the amino acid homocysteine, which can be disruptive. Low folate contributes to a greater risk of depression, including postnatal depression in women.

SUGGESTED SERVING

Enjoy a variety of nutrient-rich legumes. If you eat a plant-based diet, eat 3 rounded tablespoons of cooked legumes each day.

HOW TO ENJOY

Dried peas have been a pantry mainstay since early times and are excellent in soups, stews, dips, and dahls. They are best soaked for a minimum of 6 hours before use.

Eat with garlic to promote healthy blood flow to the brain.
➠*Make a fresh pea and garlic soup.*
Combine with sage, another memory-boosting ingredient.
➠*Blend cooked dried peas with sage for a delicious dip.*
Eat with anti-inflammatory, antioxidant turmeric to support brain health.
➠*Use frozen peas to make pea, sweet potato, and turmeric samosas.*

PERFECTLY FRESH PEAS

Frozen peas have more vitamins and minerals than canned. Fresh are best eaten on the day of purchase.

BLACK BEAN

Black beans, also known as turtle beans, are native to the Americas, where they have long been a staple food. These small, oval, and satiny beans are packed full of brain-supporting nutrients. In particular, black beans are a source of phytonutrients called anthocyanins, powerful antioxidants that have a valuable protective role in the brain.

BENEFITS

As well as providing magnesium, iron, and folate, black beans have an excellent mix of protein and fiber, which helps regulate blood sugar levels, avoiding fluctuations that can lead to "brain fog" and low mood. Black beans are also a good source of molybdenum and copper, both helpful for mental health.

Magnesium is a vital nutrient in supporting the brain's ability to process information and memory. It has a calming effect on the body and adequate amounts in the diet can make it easier for the body to cope with stress. In addition, magnesium helps convert food into energy—the brain uses more energy than any other organ.

Iron supports the synthesis and maintenance of the myelin sheaths that form around nerves in the brain; insufficient myelin is linked to a progressive brain function loss. Without adequate iron, we lack energy, which can lead to feelings of depression.

Folate deficiency can decrease serotonin levels in the brain and has been linked to depression.

SUGGESTED SERVING

Enjoy a variety of nutrient-rich legumes. If you eat a plant-based diet, eat 3 rounded tablespoons of cooked legumes each day.

HOW TO ENJOY

Soak black beans overnight and rinse well before cooking. For convenience, keep a can of black beans in the cupboard, as it can quickly be turned into salads, dips, burritos, and soups. You don't need to combine plant proteins at every meal as long as you eat a variety of proteins during the day.

Enjoy in a stew.
➡️ *Make a black bean and sweet potato stew and serve with rice for the perfect complete protein combination. Add leftover black bean stew to an energizing and mood-uplifting salad bowl with spinach, sweetcorn, red onion, and avocado.*

Eat with chili to stimulate circulation and support a healthy flow of blood to the brain.
➡️ *Make a black bean and chili soup.*

CHICKPEA

Also known as garbanzo, chickpeas are one of the most popular and widely grown legumes globally. These rounded legumes are generally beige, but black, brown, green, and red varieties also exist. Whether dried or in a flour called "gram," chickpeas have been central to numerous food cultures, especially in the Middle East, for thousands of years.

BENEFITS

Chickpeas are an excellent source of plant-based protein as well as fiber, keeping you fuller for longer. They are also high in minerals and vitamins, including folate, iron, and zinc. In addition, chickpeas contain phytosterols, which help protect the brain from conditions such as Alzheimer's disease.

Fiber in chickpeas is mostly insoluble, which passes undigested into the colon. Here, bacteria break down insoluble fiber into several short-chain fatty acids, including butyric acid, which provides energy for the cells lining our colon. Butyric acid is also thought to improve brain health via the gut–brain axis.

Folate helps block the build-up of the amino acid homocysteine in the blood. Homocysteine can slow down the flow of nutrients to the brain, increasing the risk of depression.

Iron is required for energy, which helps promote positivity. Eating iron-rich foods such as chickpeas provides red blood cells with oxygen. If you don't have enough iron in your blood, you are more likely to experience low mood and irritability.

Zinc in chickpeas helps increase serotonin uptake. Adequate levels of serotonin in the brain help to elevate mood and increase positive feelings.

" Chickpeas are a good source of plant-based protein and fiber, keeping you fuller longer."

SUGGESTED SERVING

Enjoy a variety of nutrient-rich legumes. If you eat a plant-based diet, eat 3 rounded tablespoons of cooked legumes each day.

HOW TO ENJOY

Soak dried chickpeas for 12 hours, rinsing before use. Add sprouted chickpeas (see p.170) to salads or make into dips. Use canned chickpeas in various dishes.

Make a high-fiber chickpea curry.
➡ *Add rainbow chard and butternut squash and serve with brown rice.*
Try a gut-nourishing combination.
➡ *Toss mashed chickpeas with red miso. Serve on rye toast with avocado.*
Try with mustard seeds to stimulate circulation and rosemary for focus.
➡ *Toss spinach and chickpeas in an olive oil, tamari, mustard seed, and rosemary dressing.*

SOYBEAN

Soybeans have been eaten for thousands of years. Today, the potential health benefits of soybeans can be lost by the way they are prepared. Many products do not contain the whole bean and are not fermented. Look for whole, traditionally fermented soybean products such as miso and tempeh and avoid foods such as soy milk and oil or textured soy protein.

BENEFITS

While legumes are usually low in the amino acid methionine, soybeans contain this and are the one legume that is a complete protein, with all nine essential amino acids. Good-quality protein is key for mental health, as are the essential brain nutrients molybdenum, copper, manganese, iron, magnesium, potassium, and vitamin K, all found in soy and made more bioavailable through the process of fermentation.

Protein plays a critical role in the body, which needs a small amount of good-quality protein continuously for optimal brain function. Protein in soy can be difficult to digest. Fermenting the beans pre-digests the complex protein into amino acids, making it much easier to absorb. Amino acids are needed to form neurotransmitters, chemicals that relay messages in the brain and throughout the body.

Vitamin K is a fat-soluble vitamin found in plant foods as vitamin K1 and foods of animal origin as K2. Vitamin K2 is found in high concentrations in the brain, where it plays a key role in the nervous system. Certain microorganisms in fermented plant foods can convert K1 to K2; the best example is natto, a traditional fermented soy dish.

SUGGESTED SERVING

Enjoy a miso soup, made from a teaspoon of paste, daily. Include 3½oz (100g) tempeh or natto once or twice a week as part of a variety of legumes.

HOW TO ENJOY

Eating fermented soy foods such as tempeh, natto, and miso as well as seasoning with tamari are health-promoting ways to enjoy soybeans.

Make a pick-me-up miso soup that helps preserve beneficial gut bacteria, in turn supporting mental health via the gut–brain axis.
➡ *Use unpasteurized red miso paste. Mix with a little cold water first then add hot water.*

Make a mood-lifting dip for crudités.
➡ *Mix sweet miso, tahini, ginger, chili, and lemon juice with a little water.*
Add tamari to immune-boosting foods. Traditionally, fermented tamari contains no wheat and is a source of vitamin B3 and tryptophan, both required for serotonin synthesis.
➡ *Eat with wilted greens and shiitake.*
Enjoy in a brain-supporting salad bowl.
➡ *Toss marinated, grilled tempeh with watercress, endive, apple, and walnuts.*

WHEN TO AVOID

Allergy to soybeans is a common food allergy. Those with a soy allergy can react to other legumes, too. Some are also intolerant of soybeans. Fermenting soy reduces potential risks.

RECIPE

Miso dressing

Make a delicious dressing. Mix 1 teaspoon sweet or yellow miso with a small bunch of snipped chives, 1 teaspoon Meaux mustard, 2 tablespoons water, and 2 tablespoons olive oil. Drizzle over salad leaves.

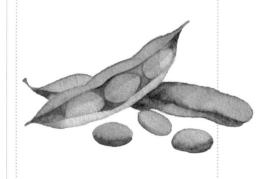

GRAINS

Grains belong to the grass family, which includes the major cereals such as rye, wheat, rice, oats, and barley, and have been a staple part of our diets for thousands of years. Whole grains have three components: the fiber-rich bran; the germ, with most vitamins, minerals, and fat; and the starchy endosperm. Quinoa, amaranth, buckwheat, and wild rice belong to a different family and are "pseudo-cereals."

OAT

Different oats flourish in different regions: common oats are grown in cool, temperate areas, while more heat-tolerant red oats are grown in warmer climes. Oats are the best wholegrain for lowering blood cholesterol levels and improving high blood pressure. Also, because being diagnosed with cardiovascular disease has been linked to higher incidence of anxiety and depression, oats are a supportive food for mental wellness.

BENEFITS

Oats are a good source of manganese and molybdenum, both of which support antioxidant activity, as well as B vitamins and phosphorus, needed to produce energy from our food. They also provide iron, zinc, and copper, all of which play an important role in brain health. Oats are an excellent source of soluble and insoluble fiber. They contain more soluble fiber than any other grain, mostly in the form of beta-glucans.

Beta-glucans are a kind of soluble fiber that turns into a thick, viscous gel in the body. This gel slows the digestion of carbohydrates, helping to avoid spikes in blood sugar levels that can lead to irritability and mood swings. "Brain fog," or confusion, also often occurs as a response to fluctuating sugar levels. In the large intestine, beta-glucans provide food for the beneficial bacteria that support a healthy gut. Millions of nerves and neurons run between the gut and the brain, and research has established that a healthy gut in turn promotes mental well-being.

Copper is important for producing hemoglobin, which is needed to carry oxygen to the brain and all around the body.

SUGGESTED SERVING

Enjoy a variety of whole grains in your daily diet. Include a total of at least 1¾oz (50g) spread over 3 meals.

HOW TO ENJOY

Oats are available as whole grains known as oat groats, rolled into flakes, cut into oatmeal, or ground into flour. Incredibly versatile, their soft subtle flavor can be used in sweet or savory dishes.

Treat yourself to a batch of granola bars for a sustained energy snack.
➼ *See recipe, below.*

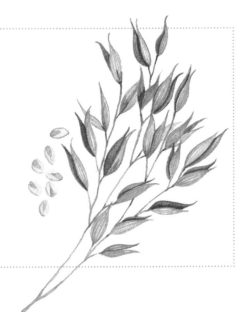

RECIPE

Oat granola bars

Chop 7oz (200g) figs. Add 5½oz (150g) chopped almonds, 4½oz (125g) oats, and 1oz (30g) each hemp and chia seeds. Stir in 3fl oz (90ml) warm maple syrup and 2oz (60g) almond butter. Chill in a lined tin. Cut into bars.

Enjoy oats with fruit for beneficial phytonutrients and add cardamom to lift the spirits.

➡ *Top flaked oatmeal with seasonal fruits and cardamom. Or try a savory porridge with chili and avocado, both of which support blood flow to the brain, and shelled hemp seeds for beneficial fats and protein.*

Eat with gut-nourishing yogurt.

➡ *Soak whole oats overnight in water. Add a squeeze of lemon, strain, and serve with berries and live yogurt.*

WHEN TO AVOID

Oats are usually tolerated by celiacs if processed in a gluten-free environment. Some people, however, are sensitive to the protein in oats.

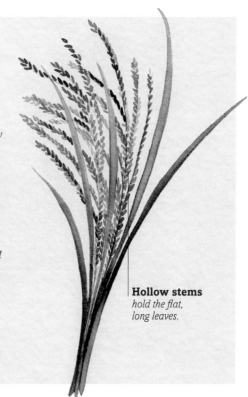

FOCUS ON

Rice

PROFILE
This staple food crop, especially popular in Africa and Asia, is cultivated best in areas with high rainfall.

PROPERTIES
Brown, whole-grain rice can play an important role in helping to control the blood sugar level spikes that can lead to mood swings, while fiber in brown rice can help to keep cholesterol under control.

Hollow stems *hold the flat, long leaves.*

RICE

Rice is an ancient grain and a staple food for many people in the world. Rice is classified according to the degree of milling that it undergoes. While whole-grain, or brown, rice retains its nutrient-rich bran and germ, white rice is milled and polished, with the nutrient-rich bran and germ removed. Most varieties are available as brown rice. In addition, there are red and black rice, both of which are considered whole grains rich in phytonutrients.

BENEFITS

Choosing whole grain or brown rice over white rice retains the minerals and vitamins in the bran and germ. These include B vitamins and selenium, magnesium, and phosphorus. Brown rice has three times the amount of fiber of white rice. Wild rice is not strictly rice but is very similar and considered a pseudo-grain. It is especially high in B vitamins and fiber.

Selenium is vital for the development and functioning of gamma aminobutyric acid (GABA), a neurotransmitter that facilitates communication between brain cells. Selenium is linked to our emotional and mental well-being, and low levels are associated with anxiety, confusion, and low mood.

Magnesium stimulates tiny electrical switches in the brain. If these don't work, then the brain's ability to process information and memory cannot function. Plenty of magnesium in the diet helps promote positivity.

Phosphorous is required to help provide energy for the brain. A deficiency can lead to anxiety and difficulty concentrating.

Fiber in whole-grain rice is mostly insoluble, which helps speed up the movement and processing of waste. Both soluble and insoluble fiber help to keep the gut healthy, in turn promoting brain health.

SUGGESTED SERVING

Enjoy a variety of whole grains in your daily diet. Include a total of at least 2oz (60g) dry weight spread over 3 meals.

HOW TO ENJOY

Rice is usually categorized as short-, medium-, or long-grain. Short-grain has the highest starch content, making sticky rice; long-grain is fluffier. Resistant starch, beneficial for gut health, forms when rice is reheated. Refrigerate cooked rice no longer than 2 days and reheat thoroughly.

Enjoy a brain-supporting sushi snack.

➡ *Make with nori, brown rice, and either fish or vegetables.*

Ferment for a healthy gut.

➡ *Ferment with lentils to make the classic "idli" batter for dosa.*

Make anti-inflammatory, antioxidant soup.

➡ *Make a rice and chicken soup with turmeric and garlic.*

RYE

This important cereal crop is grown throughout the world. The most common use of rye grain is as a flour for baking. It is not easy to separate the germ and bran from the endosperm of rye, so the flour usually retains a large quantity of nutrients. Its high fiber content helps digestive health—both the endosperm and bran in rye are high in fiber.

BENEFITS

Rye is a good source of manganese, phosphorus, copper, and pantothenic acid. It is thought to have several potential health benefits, including helping to prevent the onset of diabetes. Insulin signaling is essential for brain health, and people with diabetes are at increased risk of mood disorders, cognitive impairment, and dementia.

The fiber in rye is mostly insoluble, which remains more or less unchanged as it moves through the digestive tract. As this type of fiber passes through the intestines, it collects byproducts of digestion

" Insoluble fiber in rye gives a feeling of fullness that can help promote weight loss."

RECIPE

Amaranth stuffing

Make this delicious stuffing to fill baby squash or peppers. Soften 2 finely sliced shallots in olive oil. Add 6 finely sliced sage leaves and a handful of soaked sunflower seeds. Stir in 7oz (200g) cooked amaranth, 1 tbsp lemon juice, and season. Use to stuff roast pepper halves or a baby roast squash.

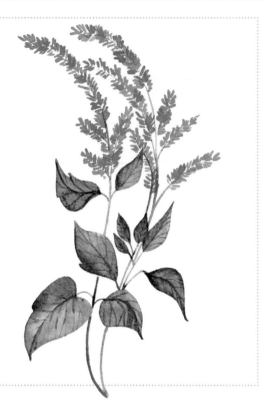

and absorbs water to form a soft stool. Its presence speeds up the movement and processing of waste, helping to prevent constipation. The water absorption of insoluble fiber gives a feeling of satiety, making rye helpful for weight loss. Being overweight can lead to negative emotions.

Copper is a catalyst for certain enzymes that control neurotransmitters, such as the "feel good" hormone dopamine.

Pantothenic acid (vitamin B5) is required to produce energy from food. Through its essential role in synthesizing the neurotransmitter acetylcholine, pantothenic acid boosts memory and helps reduce "brain fog."

SUGGESTED SERVING

Enjoy a variety of whole grains in your daily diet. Include a total of at least 2oz (60g) spread over 3 meals.

HOW TO ENJOY

Rye is traditionally used in bread, but the whole berries can also be used in salads, casseroles, and soups. Rye flour contains less gluten than wheat flour and is heavier and darker than most other flours. Choose artisan long-fermented rye bread, which is easiest to digest. Dark rye bread contains more nutrients than light rye and has a richer, earthier flavor.

Eat a rye toast brain-supporting snack.
➡ *Top with wilted green leaves, sauerkraut, and a poached egg.*

Enjoy a lebkuchen with a glass of stress-relieving lemon balm tea.
➡ *Lebkuchen, the German gingerbread cookie, is traditionally made with spices and rye flour.*

WHEN TO AVOID

Rye contains gluten, so is not suitable for celiacs. Some people with gluten intolerance may be able to tolerate rye.

QUINOA

Quinoa originated in the Andes and was a staple crop of the Incan Empire. It is often referred to as a pseudo-grain because technically it is a seed rather than a grain. There are hundreds of different cultivated varieties and it comes in many colors: orange, red, pink, purple, white, and black. All are nutrient-rich and also gluten-free, so are an excellent choice where there is gluten intolerance.

BENEFITS

Quinoa contains all nine essential amino acids, making it an excellent protein alternative for a vegan diet. It is also high in fiber and minerals such as zinc and magnesium, along with B vitamins, which help convert the food we eat to fuel for energy. This gluten-free ingredient is easy to digest.

Protein is critical for brain health. Amino acids, the building blocks of protein, perform different essential tasks in the brain. For example, the amino acid tryptophan is essential in serotonin production, and tyrosine promotes the creation of norepinephrine and dopamine, two neurotransmitters that boost focus and energy. Protein deficiency can negatively affect mood, emotions, and cognitive function and has been linked to ADHD and anxiety.

Magnesium plays a key role in neurological health. It is thought to stop stress hormones from entering the brain, so it has a calming effect, helping reduce stress and anxiety.

Zinc is a catalyst for a number of critical enzymes, many of which are found in the brain. It is required for optimal brain health and cognition and low levels are associated with depression.

SUGGESTED SERVING

Enjoy a variety of whole grains in your daily diet. Include a total of at least 2oz (60g) dry weight spread over 3 meals.

HOW TO ENJOY

Quinoa cooks quickly to produce an easily digested, nutty-flavored grain. Use it to stuff vegetables such as peppers and mushrooms, add to a salad bowl, or eat as porridge. It is best to rinse it before use to remove a naturally bitter compound that protects the seed from predators.

Eat with antioxidant-rich fruit.
➡ *Cook in coconut milk and stir in seeds and fruits for a porridge.*
Sprout to increase the nutrient content (see p.170).
➡ *Toss sprouted seeds into salads.*

AMARANTH

This ancient grain was cultivated by the Aztecs more than 8,000 years ago. The tall amaranth plant with its vivid red or gold flowers and tiny seed is now grown on many continents and has become popular in gluten-free baking. Amaranth contains excellent protein and has a nutty flavor and grassy aroma.

BENEFITS

Amaranth is a good source of vitamin B6, which helps stabilize mood. It is also high in magnesium and iron. The protein quality in amaranth is better than in most whole grains, which are low in the amino acid lysine.

Protein is essential for the growth and repair of all cells and tissues in the body and is vital for the immune system, as it is needed to form antibodies that fight infection. Our hormones are also made from protein and these chemical messengers play a key role in brain health. Good-quality protein in the diet optimizes brain function and reduces inflammation, improving mental clarity and memory.

Magnesium, involved in many brain chemistry reactions, calms nerves and relaxes muscles. Low levels of magnesium in the diet are linked to depression and anxiety.

Iron plays a crucial role in transporting oxygen to tissues in all parts of the body. Iron is required in every cell to make energy and a diet low in iron leads to fatigue, poor concentration, and impaired memory. People with iron deficiency are more prone to depression. Iron is also a component in antioxidants that protect white blood cells that are integral to our immune systems.

SUGGESTED SERVING

Enjoy a variety of whole grains in your daily diet. Include a total of at least 60g (2oz) dry weight spread over 3 meals.

HOW TO ENJOY

This golden grain cooks to a porridgelike consistency. You can also toast the seeds in a hot pan, tossing all the time until they begin to pop, and use in salads or add to soups, biscuits, and bread.

Make an anti-inflammatory salad.
➡ *Mix cooked amaranth with wilted green leaves to reduce inflammation and support healthy brain function.*
Make amaranth stuffing with vitamin E-rich sunflower seeds and memory-supporting sage.
➡ *See recipe, opposite.*
Cook with immune-supporting, anti-inflammatory ingredients.
➡ *Make an amaranth risotto with shiitake mushrooms, red onions, garlic, and parsley.*

MEAT

Fresh, unprocessed meat is a "whole" food and a good source of minerals, amino acids, and fats to support mental well-being. How an animal is reared affects the quality of its meat. Those reared in organic and biodynamic conditions have less stress, better diets, and produce nutritionally superior meat.

GRASS-FED BEEF

Raising beef animals exclusively on pasture provides health benefits to the cattle and, if eaten in moderation, to humans. Pasture-fed beef adds excellent quality protein to the diet, and because of the grass diet, it contains a high content of antioxidant and anti-inflammatory beta-carotene. It also contains conjugated linoleic acid (CLA), a polyunsaturated fat that helps lower inflammation.

BENEFITS

One hundred percent pasture-fed beef is lower in total fat and with a much better omega 3:6 ratio than grain-fed beef. It is a good source of vitamin B12 and choline as well as the essential minerals selenium, zinc, iron, and potassium, important for brain health.

Choline is a water-soluble nutrient required for the health of cell membranes. It is important for liver function, brain development, and the nervous system. Choline is needed to produce the neurotransmitter acetylcholine, whose role in cognition includes reasoning, concentration, and focus, as well as helping regulate memory and mood.

Vitamin B12 is an essential water-soluble vitamin abundant in grass-fed beef. It plays a role in the metabolism of almost every cell in the body, including in the synthesis of myelin, the fatty layer that surrounds our nerve cells and is essential for the synthesis of DNA and RNA and neurotransmitters that affect cognition. Vitamin B12 is also needed to regulate the amino acid homocysteine, preventing high levels that can lead to blood vessel damage.

SUGGESTED SERVING

Eat fresh, unprocessed meat products from animals that have been raised in higher welfare, pasture-fed, and, preferably organic, systems. Meat is generally higher in fat so keep portions to around 4½oz (125g) and try to limit to once or twice a week.

HOW TO ENJOY

High-heat cooking methods such as grilling and barbecuing are best avoided. High temperatures can lead to the production of compounds called advanced glycation end products (AGEs), which are linked to various diseases. Slow, low-heat cooking methods are therefore best for beef—and produce delicious, tender results.

Make a one-pot stew in a slow cooker or crockpot.
➡*See recipe, left.*

RECIPE

Slow-cooked beef

Place a grass-fed beef steak, some rosemary sprigs, chopped garlic, onions, celery, carrots, and turnips, tomato purée, and stock into the pot and cook on low heat for up to 10 hours.

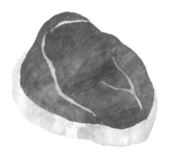

WILD VENISON

Wild venison is lean, red meat from deer. It is lower in fat and calories than beef and contains a higher amount of good-quality protein than any other red meat. Deer browsing for food in the wild eat various leaves, shoots, nuts, and berries, resulting in nutrient-rich flesh, high in essential minerals and vitamins. If you are unable to source wild, then farmed venison is an excellent alternative.

BENEFITS

Wild venison is particularly rich in iron and selenium. It is also a good source of the B vitamin family, all of which are critical in brain chemistry. In addition, venison contains a good amount of zinc and omega-3 essential fatty acids, with an excellent ratio of omega 6:3.

The range of B vitamins in venison helps to produce much-needed energy for the brain, which increases mental clarity and alertness and aids memory.

Protein plays a critical role throughout the body, and the excellent quality protein that is found in venison helps to optimize brain function. Chemical neurotransmitters in the brain require protein daily to function properly, as do many of the hormones and enzymes throughout our bodies. Cognitive function is impaired without adequate high-quality sources of protein.

Zinc is particularly important for optimum brain health, and wild venison is an excellent source of this essential mineral. Zinc ensures adequate serotonin levels in your brain and low levels of zinc are linked to depression. Zinc is also required for effective memory.

Iron is one of the essential minerals for brain function. It is a component of hemoglobin, transporting oxygen and carbon dioxide to and from cells around the body. Iron is also necessary for the synthesis of serotonin, which promotes a positive mood; and dopamine, which serves as a chemical messenger between neurons and enhances focus, attention, memory, and sleep.

Selenium is needed by our bodies for the functioning of the neurotransmitter gamma aminobutyric acid (GABA), which supports neural messaging. Low levels of selenium are linked to anxiety and confusion.

SUGGESTED SERVING

Though venison has less fat and fewer calories than other types of red meat, meat of any kind is best limited to portions of about 4½oz (125g) once or twice a week.

HOW TO ENJOY

Venison is very lean and therefore is best cooked as gently as possible, using methods that preserve the maximum amount of minerals and B vitamins. Try pan-frying venison steaks gently but quickly, or cook a shoulder or leg of venison slowly in a casserole—the B vitamins will leach into the liquid, but most of the vitamins will be retained in the juices of the casserole and enjoyed in the meal.

Enjoy a venison steak with red cabbage sauerkraut. The cabbage provides a rich source of phytonutrients, and the enzymes in the sauerkraut will help the body to digest the meat efficiently.
➡ *Very gently pan-fry a small fillet steak, keeping it rare to medium-rare. If it is cooked any longer, a venison steak will become tough. Serve with delicious red cabbage sauerkraut.*

" Good-quality protein, such as that found in wild venison, plays a critical role in brain health, helping neurotransmitters to function properly."

FISH

Fish and other types of seafood are credited with providing our human ancestors with the high-quality nutrition crucial for the evolution of our brains and advanced cognitive abilities. Choosing fish sourced from sustainable fisheries helps ensure that we, and future generations, can continue to benefit from the nutrition that comes from the sea.

SARDINE

Sardines are small saltwater fish. Tinned sardines contain similar nutrition as freshly caught and have the advantage of being very easy to use. Choose sustainably sourced fish packed in tins that are free from bisphenol A (BPA), a chemical added to packaging that can leach into food.

BENEFITS

Sardines are rich in omega-3 essential fatty acids for brain health, as well as vitamin D, which protects the brain through its anti-inflammatory and immune-boosting properties. They are also an excellent source of vitamin B12, selenium, and protein.

Vitamin B12 is a crucial vitamin for the brain and nervous tissues throughout the body. It is required to produce vital neurotransmitters, including dopamine, which plays a key role in how we think and focus and how we experience pleasure. Higher levels of B12 are linked to improved memory, mental clarity, and more balanced moods.

Selenium is a trace mineral with antioxidant properties. While found in a variety of foods, including nuts, seeds, and mushrooms, sardines are an exceptionally good source. Selenium is required for thyroid hormone synthesis and metabolism. A deficiency in selenium, which fails to meet the needs of the thyroid, has been linked to a greater risk of anxiety and depression.

Protein is vital to our brain health. Proteins are made up of amino acids, nine of which are essential and must be sourced from our diet daily. A lack of these essential amino acids depletes the chemicals in the brain that control our energy levels, thoughts, and feelings, and can lead to fatigue and depression.

FIRMER FLESH

Salmon that swim freely in the sea, fleeing from predators and sourcing their own food, have denser muscle fibers than farmed salmon.

SUGGESTED SERVING

Eat a 5oz (140g) portion of either sardines or another oily fish such as salmon twice a week.

HOW TO ENJOY

Enjoy fresh sardines whenever possible, but keep a couple of tins in the cupboard as a quick and easy alternative.

Start the day with sardines to give you sustained energy throughout the morning.
➡ *Eat tinned sardines on sprouted spelt toast with watercress.*

Combine with focusing herbs and immune-supporting garlic.
➡ *Roast fresh sardines with rosemary and garlic.*

Make a nutrient-dense salad for brain health.
➡ *Toss some tinned sardines with a good handful of green leaves, a red onion, artichoke hearts, and a garlic–chili dressing.*

Enjoy with tomatoes. The lycopene in tomatoes and the fats in sardines are a powerful combination to protect and nourish the brain.
➡ *Grill fresh sardines and toss with seared cherry tomatoes cooked with fresh mint.*

WILD ALASKAN SALMON

Alaska ranks as one of the world's healthiest and best-managed fisheries. The management is based on minimal damage to the environment and the long-term health of its fish stocks. The nutrient composition of wild and farmed salmon differ greatly. A key difference is the fatty acid profile. This is much healthier in wild-caught salmon, which has a richer concentration of essential omega-3 fatty acids.

BENEFITS

As well as being an excellent source of omega-3 fatty acids, essential for mental well-being, salmon is also a good source of protein and vitamin B12, both needed to produce key neurotransmitters, and selenium and vitamin D, which support the health of the immune system.

Omega-3 is a family of fatty acids. Our brain needs specific types of omega-3s to function optimally. Omega-3 from plants is found in the form of alpha-linolenic acid (ALA), which the body must convert into the longer chain fatty acids, eiocosapentaenoic acid (EPA) and docosahexaenoic acid (DHA), vital for normal brain function. For many people, the conversion of ALA to EPA and DHA in the body is not optimal. Oily fish contains preformed, or ready formed, EPA and DHA, which is why it is so beneficial for our health. Salmon, in particular, contains high concentrations of these fatty acids. EPA and DHA are crucial for the development of the brain and nervous system and these long-chain fatty acids support positive mood, helping to increase our sense of well-being.

RECIPE

Salmon salad

Poach or grill salmon fillets. Flake the cooked salmon and place in a bowl with olives, tomatoes, peppers, and basil. Drizzle with an olive oil dressing and toss all the ingredients together.

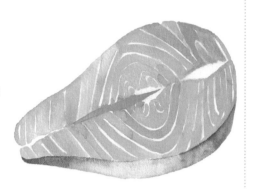

Obtaining adequate amounts of DHA and EPA from our diets is associated with a reduced risk of depression.

SUGGESTED SERVING

Eat a 5oz (140g) portion of either salmon or another oily fish such as sardines twice a week.

HOW TO ENJOY

There are plenty of nutritious ways to cook salmon fillets, such as grilling, baking, steaming, or poaching. If salmon is ultra fresh, try sushi or gravlax.

Combine salmon with greens. The vitamin B12 in salmon and the folate in greens work together to break down the compound homocysteine, high levels of which are linked to mental disorders.
➡ *Grill salmon and serve on a bed of wilted greens.*

Try with spices and buckwheat to boost immunity and lift mood.
➡ *Enjoy steamed salmon with buckwheat noodles, turmeric, and ginger.*

Enjoy a brain-nourishing fish salad for a sustaining, nutrient-dense dish.
➡ *See recipe, above.*

Make a salmon chowder for a bowl of comfort on a cold winter's night.
➡ *Switch cream for coconut milk to make a creamy dish with antioxidant properties.*

" *Sardines are a rich source of the mineral selenium, needed for a healthy thyroid, which in turn supports a balanced mood.* "

CHICKEN AND EGGS

Adequate intake of protein is essential for our mental well-being and both poultry and eggs are protein powerhouses. Meat from higher-welfare organic and free-range birds can be up to 50 percent lower in fat, while organic and free-range eggs are higher in vitamins, including vitamin D, and long-chain omega-3 fatty acids.

CHICKEN

Chickens reared for meat are called broilers; the most important consideration is ensuring you eat an organic pasture-fed bird. Aside from the obvious animal welfare issues, these chicken are free from antibiotics and other chemicals, making them much healthier to eat. Although more expensive, you do not have to eat much to benefit from the superior nutrition.

BENEFITS

Chicken is an excellent source of protein, and, with the exception of biotin, contains all of the B vitamins, which play an important role in healthy cognition—it is exceptionally high in vitamin B3. Chicken also provides a range of minerals, including iron, zinc, and selenium, and is a good source of the important brain nutrient, choline.

Protein is an essential component of every cell in the body and key for optimal brain function. It breaks down into amino acids, which are the critical building blocks of neurochemicals in the brain. Without protein enzymes from our diets, hormones and neurotransmitters would be unable to accomplish their numerous tasks.

Selenium is an essential brain mineral and chicken is an excellent source of this nutrient. In the brain, selenium acts as an antioxidant, helping prevent inflammation. Dopamine, the "feel-good" neurotransmitter, is dependent on selenium and the neurotransmitter acetylcholine, critical for memory, reasoning, and concentration, also relies on this mineral. Low levels of selenium have been linked to anxiety and depression.

Vitamin B3, also known as niacin, plays a role in the signaling between nerve cells—efficient signaling supports mental agility. Niacin is required for serotonin metabolism and, along with other B vitamins, niacin helps produce the energy needed for our brains to function.

SUGGESTED SERVING

Eat up to 8oz (225g) raw weight of chicken a week (not including chicken bone broth).

HOW TO ENJOY

The best way to buy chicken is whole. Any meat or bones that are not used right away can then be frozen, either raw or cooked.

Rustle up a colorful nutrient-dense chicken salad.
➡ *Toss cooked chicken pieces with avocado, ribbons of carrot, pomegranate seeds, baby spinach, mint, and some chili dressing.*
Ease anxiety with a comforting, slow-cooked, chicken stew.
➡ *Pack with plenty of vegetables of your choice and add ginger and turmeric.*

" Choline in eggs is a building block for brain chemicals that support memory and concentration."

Make a bone broth. This is full of nutrients for gut health, supporting brain health via the gut–brain axis.
➡️*Place the bones from a roast chicken in a pot. Cover with water, add herbs as desired, and some wine or cider vinegar and simmer slowly.*

EGG

Chickens bred for eggs are called layers, and generally, they lay an egg a day. Eggs are a nutrient-dense food, with most of the nutrients found in the yolk, while the white is mostly protein. Egg yolks contain some beneficial omega-3 fats, depending on the food the chicken has eaten. Studies show chickens allowed to roam and feed on natural pasture have increased amounts of omega-3 fats in their eggs.

BENEFITS

Eggs are a good source of several nutrients linked to mental health and well-being. As well as being an excellent source of choline and vitamin B12, they also provide high-quality protein, are a good source of selenium, and contain biotin, essential for maintaining a healthy nervous system.

Choline plays a critical role throughout the body by maintaining the structural integrity of all cell membranes. Egg yolks are one of the best sources of this nutrient. One egg provides between 25 and 30 percent of our daily needs. Choline is a vital building block for acetylcholine, a brain chemical that is important for memory and our ability to focus. The brains of people with Alzheimer's disease have been found to have lower levels of acetylcholine than in those without the disease.

RECIPE

Garlic aioli

Grind 2 garlic cloves to a paste with ½ tsp salt. Add 2 egg yolks and whisk together. Slowly add 6fl oz (175ml) olive oil, whisking constantly until the mixture thickens. Finish with a squeeze of lemon. Enjoy as a dip for lightly steamed or raw broccoli florets.

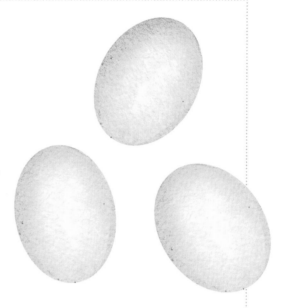

Vitamin D3 is found in egg yolks. Adequate levels have been linked to a reduced risk of depression.

Vitamin B12, also known as cobalamin, helps regulate the amino acid homocysteine in the body, high levels of which are linked to inflammation and even brain damage. B12 is also needed for the synthesis of neurotransmitters that affect our alertness, cognition, and memory. Low levels can lead to anxiety and low mood.

SUGGESTED SERVING

Enjoy an egg a day as part of a healthy diet full of green leaves and different colorful vegetables.

HOW TO ENJOY

Eggs are one of the most versatile and widely used ingredients. If you are short on time, poached, boiled, or scrambled eggs are quick to prepare. Alternatively, eggs can be turned into pancakes, frittatas, or omelettes, and make a delicious addition to salads.

Make shakshuka. This brightly colored traditional north African dish is packed with protein and essential vitamins and minerals needed for brain health and therefore our mental well-being.
➡️*Cook the traditional dish with red peppers, tomatoes, onions, garlic, and herbs, with a baked egg nestled in the middle.*

Enjoy an energizing protein snack.
➡️*Try a hard-boiled egg dipped in dukkah, a traditional condiment made with nuts, herbs, and spices.*

Enjoy a rich, garlicky aioli. The choline in eggs, monounsaturated fat in olive oil, and vitamin K in broccoli all help to support memory and improve concentration.
➡️*See recipe, above.*

WHEN TO AVOID
Both egg yolks and whites contain proteins that can cause allergies, but an allergy to egg whites is the most common, in which case it is possible to eat the yolk. Some people are intolerant to eggs.

DAIRY, FATS, AND OILS

In moderation, dairy products—not just from cows, but from goats and sheep, too—can provide healthy fats and a range of beneficial minerals such as calcium. Fermented dairy products add beneficial bacteria to our guts and can be easier to digest. Fats derived from dairy and vegetable sources are also essential for maintaining the health of the brain and nervous system.

YOGURT AND KEFIR

Yogurt is made using two active lactic acid-producing bacteria cultures and is excellent for providing beneficial gut bacteria. Kefir, a fermented milk drink, is made from white gelatinous clumps of micro-organisms called milk kefir grains. Kefir contains more strains of bacteria than yogurt, promoting the growth of beneficial bacteria and introducing new strains to the gut microbiome. Both yogurt and kefir support gut health, which in turn influences mood and overall cognitive function.

BENEFITS

Yogurt and kefir share a diverse range of nutrients critical to brain function: the B vitamin (including B12), zinc, iodine, calcium, phosphorous, and protein. The process of fermenting converts milk protein into an easily digestible form.

Vitamin B12, in its natural form, is found only in foods of animal origin. It is needed to regulate the amino acid homocysteine, raised levels of which are linked to inflammation, declining memory, and poor concentration. B12 is a catalyst in the synthesis of neurotransmitters that affect alertness and mood.

Iodine is an essential trace mineral that combines with the amino acid tyrosine to form thyroid hormones. Thyroid hormone receptors in our brains help regulate the production of all crucial neurotransmitters that keep us centered and alert.

Calcium is crucial to the electrical signaling in the brain and plays a critical role in saving and retrieving memory. It is a "sedative mineral," so-called because it exerts a calming effect on conditions such as anxiety.

Phosphorous is needed to make adenosine triphosphate (ATP), a molecule that stores and transfers energy and regulates communication between neurotransmitters.

SUGGESTED SERVING

If dairy tolerant, fermented foods offer good nutrition. A daily glass of kefir or bowl of yogurt supports the gut microbiome.

HOW TO ENJOY

Make your own yogurt or kefir. Once you have milk kefir grains, this is effortless,

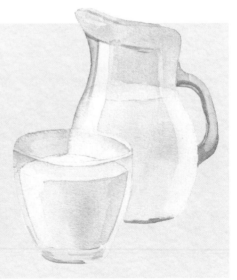

FOCUS ON

Kefir

PROFILE
This milklike drink originated in Russia and Eastern Europe.

PROPERTIES
Kefir is linked with improved cardiovascular health and helps to balance blood sugar levels, avoiding energy spikes.

" Yogurt is high in calcium, a calming mineral that helps to reduce anxiety. "

taking just 24 hours at room temperature. When looked after, milk kefir grains will last for life. Generally, milk kefir is enjoyed as a drink on its own or in smoothies. Yogurt can be cultured with the addition of a live yogurt bacteria, using equipment that allows a steady temperature of about 110°F (43°C).

Eat with fresh fruit. The protein and fat in the yogurt help counter sugar spikes from the fruit.
➡ *Add yogurt to fruit smoothies.*
Make a soft yogurt cheese like labneh.
➡ *Add a pinch of salt to full-fat yogurt. Place in a muslin cloth over a bowl. Leave for 24–48 hours for the whey to strain through.*

WHEN TO AVOID
Yogurt and kefir can cause adverse effects for those with a milk allergy or who are lactose intolerant. However, some can tolerate fermented products such as kefir and yogurt despite an intolerance or allergy to milk.

A LONG HISTORY
References to yogurt date back to 6000BC in Indian Ayurvedic texts. When eaten with honey, it was called "the food of the gods."

BUTTER

Butter, eaten in moderation as part of an overall healthy diet with plenty of fruit and vegetables, can provide some important nutrients. The nutritional value of butter is affected by a cow's diet. Cows that are 100 percent grass fed produce butter with the highest concentration of vitamins A, D3, and K2, and with a much better balance of omega 3:6 than grain-fed cows. Traditionally, butter was made from lacto-cultured cream—the best choice nutritionally.

BENEFITS

Vitamin A in butter promotes learning and memory and vitamin K2 plays a vital role in controlling inflammation. About 12 percent of the saturated fats in butter are short-chain fatty acids, including butyric acid, which reduces inflammation.

Vitamin D3 is involved in the synthesis of the neurotransmitters gamma aminobutyric acid (GABA), which helps reduce stress, lower anxiety, and calm the body and mind; glutamate, which plays an important role in learning and forming memories; and dopamine, which aids memory, attention, focus, and sleep. Vitamin D3, along with omega-3 (also found in butter), is needed to synthesize serotonin, the neurotransmitter that lifts mood. While the benefits of vitamin D3 from butter are limited by the

recommended amount of saturated fat, butter does provide a natural source of this vitamin.
Butyric acid is a potent anti-inflammatory that aids digestion and improves gut health. It forms part of the calming neurotransmitter GABA. Dietary butyric acid has a beneficial effect on gut health. Butyric acid is also made in the gut as a by-product from bacteria fermenting insoluble fiber for energy. If there is a reduction in the beneficial bacteria in the gut, less butyric acid is produced.

SUGGESTED SERVING

Less than 10 percent of daily calories should come from saturated fat. For a diet of 2000 calories a day, this equates to ¾oz (22g) a day. 1oz (30g) butter contains about ½oz (18g) saturated fat.

HOW TO ENJOY

Including butter (or any fat) with vegetables helps the body absorb valuable phytonutrients such as lycopene and beta-carotene.

Toss with green vegetables.
➡ *Melt a pat of butter over lightly steamed or roasted vegetables.*
Make ghee, a staple in Indian culture. In Ayurvedic medicine, this "golden liquid" is revered and used as a carrier for healing herbs. Ghee has a much higher smoke point than butter, making it more suitable for cooking.
➡ *Very gently melt unsalted, organic butter from grass-fed cows. Foam will accumulate on the top and milk solids will drop to the bottom. Cook gently for up to an hour (depending on the quantity) until the solids on the bottom brown. Skim off the top layer of foam and pour the central layer through a very fine sieve. Toss the milk solids and store the liquid ghee in a clean glass jar.*

COCONUT OIL

Coconut oil has become a popular alternative fat to dairy. Extra virgin coconut oil has negligible amounts of vitamins and minerals compared to butter, but contains polyphenols with antioxidant properties, supportive for our brain cells that use a lot of oxygen and are particularly vulnerable to oxidative damage. Coconut oil, like butter, is a saturated fat, despite being called an oil.

BENEFITS

Coconut oil contains medium-chain fatty acids with potential health benefits. However, much of this research has been done on 100 percent medium-chain triglyceride (MCT) oils, whereas only about 15 percent of the fats in coconut oil are MCTs. An important benefit of coconut oil is its resistance to oxidation at high temperatures—oxidized fats are harmful to mental health and well-being.

Medium-chain fatty acids are easily absorbed in the digestive tract without needing to be combined with bile and digestive enzymes. They are then converted to ketones in the liver. With mild cognitive impairment and Alzheimer's disease, there is a

dramatic decline in the brain's ability to use glucose. Research suggests that the uptake of ketones as an energy source is not impaired, making MCTs an alternative fuel for the brain.

SUGGESTED SERVING

Less than 10 percent of daily calories should come from saturated fat. For a diet of 2000 calories a day, this equates to ¾oz (22g) a day. 1oz (30g) coconut oil has a scant 1oz (25g) of saturated fat.

HOW TO ENJOY

Choose extra virgin, cold-pressed coconut oil to benefit from the polyphenols. Coconut oil can be used for high-temperature cooking. However, even though the oil is resistant to oxidization, it should not be heated above 350°F (180°C).

Toss with vegetables to make fat-soluble nutrients more available.
➥*Melt coconut oil over steamed and roasted vegetables.*

" *Extra virgin olive oil provides anti-inflammatory plant compounds.* **"**

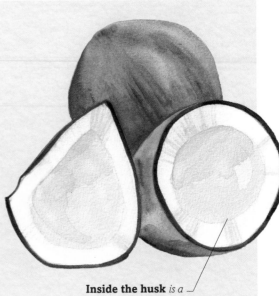
OLIVE OIL

Olive oil comes from one of the oldest cultivated trees in the world. The healthiest kind of olive oil to buy is extra virgin cold-pressed oil, which is obtained from the first pressing of olives, without the use of any chemicals or heat processes. This ensures the oil still contains all its important antioxidant and anti-inflammatory ingredients, which are known to help prevent memory loss and slow a decline in brain function.

BENEFITS

The predominant fat in olive oil is the monounsaturated fat, oleic acid, which provides various benefits for the brain. Olive oil is a good source of antioxidant vitamin E and extra virgin olive oil is an excellent source of polyphenol plant compounds, which have anti-inflammatory benefits.

Vitamin E is a fat-soluble vitamin. As a potent antioxidant, it plays a role in protecting cells in the brain from oxidative stress caused by free radical damage. Neurons that are built largely from cholesterol and polyunsaturated fats are highly susceptible to oxidative damage, so vitamin E is an important nutrient to ensure that neurons are able to function well and send messages to other cells around the body.

Oleic acid is one of the fats in the myelin sheath that twists around the nerves and insulates them, enabling quick transfer of information. It is thought to help control harmful inflammation, to play a potential role in controlling blood pressure, and improve the functioning of blood vessels, ensuring a good flow of blood to the brain. Several studies show that consuming oleic acid can reduce the risk of stroke.

SUGGESTED SERVING

A tablespoon of olive oil every day will provide your daily requirement of oleic acid. No more than 30 percent of your daily calories should come from fat. For a diet of 2000 calories a day, this equates to 2¼oz (66g) total fat. 1 tablespoon of olive oil is ½oz (14g).

HOW TO ENJOY

Extra virgin olive oil is not suitable for high-heat cooking. If you do use it to cook with, try combining the oil with an equal amount of water, steam the veggies first, then briefly sauté in the oil and water, which protects the oil from oxidation.

The oil will help the body absorb fat-soluble nutrients in vegetables.
➡ *Use as a salad dressing or toss vegetables in oil after steaming.*
Try an olive oil bread dip.
➡ *See recipe, right.*

HEMP OIL

Hemp has a very long history as a medicinal food. The oil, made from the hemp plant's seeds, contains several minerals, vitamins, and polyunsaturated fats that are critical for mental health and well-being. Hemp oil contains fatty acids that are essential for the optimal composition of the high fat content of the brain.

BENEFITS

Hemp oil contains antioxidants vitamin E and beta-carotene as well as important minerals for brain health, including zinc, iron, and magnesium. It provides a good ratio of the two essential fatty acids: omega-6 at about 60 percent of its fat, and omega-3, at about 20 percent. A 3:1 ratio is generally considered the perfect balance. Hemp oil is also a good source of gamma-linolenic acid, used to make prostaglandins, short-lived hormonelike chemicals that control inflammation.

Omega-3 and omega-6 fatty acids must come from the diet, as our bodies are unable to make them. The ratio of omega-3 to omega-6 is critical to overall health, and hemp oil has the optimum 1:3 ratio. DHA and EPA from the omega-3 fatty acid family are essential for reducing inflammation in the body, supporting learning and memory, and the repair and growth of new brain cells.

SUGGESTED SERVING

A tablespoon of hemp oil every day will more than meet the daily requirements of omega-6 and omega-3 essential fatty acids. No more than 30 percent of your daily calories should come from fat. For a diet of 2000 calories a day, this equates to 2¼oz (66g) total fat. 1 tablespoon of hemp oil is ½oz (14g).

HOW TO ENJOY

Hemp oil is damaged by heat, so it is not suitable for cooking. Adding the oil to vegetables increases the bioavailability of the fat-soluble nutrients in them for the body. Store hemp oil in the fridge to protect the polyunsaturated fats from light, air, and heat.

Combine with vegetables and salad leaves to add a nutty flavor and help the absorption of fat-soluble nutrients in the body.
➡ *Use in a salad dressing or toss cooked vegetables in oil after steaming.*

RECIPE
Olive oil dip

Mix 3 crushed garlic cloves, ½ tsp each finely chopped thyme and rosemary, ¼ tsp chili flakes, ¼ tsp freshly ground black pepper, a pinch of salt, and 1 tbsp balsamic vinegar. Add 9fl oz (250ml) extra virgin olive oil.

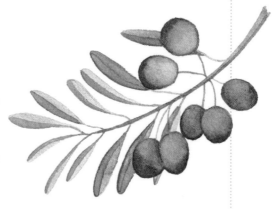

RECIPES FOR MENTAL WELLNESS

SNACKS

Healthy snacks can be an excellent way to balance blood sugar levels over the course of the day, providing sustaining nutrients that help the body to avoid sugar dips, in turn keeping our moods balanced and warding off feelings of irritability and fatigue. Nut butters and oils provide healthy, brain-nourishing fats, while natural ingredients such as blueberries and honey add a pleasing sweetness.

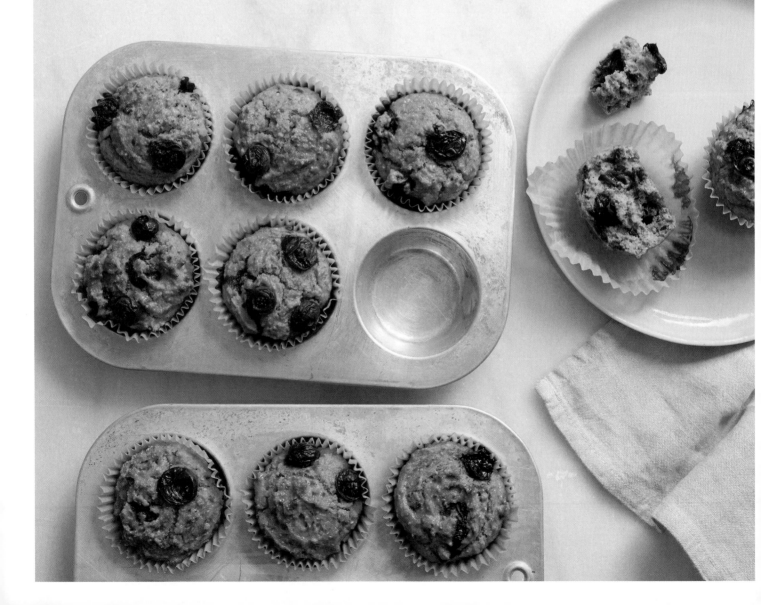

1

Sprouted spelt and blueberry muffins

The sprouting process increases the availability of nutrients and also makes it easier for the body to digest the grain, which supports gut, and in turn, brain health. Adding blueberries and cacao nibs provides calming and uplifting nutrients.

MAKES **12** | PREP TIME **10 MINS**
BAKE TIME **20 MINS**

Preheat the oven to 375°F (190°C). Place paper muffin liners in a 12-hole muffin tin. Combine **8oz (225g) sprouted spelt flour, 2 tsp baking powder, 1¾oz (50g) chia seeds,** and **2 tbsp raw cacao nibs.** Mix together **2 eggs, 7fl oz (200ml) yogurt, 4 tbsp olive oil,** and **3 tbsp honey**. Gently combine the dry and wet mixtures and stir in **3½oz (100g) blueberries**. Divide the mixture between the liners and bake for 20 minutes, or until they are golden, risen, and cooked through.

2

Dulse oatcakes

The iron, zinc, and B vitamins in oats combine with mineral-rich dulse to provide a nutrient-dense snack and sustained energy to help ensure healthy brain function and provide "get up and go" when feeling lethargic in body and mind.

MAKES **12** | PREP TIME **10 MINS**
BAKE TIME **20 MINS**

Preheat the oven to 375°F (190°C). Place **8oz (225g) oatmeal**, a **pinch of fine sea salt**, and **1 heaping tbsp dulse flakes** in a bowl. Add **2 tbsp olive oil**, then, stirring, add **3½–5fl oz (100–150ml) hot water** for a soft dough. With your hands, roll the dough into a ball and dust well with extra oatmeal. On an oiled flat baking tray, roll out the dough into a 10in (25cm) circle. Cut into 12 wedges and bake for 20 minutes, or until crisp.

3

Uplifting sweetmeats

These nutty sweetmeats are a brain-nourishing treat. Walnuts, hemp, and linseed provide omega-3 fatty acids, an essential brain fat that supports healthy cognition; while almond contains calming magnesium, and cacao has mood-boosting compounds.

MAKES **20** | PREP TIME **10–15 MINS**

Place **3½oz (100g) chopped walnuts** in a food processor with **1 tbsp ground linseed, 1 tbsp cacao, 1 tbsp honey,** and **2 tbsp almond butter**. Blend all the ingredients, then divide and roll into 20 balls. Place **2oz (50g) shelled hemp seeds** on a plate and roll each ball in the seeds. Store in an airtight container for up to a week in the fridge.

NUTS

While all nuts are packed full of beneficial fats, proteins, minerals, vitamins, and phytonutrients, each type of nut has a unique nutritional profile. Walnuts, almonds, and hazelnuts are a particularly good choice for supporting healthy brain function. A common belief is that eating nuts causes weight gain, but research disputes this. Regularly eating nuts improves our overall health.

WALNUT

Walnuts have a long culinary history and are available all year long. They contain several unique and powerful antioxidants that are critical to our health and play an important part in the way we age in both body and mind.

BENEFITS

Walnuts provide some key nutrients for supporting healthy brain function. Vitamin E, alpha-linolenic acid (ALA), and the antioxidant juglone have neuroprotective properties. Walnuts also contain manganese, the B vitamin complex, and a wide variety of flavonoid phytonutrients.

Vitamin E is a key fat-soluble vitamin involved in many neurological processes. Vitamin E is actually an umbrella term for eight different types of the vitamin. Walnuts have a type that acts against specific free radicals that can lead to degenerative brain disorders. Vitamin E also protects the fats that line the outside of every cell of our body.

Alpha-linolenic acid (ALA) is an omega-3 fatty acid that our bodies cannot make so it has to come from our diets. It converts to the long-chain fatty acid EPA, which in turn converts to DHA, two essential brain fats.

Juglone is an antioxidant that promotes a healthy intestinal lining, promoting brain health via the gut–brain axis.

SUGGESTED SERVING

Eating 1oz (30g) of walnuts or mixed nuts each day is beneficial to the brain.

HOW TO ENJOY

Walnuts are an excellent substitute for harmful sugary snacks. Their nutrients are at their best when eaten raw. Store in an airtight container in the fridge.

Enjoy a mood-boosting salad.
➡ *Toss brain-supporting walnuts into a hydrating green leaf salad.*
Whip up a nutty pesto.
➡ *In a food processor, finely chop 3½oz (100g) each walnuts and arugula, 2 spring onions, and 2 garlic cloves. Drizzle in 6 tablespoons walnut oil and 3 tablespoons olive oil and season.*

WHEN TO AVOID
Nut allergies are common; reactions can be severe and even life-threatening. If you are allergic to any nut, make sure there is no trace in anything you eat.

RECIPE

Almond dip

Puree 3½oz (100g) almonds, 4fl oz (120ml) water, the juice of 1 lemon, 1 tsp wholeseed mustard, and 5fl oz (150ml) olive oil. Add salt, pepper, and a pinch of paprika and enjoy as a mood-supporting and energizing vegetable dip.

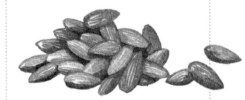

" *Walnuts contain powerful antioxidants that play a part in how we age.* "

HAZELNUT

Hazelnuts have been eaten for thousands of years. When picked and stored in bygone times, they would have provided valuable protein and fats in the colder months. Full of brain-nourishing nutrients, today hazelnuts are eaten worldwide.

BENEFITS

Hazelnuts are higher in folate than any other nut, and are a good source of monounsaturated fatty acids, both of which have a positive effect on cognitive function. Hazelnuts also contain important B vitamins such as riboflavin, niacin, and thiamine, and are a good source of vitamin E and manganese.

Folate is necessary for cells to function. It also helps convert the amino acid homocysteine into the powerful antioxidant glutathione and the compound S-adenosyl methionine (SAMe), which is thought to help protect against depression. If homocysteine is not converted efficiently, elevated levels are a risk factor for neurological conditions and symptoms of depression.

Monounsaturated fatty acids (MUFAs) help to stabilize blood sugar, in turn helping to balance mood and reduce anxiety. MUFAs increase the production and release of the neurotransmitter acetylcholine. This important neurotransmitter is found in many brain neurons and plays a key role in memory. Loss of acetylcholine is associated with the onset of Alzheimer's disease.

SUGGESTED SERVING

A 1oz (30g) handful of hazelnuts, or mixed nuts, a day is a nourishing choice of snack.

HOW TO ENJOY

Raw hazelnuts have the highest nutritional benefits, although roasted are delicious. Buy them whole and unroasted with the skin intact.

Dry-roast hazelnuts.
➡️*To protect the nutrients, dry roast hazelnuts no higher than 170°F (76°C). When the skins begin to crack, pour onto a dishtowel and gently rub until the skins flake off.*
Add a nutty crunch to salads.
➡️*Pair roasted hazelnuts with green beans, fennel, spinach, and radicchio.*
Whizz up a folate-boosting smoothie.
➡️*Soak ½oz (15g) raw hazelnuts overnight, drain, rinse, and puree with 3½fl oz (100ml) water, ½ tsp raw cacao, ¼ teaspoon vanilla extract, and a handful of blueberries.*

WHEN TO AVOID

Nut allergies are common; reactions can be severe and even life-threatening. If you are allergic to any nut, make sure there is no trace in anything you eat.

ALMOND

One of our most popular nuts, almonds contain plenty of protective nutrients for brain health. A 2016 study concluded that raw and roasted almonds were prebiotic, supporting the gut microbiome.

BENEFITS

As well as vitamin E, biotin, magnesium, and oleic fatty acid, almonds also provide manganese and copper, which help synthesize an enzyme, superoxide dismutase, that disarms damaging toxins.

Oleic acid, a monounsaturated fatty acid, has a positive effect on cognitive

A GOOD SOAK

Phytic acid in nuts affects mineral absorption and enzyme inhibitors can unsettle digestion. Soak in salted water overnight to neutralize both.

function. Oleic acid in olives is thought to contribute to the longevity associated with the Mediterranean diet.

Vitamin E has impressive antioxidant abilities that help neutralize toxic by-products produced by the brain.

Biotin, in synergy with other B vitamins, helps convert food to energy. It is thought to help improve focus and promote a positive outlook.

Magnesium is involved in many chemical brain reactions and low levels are linked to depression. It supports the brain's ability to process and remember information.

SUGGESTED SERVING

Enjoy a handful, or 1oz (30g), of almonds or mixed nuts a day to reap the benefits.

HOW TO ENJOY

As well as adding to dishes for extra bite, there are plenty of ways to enjoy almonds.

Puree for a quick and easy savory dip.
➡️*See recipe, opposite.*
Grind into a gluten-free flour for cakes.
➡️*Bake with eggs, honey, olive oil, and cooked pulped oranges for a citrus boost.*

WHEN TO AVOID

Almonds are a tree nut, one of the eight most common allergies. If allergic, ensure there is no trace in any food.

SEEDS

Seeds hold the potency for new life and are a treasure trove of nutrients. They contain supportive phytonutrients, which nourish the nervous system, and many seeds are packed full of omega oils, which are essential for health and vitality. Including seeds in your diet regularly is a simple way of providing the brain with a wide range of protective and nourishing nutrients.

HEMP SEED

The hemp seed is a small, hard shell that contains a soft nut. The shelled seed is the easiest and tastiest way to eat this nutritious gem, which is well balanced in proteins and fats. Different products are produced using the whole seeds, including hemp oil (see p.161), which is an excellent source of essential fatty acids, and hemp flour, which is high in protein and fiber.

BENEFITS

Hemp protein contains all nine essential amino acids and the fats in hemp are in a healthy ratio of omega-3 and omega-6 essential fatty acids. In addition, the seeds contain beta-carotene and vitamin E, both powerful antioxidants. Hemp is also a good source of many minerals, including magnesium, iron, calcium, manganese, zinc, and copper, all of which help maintain a healthy brain.

The protein in shelled hemp is about 30 percent and is of a very high quality, containing all the essential amino acids. The seed is composed of two primary proteins, edistin and albumin, which are easily digested, absorbed, and utilized by the body. Hemp is also a good source of the protein glutamic acid. In the body, glutamic acid turns into glutamate, which helps the nerve ends send and receive messages.

The fat content in shelled hemp seeds is about 50 percent. The seeds provide a ratio of the two essential fatty acids, linoleic acid and alpha-linolenic acid (ALA), in a ratio that is considered optimal for human nutrition. Hemp is one of only a few natural sources of gamma-linolenic acid (GLA), which helps to prevent inflammation in the body.

SUGGESTED SERVING

Enjoy 2–3 tablespoons of shelled hemp seeds every day as part of a healthy, balanced diet.

HOW TO ENJOY

The shelled seeds are versatile and easy to add to cooked and raw ingredients.

Enjoy the seeds throughout the day.
➡️ *Sprinkle over fruits and vegetables or your morning oatmeal, mix into natural yogurt for a gut-supporting breakfast or snack, or add to grain dishes just before serving.*
Blitz the shelled seed into a cream or milk, or make your own hemp cream.
➡️ *See recipe, opposite.*
Add a crunch to nourishing bakes.
➡️ *Add the whole seeds to homemade granola bars, muffins, and breads.*
Use the oil as a dressing. Due to its high polyunsaturated fat content, hemp oil is unsuitable for using with heat in cooking.
➡️ *Drizzle over salads and rice dishes.*

"Hemp seeds are an excellent source of healthy proteins—containing all nine essential amino acids—and omega fats."

RECIPE

Hemp cream

Place 4½oz (125g) shelled hemp seeds, 3½fl oz (100ml) water, ¼ teaspoon chili powder, and 1 chopped garlic clove in a food processor. Process until smooth and creamy. Swirl on top of soup or drizzle over wilted greens.

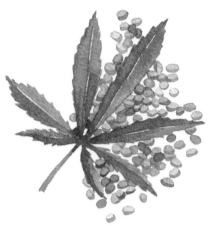

sunflower, pumpkin, poppy, and chia, and keep them in a jar in the fridge to add to your breakfast bowl.

Combine with seaweed for a mineral- and vitamin-rich condiment.
➡ *Grind sunflower seeds and mix with dulse flakes.*

Sprouted sunflower seeds contain more readily available and absorbable nutrients than the seeds alone. They are fresh, juicy, crunchy, and bursting with flavor.
➡ *Toss sprouted sunflower seeds into salads and use them in wraps.*

SUNFLOWER SEED

Sunflowers produce a nutritious seed that supports all-around good health. The seeds are high in beneficial fatty acids, mainly omega-6 linoleic acid and omega-9 oleic acid. The oil should be used in moderation in cooking, as it is high in omega-6 but low in omega-3. For massage, the vitamin E supports glowing skin.

BENEFITS

Sunflower seeds have anti-inflammatory benefits and are a good source of protein. They are packed full of vitamins and minerals including vitamin E, selenium, and magnesium, which are particularly important for brain health.

Vitamin E is a potent antioxidant that plays a crucial role in protecting the brain's high-fat content and helps prevent inflammatory conditions in the brain. As a fat-soluble vitamin, the fat in sunflower seeds helps to ensure that vitamin E is absorbed.

Selenium helps the immune system to fight inflammation and infection. Maintaining a healthy immune system supports a healthy brain, suggesting a diet rich in selenium

could play a signficant role in maintaining good mental health.

Magnesium is critical for healthy brain function. Many people are deficient in magnesium and it is further depleted through periods of stress and anxiety. Research shows that low levels of magnesium are associated with depression. Including plenty of seeds and dark green leafy vegetables will help ensure sufficient levels of magnesium in your diet.

SUGGESTED SERVING

Enjoy a handful of mixed seeds daily or eat a 1oz (30g) serving of sunflower seeds only each day. Alternatively, eat 1–2oz (30–60g) of sprouted sunflower seeds daily.

HOW TO ENJOY

Try soaking sunflower seeds before eating to remove enzyme inhibitors. Or sprout the seeds (see p.170).

Make a sunflower seed pâté full of healthy fats.
➡ *Blend soaked sunflower seeds, sundried tomatoes, basil, and olive oil.*

Keep a nutrient-dense seed mix handy to enjoy with your breakfast.
➡ *Mix together a variety of seeds:*

PUMPKIN SEED

When you scoop the seeds out of a pumpkin, be sure to save them because they are densely packed with nutrients. The seeds can be eaten with or without the shell. In Mexico, for example, the whole seed is roasted with spices. Some varieties produce seeds without shells and some pumpkins are grown for their seeds only. Generally, the pumpkin seeds we buy are shelled.

BENEFITS

Pumpkin seeds are high in magnesium and are also a good source of both zinc and iron. The seeds also contain vitamin E in a variety of forms. In addition, pumpkin seeds are a rich source of protein, particularly tryptophan. This is an amino acid that converts to serotonin in the brain, helping to regulate mood and also playing a role in promoting restful sleep.

Magnesium calms nerves and relaxes muscles. It is involved in many brain chemistry reactions. Low levels of magnesium in the diet are linked to depression and anxiety.

➤ CONTINUED...

Iron is crucial for transporting oxygen to tissues all around the body and is needed by every cell to make energy. Low iron levels in the diet lead to fatigue, lack of focus, and impaired memory. People with iron deficiency are also more prone to depression.

Zinc cannot be stored in our bodies so we need to include good sources in our diet regularly. It supports a robust immune system and the brain needs zinc to synthesize mood-regulating serotonin; people with low levels are at a greater risk of depression.

SUGGESTED SERVING

Enjoy a handful of pumpkin seeds 2–3 times a week.

HOW TO ENJOY

Versatile pumpkin seeds are a flavorful addition to a variety of dishes.

Make a seed mix to add to your breakfast bowl.
➡ *See sunflower seeds, p167.*
Add texture to side dishes and snacks.
➡ *Add to quinoa, couscous, and rice, or bake seeds into breakfast muffins.*
Make a crunchy topping for salads and soups.
➡ *Season and toast in the oven on medium heat for a few minutes.*

A CONSTANT TEMPERATURE

Temperature fluctuations can cause flaxseeds to turn rancid more quickly. Store an airtight container in a cool place.

> *"Cacao stimulates the release of neurotransmitters in the brain that help to promote positive emotions."*

FLAXSEED

Flaxseed, also known as linseed, has been used as food and medicine for thousands of years. The small seeds are an excellent source of the essential omega-3 fatty acid, alpha-linolenic acid. They also contain a good amount of both soluble and insoluble fiber. Flaxseed is either golden or brown and both varieties have similar nutritional properties. The seeds are made into a delicious oil.

BENEFITS

The high content of essential fatty acids, fiber, and the phytonutrients known as lignans, makes flaxseed a particularly beneficial food for gastro-intestinal health, helping to guard against diabetes and support brain development.

Alpha-linolenic acid (ALA) is an essential omega-3 fatty acid that we have to get from our diet. Flaxseed is one of the richest sources of this healthy, anti-inflammatory fat. To maximize its anti-inflammatory benefits, our bodies must convert ALA into the more active forms of docosahexaenoic acid (DHA) and eicosapentaenoic acid (EPA). This is particularly important for vegetarians and vegans who are unable to obtain preformed DHA and EPA from animal sources. Nutrients that enhance this conversion include protein, B vitamins, calcium, zinc, and magnesium. DHA is critical in pre- and postnatal brain development, while EPA is linked to balanced moods.

Lignans, a group of chemical compounds with antioxidant properties, are found in many plants, but the highest concentration is found in flaxseed. Lignans are well-known for balancing hormones, in turn helping to promote positivity and a sense of well-being.

SUGGESTED SERVING

Eat 1–2 tablespoons of ground flaxseed a day or 1 tablespoon of flaxseed oil.

HOW TO ENJOY

Grind the seeds before using, as the whole seeds pass through the body without being digested, wasting valuable nutrition. It is best to buy whole seeds and grind them just before use, because once ground, they are prone to oxidation and spoilage. Cold-pressed flaxseed oil should have a delicious, fresh nutty taste; if this is not the case, it has turned rancid.

Add to breakfast, snacks, and drinks for an easy nutrient boost.
➡ *Scatter the ground seeds on oats and fruits, or add to smoothies.*
Use as an egg replacer, particularly useful for vegan cooking.
➡ *To replace an egg, combine 1 tbsp ground flaxseed with 3 tbsp water. Let stand for 10–15 minutes to thicken before using.*

CACAO SEED

Cacao seeds (often called beans) come from the large pods of the cacao tree. After harvesting, the pods are split open, and the seeds, covered in a white pulp, are left to ferment. Conventional chocolate-making roasts the seeds at high temperatures. Raw cacao, which provides the maximum nutrition, is made by drying the raw seeds at temperatures around 113°F (45°C). The husks are then removed and the seed broken into nibs.

BENEFITS

Raw cacao is full of nutrients that support brain health, including manganese, iron, copper, and, in particular, magnesium. Cacao is also an excellent source of flavonoids, which support our brain health in a variety of ways.

Cacao stimulates the brain to release neurotransmitters that, in turn, can trigger positive emotions. Phenylethylamine, which is found in cacao, combines with dopamine to produce a mild antidepressant effect.

Magnesium is vital for our mental health. It relaxes muscles and has a calming effect on the body and mind. Obtaining plenty of magnesium from our diet is critical to help us cope with stress. Deficiencies in magnesium have been linked to a wide range of brain disorders, including anxiety and depression. Cacao is a fantastic source of this stress-busting mineral.

Flavonoids in cacao nibs are potent antioxidants with anti-inflammatory and immune-supporting benefits. Including this antioxidant in the diet helps support brain health. Flavonoids support a healthy blood flow to the brain, which in turn can help to improve and support memory and lower the risk of dementia.

Iron is vital for making hemoglobin, needed to carry oxygen around the body, ensuring that vital organs such as the brain function at their best. Iron plays an essential role in the processes of thinking, reasoning, and memory, and a deficiency is linked to a higher risk of depression.

SUGGESTED SERVING

Include up to 1oz (30g) of cacao nibs daily in your diet.

HOW TO ENJOY

Cacao nibs have a different taste than more commercially processed chocolate, especially processed milk chocolate. While the nibs do taste chocolatey, they also have a slightly bitter flavor. The nibs are easy to incorporate into the diet, for example, in smoothies, breakfast dishes, and desserts.

The iron in cacao is absorbed more efficiently when it is eaten together with vitamin C.
➥*Combine cacao nibs with orange segments for a refreshing snack.*
Enjoy with hemp milk and oats for a calming and mood-lifting porridge.
➥*Soak cacao nibs and oats in hemp milk overnight.*
Make a batch of brain-supporting energy balls.
➥*Blend chopped walnuts, raisins, almond butter, shelled hemp seeds, and cacao nibs. Roll into small balls.*

WHEN TO AVOID

Cacao contains theobromine—a nervous system stimulant that affects the body in a similar way to caffeine. Cacao may cause you to have anxiety or affect your sleep, especially if you are sensitive to caffeine. During the third trimester of pregnancy, seek professional advice about limiting or omitting cacao until your baby is born.

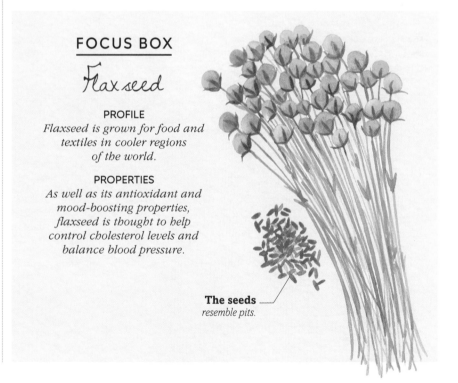

FOCUS BOX

Flax seed

PROFILE
Flaxseed is grown for food and textiles in cooler regions of the world.

PROPERTIES
As well as its antioxidant and mood-boosting properties, flaxseed is thought to help control cholesterol levels and balance blood pressure.

The seeds
resemble pits.

SPROUTS

Soaking seeds helps them to germinate and burst into life, transforming into sprouts, which are superbly suited to our nutritional needs. The sprouting process leads to increased enzyme activity, which converts starches into simple sugars, complex proteins into amino acids, and fats into fatty acids. This makes the seed much easier to digest and enhances the bioavailability of minerals and nutrients.

MUNG BEAN SPROUTS

Nutrient-dense sprouted mung beans are among the most common sprouts enjoyed. They contain a significant amount of mainly soluble fiber, which supports the health of the gut and, in turn, our brain health.

BENEFITS

Sprouting significantly increases the vitamin C content of mung beans. A 3½oz (100g) portion of sprouts provides 21mg of vitamin C—about a quarter of our daily needs. The sprouting process also dramatically increases the availability of beneficial phytonutrients and antioxidants.

Vitamin C, a vital antioxidant molecule in the brain, protects the body's cells from the damaging action of free radicals—the unstable molecules that harm our cells. Without antioxidants to neutralize free radicals, these harmful compounds attach to healthy cells, causing damage and inflammation. Vitamin C must be obtained from the diet every day.

Phytonutrients are chemicals made by plants, many of which give plants their color, taste, and aroma.

Essentially, they are the plant's immune system—when we eat the plant, we harness their benefits. Many have high free radical scavenging abilities. Sprouting seeds increases their phytonutrient content. In the case of mung beans, there is a significant difference between the bean and the sprout.

SUGGESTED SERVING

Many sprouted seeds are beneficial, including mung, lentil, broccoli, radish, sunflower, buckwheat, and quinoa. Try to include a portion—a large handful—of one of these each day in your diet.

HOW TO ENJOY

Soak seeds overnight (6–12 hours) in filtered water in a bottle with a mesh lid. Drain, rinse thoroughly, and leave angled to drain. Rinse the seeds 2–3 times daily and keep them well-drained. They will be ready in 2–4 days when the sprout is ¼in (5mm) long. Store in the fridge in a sealed container for up to 3 days. It is essential to wash sprouts well before eating.

Enjoy raw in a salad.
➡ *In a bowl, combine 2½oz (75g) sprouted mung beans, 2½oz (75g) sunflower seeds with 1 each seeded and diced red and yellow pepper.*

RECIPE

Breakfast bowl

Put 2 tbsp sprouted buckwheat and 2 tsp each of pumpkin and sunflower seeds in a bowl. Add 1 tsp honey and 4fl oz (125ml) hemp milk. Soak overnight then top with diced apple or berries and 2 tsp ground flaxseed.

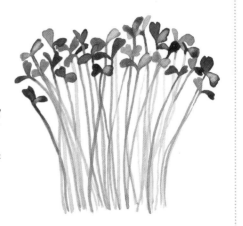

" Buckwheat sprouts are a good source of plant-based protein, essential for the repair of cells."

Whisk 2 tbsp extra virgin olive oil with ½ tsp fennel seeds, 2 tsp fresh ginger, and 2 tsp tamari. Pour over the sprouts and peppers and toss all the ingredients together.

BUCKWHEAT SPROUTS

Despite its name, buckwheat is not related to wheat and belongs to a completely different family that includes sorrel and rhubarb. Buckwheat is gluten-free, so is an excellent alternative for those who avoid cereal grains. To sprout buckwheat seeds, buy the raw hulled variety, often referred to as "groats," not the Russian-style toasted buckwheat, which will not sprout.

BENEFITS

Buckwheat is a fantastic source of plant-based protein in an easily digestible form. It is also an excellent source of rutin, a bioflavonoid with antioxidant properties. Sprouting buckwheat increases rutin from 13.66 to 283.43mg per 3½oz (100g). In addition, buckwheat is packed full of nutrients that support mental wellness, including copper, manganese, magnesium, phosphorous, co-enzyme Q10, selenium, and fiber.

Protein is essential to the growth and repair of all the cells and tissues in our bodies and is needed to create enzymes and form antibodies.

Hormones are also made from protein; these chemical messengers play an essential role in brain health. Good-quality protein in the diet optimizes brain function, reduces inflammation, improves mental clarity, and boosts memory. Buckwheat contains all nine indispensable amino acids.

Rutin, a bioflavonoid in plants, helps to promote healthy interactions between hormones and is well-known for its ability to strengthen blood vessels and improve circulation. Its powerful anti-inflammatory and antioxidant properties also help protect the brain. Rutin has shown promising results in the treatment of neurodegenerative diseases such as Alzheimer's.

SUGGESTED SERVING

You can include a large handful of buckwheat sprouts as one of your daily sprouted seed portions.

HOW TO ENJOY

After sprouting buckwheat (see How to Enjoy, opposite), use it in a variety of ways.

Dehydrate and blitz into a flour.
➥*Use to make buckwheat crackers.*
Blend into a smoothie, providing easy-to-digest protein, B vitamins to lift mood, and calming magnesium.
➥*Puree a handful of sprouts, 1 banana, 9fl oz (250ml) hemp milk, and ginger and cinnamon, to taste.*
Include in a breakfast recipe.
➥*See box, opposite.*

BROCCOLI SPROUTS

As with other sprouted seeds, broccoli sprouts are highly nutritious. Juicy and with a spicy kick, they also have a high water content, keeping the body hydrated, essential for overall wellness.

BENEFITS

Adding broccoli sprouts to your meals will provide you with stress-busting vitamin C, gut-friendly soluble fiber, and anti-inflammatory sulforaphane.

Vitamin C helps reduce stress and anxiety. The highest concentration of vitamin C is found in the brain, where it is crucial for its mood-lifting effect.
Soluble fiber is fermented by bacteria in the gut to produce butyrate, a short-chain fatty acid that helps reduce inflammation and improve memory.
Sulforaphane is a beneficial compound produced when the phytochemical glucoraphanin is broken down during chewing. It has antiviral properties, reduces inflammation, detoxifies the body, and fights free radicals. There is up to 100 times more sulforaphane in sprouts than in mature broccoli.

SUGGESTED SERVING

Eat a large handful 3–4 times a week.

HOW TO ENJOY

It is best to eat broccoli sprouts at 3–4 days old. After sprouting (see How to Enjoy, opposite), wash thoroughly before use.

Include broccoli sprouts in a nori wrap or sandwich.
➥*Try a wrap with avocado, broccoli sprouts, and chili pepper.*

HERBS AND SPICES

Throughout history, herbs and spices have added depth and flavor to food. As we traveled, our palette of herbs and spices grew and we used them not only to liven up dishes but also to support health. The abundance of phytonutrients in herbs and spices can bring many positive effects, including aiding digestion, enhancing memory, and lifting low spirits.

ROSEMARY

Rosemary (*Salvia rosmarinus*) is a perennial evergreen plant with needlelike leaves. It is sometimes called the herb of remembrance for its ability to strengthen memory. It is a versatile culinary herb with potent antioxidant properties and is often used as a food preservative, particularly for meat products.

BENEFITS

Rosemary contains various minerals and vitamins, but the quantity of herb used in cooking will not contribute a significant amount of these nutrients to the diet.

BEST STORAGE

Keep rosemary fresh longer by wrapping sprigs in a damp paper towel and storing in a reusable container in the fridge.

However, rosemary is rich in phytonutrients, many with antioxidant and anti-inflammatory benefits that can help support the immune system, improve blood circulation, help with memory performance, and enhance focus. Just the aroma of rosemary has been linked to improving mood and relieving stress.

Rosmarinic acid is a polyphenol phytonutrient found in rosemary and other herbs, including lemon balm, sage, and mint. It has antioxidant, anti-inflammatory, and antimicrobial activities and is considered a cognitive stimulant that can help to improve memory. Regularly consuming polyphenols is thought to support healthy digestion, essential for the proper utilization of nutrients and for maintaining a healthy brain.

SUGGESTED SERVING

Rosemary is safe in the quantities used to flavor food. For medicinal amounts, consult a medical herbalist.

HOW TO ENJOY

Available all year round, it is easy to choose the vibrant, superior flavor of fresh over dried. Rosemary has a big character and its piney flavor marries well with beans, soups, stews, and venison. When crushed or chopped, it adds a powerfully aromatic flavor to savory and sweet dishes.

Make an aromatic infusion to dress a warm salad. Jerusalem artichokes and chestnuts with rosemary oil provides an excellent combination of brain-supporting nutrients.
➡ *Infuse rosemary in oil or vinegar. Or for a restorative blend, infuse in honey for four weeks, then add a spoonful to a bowl of fresh fruit.*
Flavor fish, meat, and potatoes.
➡ *Lay sprigs under fish or meat during cooking. See recipe opposite for potatoes.*

LEMON BALM

Lemon balm (*Melissa officinalis*) is a perennial herb related to the mint family. It has lemon-flavored minty leaves and its small white flowers attract bees—it is one of the most famous bee-loving herbs. The seventeenth-century English gardener, John Evelyn, declared lemon balm "sovereign for the brain, strengthening memory and powerfully chasing away melancholy."

BENEFITS

Lemon balm is used to reduce tension and anxiety and enhance relaxation and restful sleep. It is a potent antioxidant that helps to protect the brain cells from oxidative damage. A combination of phytonutrients in lemon balm work together to support mental wellness.

Key phytonutrients in lemon balm include citral, whose potent antioxidant and anti-inflammatory properties support brain health, and rosmarinic acid, which appears to elevate levels of the calming neurotransmitter gamma aminobutyric acid (GABA), which helps promote a good night's sleep, essential for a balanced mood.

SUGGESTED SERVING

Enjoy a daily infusion made from a small handful of fresh leaves. Also, add fresh leaves daily to salads and desserts.

HOW TO ENJOY

Lemon balm is best used fresh; add the fragrant leaves to both sweet and savory dishes. It complements fish, poultry, and vegetables, and can be added easily to salads and drinks. The most common use is in a refreshing herbal tea.

Toss into salads.
➼ *Add the lemon-flavored, minty leaves to a bowl of green leaves.*
Enjoy with vegetables.
➼ *Try with fresh peas, fava beans, and new potatoes.*
Add to a lacto-fermented lemonade for a calming, gut-friendly drink.
➼ *Add a handful of leaves.*
Enjoy in a gut-friendly yogurt.
➼ *Shred and add to live yogurt with summer fruits.*
Flavor water for a refreshing drink.
➼ *Add a few leaves to water.*

CINNAMON

Cinnamon is an aromatic spice that comes from the bark of an evergreen tree native to Sri Lanka. One of the earliest traded spices, it has a long history as a culinary spice and a medicine. There are two types: cassia cinnamon comes mainly from China, Vietnam, and Indonesia; and Ceylon cinnamon is produced in Sri Lanka. Ceylon cinnamon is superior nutritionally and therapeutically.

BENEFITS

Various studies suggest that cinnamon can help reduce harmful oxidation in the brain, improving cognition and memory. It's thought that even the sweet, spicy aroma of cinnamon alone helps boost memory. Research also suggests it may help prevent the progression of Alzheimer's disease. It contains many phytonutrients, manganese being its most notable mineral.

Manganese, an essential mineral and powerful antioxidant crucial for brain health, is vital both as a constituent and activator of enzymes. It helps enlarge veins, assisting in the efficient transportation of blood, and therefore oxygen, to tissues in the brain to support brain function.

Cinnamaldehyde, the phytonutrient that produces the flavor and aroma in cinnamon, acts as an antioxidant, neutralizing damaging free radicals that form every day. When left unchecked, free radicals can lead to degenerative diseases, including dementia. Antioxidants in cinnamon, including cinnamaldehyde, prevent unwanted inflammatory responses.

SUGGESTED SERVING

Due to the antioxidant activity and manganese content, ½ tsp a day can have beneficial effects.

HOW TO ENJOY

Uplifting cinnamon, a store-cupboard essential, is easy to use as a powder or in a stick. Sticks last longer and can also be processed to make a powder.

Add to a range of dishes.
➼ *Sprinkle powder over chopped apple with almond butter, oats, or quinoa, and use to flavor tagines.*
Make a calming and uplifting drink.
➼ *Sprinkle over hot milk.*

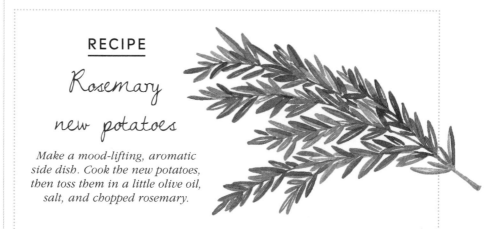

RECIPE

Rosemary new potatoes

Make a mood-lifting, aromatic side dish. Cook the new potatoes, then toss them in a little olive oil, salt, and chopped rosemary.

SUPPLEMENTS

Whole foods should ideally meet our nutritional needs, but when the body is under stress, supplements can help. An isolated nutrient does not have the same benefit as one in a whole-food context, where nutrients work synergistically. Choose "food state" supplements, which indicate they have been combined in a food "matrix" that the body recognizes and absorbs readily. See page 242 for supplement dosages.

VITAMINS

Vitamins B12, C, and D are key for mental health and well-being, providing protective antioxidants and helping neurotransmitters to function. Vitamins B12 and D are two of the most common vitamin deficiencies, while vitamin C cannot be stored in the body so daily sources are required.

VITAMIN B12

Vitamin B12 is needed for the synthesis of neurotransmitters, or brain chemicals, that affect our alertness, cognition, memory, and mood. Low levels of B12 are linked to an increased risk of depression and studies suggest that a deficiency may play a part in conditions such as dementia.

Natural sources of vitamin B12 are restricted to foods of animal origin, including cheese and eggs, as well as fortified cereals. If you eat a vegan diet, vitamin B12 supplementation is important. Older people and those who suffer from any gastrointestinal disorder are also at risk of a B12 deficiency. B12 supplements come in different forms. Those that contain methylcobalamin are the most effective. In some cases, B12 injections may be recommended.

VITAMIN C

Vitamin C is a highly effective antioxidant that protects against oxidative damage from free radicals. It is vital for healthy neurological functions.

Vitamin C is present in fruit and vegetables, but the content varies depending on where a food was grown, its maturity, storage, and cooking methods. When under stress, the body uses a considerable amount of vitamin C to control levels of our fight-or-flight hormone, cortisol, and high blood pressure so a supplement can be beneficial. For most, the recommended daily amount of 100mg a day is woefully inadequate. A therapeutic dose to support anxiety, stress, and depression is about 1000mg a day.

VITAMIN D

Vitamin D is involved in the synthesis of neurotransmitters that aid memory, lower anxiety, and help to promote good sleep.

Vitamin D occurs in different forms. The most common are Vitamin D2, originating from the yeast and plant sterol called ergosterol, and vitamin D3, from sunlight and animal sources. Vitamin D3 is thought to be most effectively metabolized by the body. The main way our bodies obtain vitamin D3 is through exposure to ultraviolet B rays from sunlight; however, factors such as the use of sunscreen and distance from the equator can limit the amount available for our bodies to absorb. Vitamin D3 is found in some foods of animal origin, the best source being oily fish, but it is hard to obtain sufficient amounts from diet alone. In the absence of adequate sunshine, supplementation is often advisable.

BEST STORAGE

Probiotics tend to have a shorter shelf life than other supplements. Buy in smaller quantities and store all supplements out of direct sunlight.

"Supplementation of certain nutrients can be beneficial when stress quickly uses up the body's supplies."

MINERALS

Iron, magnesium, and selenium help the body to carry out functions that are essential for our health and mental well-being, ensuring that cells are oxygenated and that neuron and thyroid function are regulated, allowing both to operate efficiently. Deficiencies in iron are widespread across the world. Adequate levels of magnesium and selenium should also be sought to help optimize mental well-being.

IRON

Iron is an essential mineral, involved in transporting oxygen around our bodies in the form of hemoglobin and it plays a vital role in converting food into energy to fuel the body and brain. Iron is crucial for the healthy functioning of the brain and nervous system.

There are two forms of iron: heme and non-heme. Heme iron is only found in animal-derived foods and is highly bioavailable in the body. Non-heme iron is found in plants and is less readily absorbed by the body. Absorption of non-heme iron is greatly improved in the presence of vitamin C. Iron-deficiency anemia is the most common nutritional deficiency reported worldwide. Menstruation, adolescent growth spurts, low stomach acidity, and strenuous exercise all increase the body's demand for iron.

MAGNESIUM

Magnesium regulates neuron activity and is needed to make the key antioxidant glutathione, which protects against cellular damage. It is also crucial for the normal functioning of the nerves.

Raised levels of magnesium in the brain have been shown to improve cognitive performance. Magnesium-L-threonate (MgT) is the most readily absorbed by the body. Magnesium is found in green leafy vegetables, nuts, and whole grains, all central to a healthy diet. Often, grains or nuts, or both, are omitted from the diet, and several studies show dietary sources of magnesium are lacking in the intake of older people. In these cases, supplementation can be beneficial.

SELENIUM

This trace mineral is a powerful antioxidant, providing protection against harmful free radicals. It is critical for healthy thyroid function, which impacts every cell in your body and brain.

Food sources of selenium include meat, seafood, grains, dairy products, fruits, and vegetables. However, the selenium content of food varies enormously depending on where the animal was raised or the plant grown, as many soils lack selenium. If foods highest in selenium, such as oysters, fish, Brazil nuts, and chicken, are omitted from the diet, a supplement can be helpful.

OTHER SUPPLEMENTS

Omega-3 fatty acids and probiotics play an important role in both brain health, and our gut health, which impacts and supports the health of the brain via the gut–brain axis.

OMEGA-3, EPA, AND DHA FATTY ACIDS

To perform key brain functions, omega-3 alpha-linolenic acid (ALA) must be converted into eicosapentaenoic acid (EPA) and docosahexaenoic acid (DHA).

There are plenty of plant sources of alpha-linolenic acid, including hemp seeds, linseeds, chia, and walnuts, but our diets, lifestyles, age, sex, and genetics can affect its conversion to long-chain fatty acids. EPA and DHA can be found ready-formed primarily in fatty fish. If you eat only foods of plant origin or do not eat fatty fish, an EPA and DHA supplement derived from micro algae is advisable.

PROBIOTICS

The quality and quantity of beneficial gut bacteria play an important role in mental health. The gut microbiome is delicately balanced and can be negatively impacted by a poor diet, affecting the brain via the gut–brain axis. A probiotic supplement can help restore balance.

The gut contains billions of bacteria. Research has shown that specific strains are effective at treating conditions such as anxiety and low mood. Probiotics need to be taken in sufficient amounts to make a difference. Seek advice to ensure you choose one with the best strains of bacteria and of optimal strength.

MOVEMENT AND EXERCISE

INTRODUCTION

THE ROLE OF EXERCISE

Our bodies are designed to move around, and staying active is one of the best ways to maintain physical health. If you are feeling depressed, anxious, and lacking in energy, it can be hard to motivate yourself to do even the simplest forms of exercise. However, increasing evidence shows how the body and mind are connected, so the more we do to improve our physical health, the better our mental health will be, too.

HOW ACTIVITY HELPS

Exercise supports mental health on a biological level, but it also has huge emotional and psychological benefits. Many of us don't get enough exercise, and for those suffering from depression and anxiety, the rate of physical activity tends to be even lower than average. When we do find the motivation to get moving, whether through everyday activities, organized classes, or by engaging in aerobic activity, this delivers real therapeutic benefits.

A brisk 10-minute walk around the block doesn't just stretch our legs, it also limbers up the mind, increases energy and alertness, and promotes a positive outlook. When the mind is feeling sluggish and concentration is lacking, simply completing a walking or running circuit around the park or neighborhood can bring a sense of accomplishment. Exercise can also act as a release and can bring social benefits that support mental health and well-being. A simple walk in the park,

for example, is a healthy form of exercise and can be used as a relaxing "time out" or, when done with others, becomes a supportive social activity.

More vigorous aerobic exercise that leaves us breathing hard is particularly effective in increasing circulation to the brain and muscles, supporting oxygenation of tissues throughout the body and helping to combat low energy levels and chronic fatigue.

Physical activity also promotes more restful sleep. Lack of sleep can make us more vulnerable to depression and anxiety. Being active relieves the anxiety and low mood that can affect sleep, and is also thought to help adjust our circadian rhythms, which can contribute to insomnia when out of kilter.

Movement and activity help to bolster our tolerance to stress by decreasing the activity of the sympathetic nervous system and the hypothalamic-pituitary-adrenal (HPA) axis, making the body and mind less reactive to daily stressors. It also raises levels of endorphins,

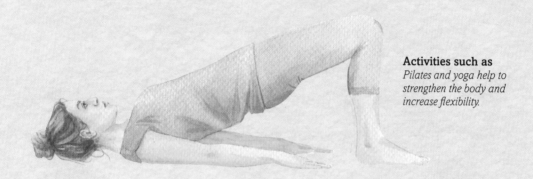

Activities such as
Pilates and yoga help to strengthen the body and increase flexibility.

feel-good brain chemicals and nature's painkillers; and serotonin, a key neurotransmitter for mood regulation.

Importantly, regular light to moderate activity fights chronic inflammation, which can be both a cause and consequence of poor physical and mental health.

YOUR EXERCISE REGIMEN

There is no one-size-fits-all exercise routine. The level of activity that works for an individual can vary from person to person and fluctuate as exercise regimens develop. Ideally, aim for about 150 minutes of moderate- to high-intensity activity per week—usually in the form of 30 minutes of exercise five times a week.

While physical activity such as household chores or taking the stairs instead of the elevator is not the same thing as exercise that involves structured and repetitive body movements, both are beneficial for physical and mental well-being and contribute to weekly activity totals.

CHOOSING AN ACTIVITY

When choosing a structured activity, opting for something you enjoy means you are more likely to stick with it. Consider your needs, too.

Alexander Technique or yoga *stretch and realign the body, making these helpful for chronic pain and stress.*

Aerobic exercise *gets blood pumping and improves oxygen intake, which helps lift a low mood and relieves feelings of sluggishness.*

T'ai chi or yogic breathing *with slow, focused movements help to restore calm when the mind is filled with anxious and distracting thoughts.*

Pilates, t'ai chi, and yoga *are ideal for those who have not been physically active for a while. These offer a way to get moving again and build strength and confidence at your own pace.*

"Regular exercise and activity have huge emotional and psychological benefits, improving our mental well-being."

AEROBIC EXERCISE

Aerobic, or cardio, exercise is any exercise that significantly raises the heart and respiratory rates. Brisk walking, swimming, running, or biking are all aerobic. Health authorities advise 30 minutes or more of aerobic exercise five or more times a week. As well as keeping bones and muscles healthy and toned, exercise has a profound influence on well-being. Many experts believe that aerobic exercise may be one of the simplest and most effective, yet often neglected, interventions in mental health care.

WHAT HAPPENS DURING AEROBIC ACTIVITY?

As the large muscles in the arms, legs, and hips are repeatedly moved during aerobic exercise, the heart starts to beat faster to pump more oxygenated blood to all the parts of the body, including the brain. Regular exercise increases physical stamina, enhancing your quality of life and decreasing the risk of diseases such as diabetes, arthritis, and coronary artery disease. Those who incorporate regular aerobic exercise into their daily routines tend to enjoy greater longevity.

THE EFFECT ON OUR MENTAL HEALTH

In addition to its clear physical benefits, aerobic exercise has been shown to lift depression, reduce the tension associated with anxiety, promote relaxation, and improve sleep. Many of these benefits are linked to neurochemical activity in the brain. Physical activity has been shown to reduce levels of stress hormones, such as adrenaline and cortisol, while also stimulating the production of endorphins, brain chemicals that act as our body's natural painkillers and which elevate mood. Vigorous exercise is also linked to increased self-esteem and feelings of self-worth, and the benefits can be enjoyed in all age groups.

"Regular exercise can help to lift depression, reduce tension and anxiety, and improve sleep patterns."

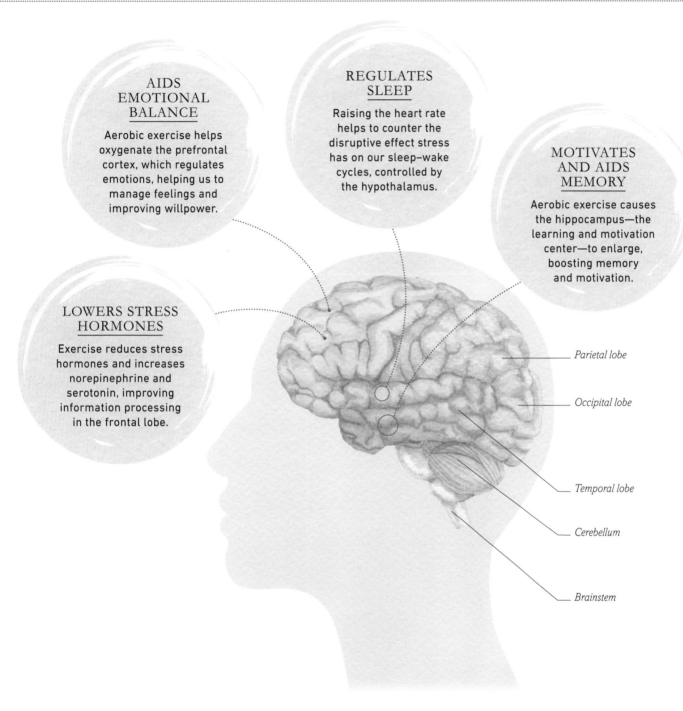

AIDS EMOTIONAL BALANCE

Aerobic exercise helps oxygenate the prefrontal cortex, which regulates emotions, helping us to manage feelings and improving willpower.

REGULATES SLEEP

Raising the heart rate helps to counter the disruptive effect stress has on our sleep–wake cycles, controlled by the hypothalamus.

MOTIVATES AND AIDS MEMORY

Aerobic exercise causes the hippocampus—the learning and motivation center—to enlarge, boosting memory and motivation.

LOWERS STRESS HORMONES

Exercise reduces stress hormones and increases norepinephrine and serotonin, improving information processing in the frontal lobe.

Parietal lobe

Occipital lobe

Temporal lobe

Cerebellum

Brainstem

HOW EXERCISE AFFECTS THE BRAIN

Regular aerobic exercise keeps all parts of the brain well oxygenated, supporting overall cognitive function. It has also been shown to enlarge and/or increase the function of certain parts of the brain responsible for particular areas, such as learning and memory, emotional and stress responses, and motivation.

EVERYDAY ACTIVITY

A whole range of activities that fall within the context of our daily lives count toward our weekly exercise targets and have tangible benefits for our health and well-being. Short bursts of activity throughout the day—such as walking, gardening, carrying groceries, vacuuming, making the bed, cleaning the car, taking the stairs instead of the elevator, and even doing stretching exercises at your desk—can easily add up to the recommended 30 minutes of low to moderate daily activity.

WHAT HAPPENS DURING EVERYDAY ACTIVITY?

There is a body of evidence that demonstrates how everyday activities can be just as beneficial as an organized exercise regimen. Everyday chores and daily activities are a low- to moderate-intensity form of exercise and, as with more formal types of exercise, they increase our circulation, lower blood pressure and cell oxygenation, and help us to lose weight.

THE EFFECT ON OUR MENTAL HEALTH

Everyday activities also have significant mental health benefits. They increase our concentration and help to reduce stress and anxiety. If you participate in team sports or exercise or take walks with friends, these also provide a sense of connection and empathy and develop our social skills. Everyday chores that are part of a regular routine also provide structure and a sense of accomplishment.

Benefits can also be related to the level of mindfulness brought to a task. For example, there is evidence that washing dishes mindfully, focusing on the smell of the soap, the water temperature, and the weight of the dishes, can reduce feelings of nervousness. Tasks help to order the mind, too. Making the bed in the morning is thought to improve productivity. And growing flowers and vegetables has an effect similar to serotonin-boosting antidepressant drugs, increasing feelings of joy and aiding the metabolism of serotonin in the parts of the brain that control mood.

"Everyday activity has significant mental health benefits, reducing anxiety and depressive thoughts."

INCREASES ENERGY

Walking for half an hour daily can make you feel less tired by the end of the day.

ENHANCES FOCUS

Going for even a short walk sharpens focus, helps creativity, and increases productivity.

IMPROVES CARDIO HEALTH

Walking 5½ miles a week can reduce the risk of a cardio-related illness by up to a third.

HELPS FIGHT ADDICTIONS

A one-hour walk five times a week has been shown to reduce cycles of addiction.

IMPROVES MOOD

Setting off on a walk can improve mood almost from the outset.

HELPS WEIGHT LOSS

A daily 30-minute walk contributes to weight loss, which in turn improves self-esteem.

LOWERS RISK OF DEPRESSION

Walking an hour a day is thought to reduce the risk of depression by 25 percent.

HOW WALKING AFFECTS BODY AND MIND

Walking regularly has measurable effects on our physical and mental health and well-being. Walking for as little as 10 minutes can improve your productivity and mood, and regularly walking for up to an hour a week can cause long-term changes to the brain that benefit mental wellness.

YOGA

The practice of yoga, which originated in India some 5,000 years ago, stems from a philosophy that takes an holistic view of health and well-being. While many refer to yoga as a form of exercise, this is somewhat misleading. Using a combination of body postures and breathing exercises, deep relaxation, and sometimes meditation, yoga helps strengthen body, mind, and spirit, building resilience in the face of the stresses and strains of everyday life.

WHAT HAPPENS DURING YOGA?

There are various types of yoga. The most common and widely available is Hatha yoga, which is relatively low-impact and focuses on flexibility, breathing techniques, and relaxation. Ashtanga yoga is more powerful and dynamic, aiming to build strength and endurance, and Iyengar yoga focuses on body alignment, using props as aids.

In all types of yoga, body postures, known as asanas, involve stretching movements to strengthen, tone, and balance the body and mind. Studies confirm that regular yoga practice can increase circulation to the nervous system, organs, and glands and improve the oxygenation of blood. Yogic breathing techniques, known as pranayamas, are cleansing and revitalizing, and studies show they help reduce production of the stress hormones noradrenaline and cortisol.

THE EFFECT ON OUR MENTAL HEALTH

Some benefits are felt quickly when taking up yoga, such as an increased ability to relax, a more positive outlook, greater body awareness, and an enhanced sense of vitality. Often, practitioners experience a reduction in insomnia and more restful sleep. Yoga has also been shown to increase the level of gamma-aminobutyric acid (GABA), a chemical in the brain that helps to regulate nerve activity. This is especially helpful for anxiety sufferers, who can have low levels of GABA. There is also evidence that yoga can help to reduce symptoms of anxiety and low mood in those suffering from depression. And, with practice, the process of meditation (see p.206), in which we continually let go of any thoughts that arrive, brings us closer to feeling centered and peaceful.

"Yoga practice promotes relaxation, a more positive outlook, and an enhanced sense of vitality."

NIYAMAS

The second limb explores self-discipline and the seeking of spiritual fulfillment through yoga, to purify body, mind, and spirit.

YAMAS

This first limb focuses on ethics, promoting a philosophy of truth, moral strength, and nonviolence in our relationships and characters.

ASANA

The third limb introduces the poses, or asanas. When body, mind, and spirit are harmonized, asanas become effortless.

SAMADHI

In the eighth, final limb, the mind merges with the point of focus and the person transcends the self, entering a state of bliss and complete absorption.

PRANAYAMA

The fourth limb, pranayama, is the practice of controlled breathing, done once asanas are mastered, in preparation for the final stages of yoga.

EIGHT LIMBS OF YOGA

The "limbs" of yoga, set out by the sage Patanjali 2,000 years ago, describe the stages of the yoga journey that help to discipline body and mind. The first limb is Yamas, and the final one Samadhi, where body, mind, and breath become fully integrated.

DHYANA

In the seventh limb, as the mind slows, a practice of meditation commences. The mind is perfectly still, quiet, and at peace.

PRATYAHARA

The fifth limb is a "turning in" of the mind, away from the senses, redirecting focus inward, away from the outside world.

DHARANA

With distractions removed, the sixth limb concentrates the mind, focusing attention on a single thought or object, to prepare for meditation.

RELAXING AND FOCUSING YOGA POSES

Stress and anxiety create tension in the body that can lead to problems such as back pain and headaches. Incorporating restful and focusing yoga poses into a regular practice allows the body to unwind and stills and quiets a busy mind.

Chronic stress takes its toll on the nervous system, triggering the fight-or-flight response and increasing the level of stress hormones in the body, which, in turn, leads to elevated breathing and heart rate.

Yoga poses designed to slow down the body and focus and ground the mind help to soothe and relieve stress by restoring balance, allowing the body and mind to relax. Attention starts to turn away from external distractions and the senses focus inward, allowing the mind to calm and become meditative and still. This, in turn, promotes balance in the endocrine and nervous systems, so the body is better able to regulate stress hormones.

STRETCHING AND BALANCING

Poses that bring the head forward and below the heart are deeply restful for the mind, while gentle stretches help to relieve problems such as back pain and tension that is held in the muscles causing stiffness and discomfort. Balancing poses focus the body and mind, helping to distract from anxious thoughts. Stillness in a pose brings awareness of areas of stiffness in the body, allowing you to breathe into these areas. If tension makes it hard to achieve a pose, props can be used to assist the body so the restorative benefits can be experienced.

KEY BENEFITS

As the body rests in a stretching pose, the mind is able to slow down and focus internally, helping to clear the mind and promote a state of relaxation. Poses that involve balance also help to enhance focus and concentration.

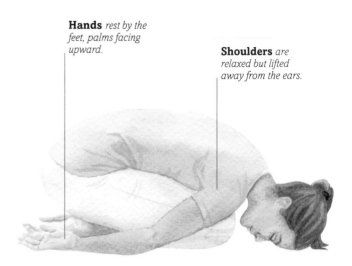

Hands *rest by the feet, palms facing upward.*

Shoulders *are relaxed but lifted away from the ears.*

CHILD'S POSE

Placing the forehead on the floor in this pose is calming and quietening. The body is gently stretched, easing tension in the back, while the abdominal muscles are massaged against the thighs, helping to soothe digestion.

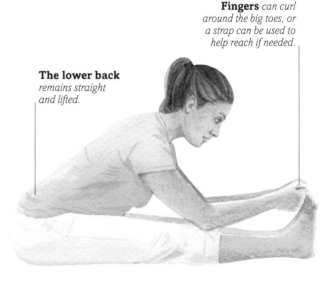

Fingers *can curl around the big toes, or a strap can be used to help reach if needed.*

The lower back *remains straight and lifted.*

FORWARD BEND

Practicing forward bends strengthens the lower back, where stress can create tension and hamper relaxation, and rests the mind. As the mind calms, breathing slows and attention is drawn inward.

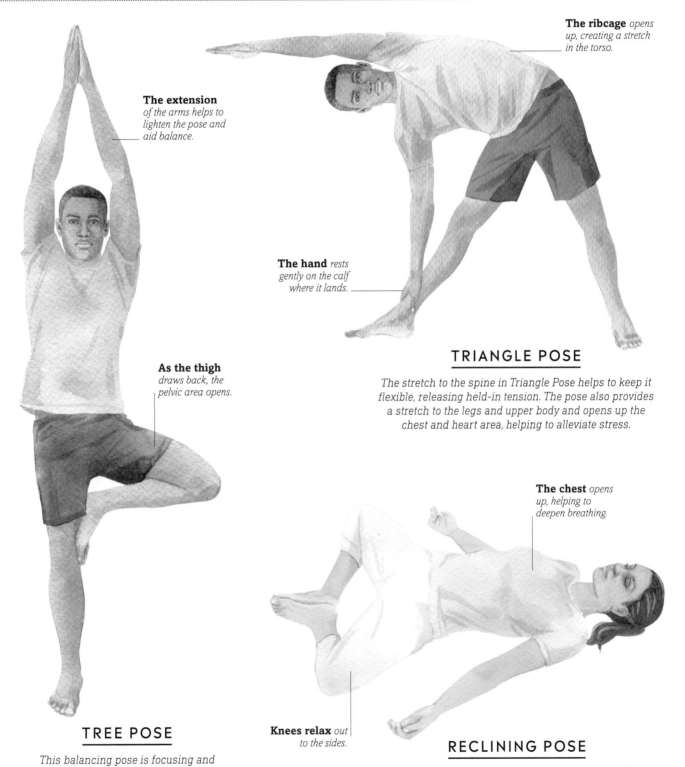

The ribcage *opens up, creating a stretch in the torso.*

The extension *of the arms helps to lighten the pose and aid balance.*

The hand *rests gently on the calf where it lands.*

As the thigh *draws back, the pelvic area opens.*

TRIANGLE POSE

The stretch to the spine in Triangle Pose helps to keep it flexible, releasing held-in tension. The pose also provides a stretch to the legs and upper body and opens up the chest and heart area, helping to alleviate stress.

The chest *opens up, helping to deepen breathing.*

TREE POSE

This balancing pose is focusing and grounding, helping to remove cycles of anxious thoughts as body and mind strive for balance and harmony. The stability in the standing leg brings a feeling of being rooted.

Knees relax *out to the sides.*

RECLINING POSE

This deeply restorative reclining pose opens the chest fully, slowing breathing and, in turn, helping to regulate blood pressure and support circulation. If needed, support under the knees can allow the body to let go completely.

ENERGIZING AND RESTORATIVE YOGA POSES

Yoga poses that stretch and strengthen help to wake up the body and restore flagging energy levels, lightening the body and lifting spirits.

Mental and physical exhaustion takes its toll, making the body feel heavy and sluggish, clouding the mind, and leaving us feeling low and irritable.

A dynamic yoga practice with poses that challenge the body to stretch up and unfurl can be intensely invigorating, stimulating blood flow around the body and oxygenating the heart, lungs, and brain so that these systems operate efficiently. In turn, the body and mind are invigorated, reducing physical fatigue and refocusing the mind so that productivity and mood are improved.

EXTENDING AND OPENING

Poses that stretch the spine and extend the limbs increase flexibility and strengthen areas of weakness, helping to remove pain and discomfort. Backbends that open up the heart chakra are especially energizing, while positions that focus on the straightness of the spine can positively impact energy levels, bringing a feeling of lightness both physically and mentally. Resting the legs against a wall allows the body to feel supported and is incredibly restorative.

KEY BENEFITS

Backbends and energetic stretches wake up the body and mind, while poses that invert the body help to restore calmness and bring a feeling of quietness, which in turn reenergizes.

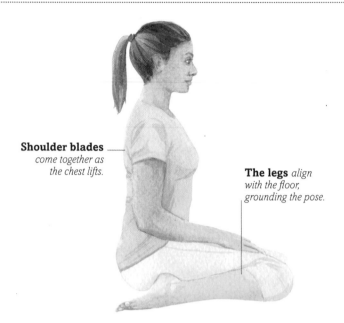

Shoulder blades *come together as the chest lifts.*

The legs *align with the floor, grounding the pose.*

SITTING "HERO" POSE

This seated pose, which moves from kneeling to sitting, helps to strengthen the spine and supports digestion, both of which boost energy levels. To ensure the lower back is lifted, it may be necessary to sit on a support.

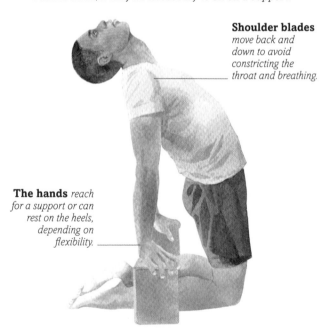

Shoulder blades *move back and down to avoid constricting the throat and breathing.*

The hands *reach for a support or can rest on the heels, depending on flexibility.*

BACKWARD BEND

Powerful backbends require a full lift of the spine before curling back. This dynamic spinal lift improves posture, which can increase confidence. The opening of the heart chakra helps release pent-up emotions.

As the hips *stretch high, the legs pull back and down.*

Shoulders lift *away from the ears and arms remain straight.*

The heels *may touch the floor or hover above, depending on flexibility.*

DOWNWARD DOG

This classic asana stretches the back and legs and increases blood flow to the head, heart, and lungs, which can calm the mind, strengthen the heart, and support the nervous system, helping to lift feelings of fatigue.

The legs *are fully supported by the wall.*

Abdominal muscles *relax and breathing slows.*

LEGS UP THE WALL

Both restorative and energizing, this inverted pose, with the legs resting against the wall, helps the body to relax while also stimulating circulation. This is a good asana for tackling insomnia to restore energy to body and mind.

The leg *is positioned at a 90-degree angle.*

The hand *can support the thigh if needed.*

LEG STRETCH

Alternate leg lifts help to strengthen and tone the leg muscles, increasing flexibility and stimulating blood flow to the legs. This can aid digestion and strengthen the back, all of which reenergizes.

PILATES

Pilates is a low-impact form of exercise that helps to strengthen muscles and improve postural alignment and flexibility. It was developed in the 1920s in the United States by Joseph Pilates, who devised a system of exercises that aimed to correct bad posture, restore vitality to the body and mind, and raise the spirit. Initially, the practice was known as "contrology," but it was renamed Pilates after its founder died.

WHAT HAPPENS DURING PILATES?

Modern Pilates involves a combination of about 50 simple, repetitive exercises performed on a mat or using different types of equipment, such as pulleys and straps. The exercises can be adapted to suit different levels of fitness and ability. The slow and controlled stretches focus on individual muscles, or groups of muscles, to improve strength and muscle tone. Regular practice can improve posture, balance, and joint mobility, as well as relieve stress and tension. This system of exercise is popular with athletes, including dancers, who use it to develop whole-body strength and flexibility and reduce the risk of injury.

THE EFFECT ON OUR MENTAL HEALTH

Studies show that Pilates can significantly reduce symptoms of depression and anxiety and help improve sleep, most likely due to beneficial changes in levels of brain chemicals such as serotonin, cortisol, and endorphins during practice. These changes, in turn, help reduce feelings of fatigue and increase energy. The focus involved in the exercises can distract from negative thought cycles, while physical benefits such as relief from back and neck pain and improved functioning of the lymphatic and circulatory systems boost energy and vitality. As a group practice, Pilates is an opportunity to socialize, which can ease symptoms of depression and anxiety.

"Focusing on precise movements in Pilates can help to distract from negative thought cycles."

CENTERING

Focusing on the center, or core, of the body helps to increase energy and stamina and can still body and mind.

RELAXATION

A conscious effort to recognize and relax areas of muscle tension can bring a feeling of calmness.

CONCENTRATION

In Pilates, the mind is trained to focus on movements, enhancing alignment and body awareness.

INTEGRATION

Using breath, alignment, and precision to perform exercises results in an integrated practice for mind and body.

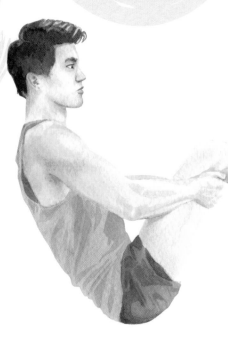

PRECISION

Each exercise is practiced with precision so correct movement becomes second nature, improving posture.

EIGHT PRINCIPLES

Modern-day Pilates marries the ethos and philosophy of Joseph Pilates with the practice that has evolved over the decades, delivering a set of core principles that inform the discipline today. These integrate mind and body, helping practitioners to find balance in both.

FLOW

Movements flow, radiating out from the core, increasing stamina and energizing physically and mentally.

BREATHING

Deep breathing from the diaphragm oxygenates the body efficiently and also triggers the release of feel-good endorphins.

ALIGNMENT

Correct posture, from head to toe, is a key part of the practice. This helps release tension and supports breathing.

PILATES FOR STRESS AND ANXIETY

When we are stressed, our shoulders tend to tense and scrunch up and our muscles tighten, which can lead to pain in the lower back. Pilates positions can help to strengthen the body to mitigate against the effects of stress.

When stress causes our muscles to tighten, this makes it harder for tissues to be oxygenated efficiently, which can lead to painful and sore muscles, exacerbating stress and tension.

Regular Pilates practice helps to strengthen and increase flexibility in the spine and improves posture, helping to stretch muscles and allow them to relax. The exertion involved in the positions here also stimulates circulation, helping well-oxygenated blood to reach and nourish all the tissues, futher reducing tension.

BACK STRENGTHENING AND TWISTING

Positions that lift the spine, whether from a sitting or lying position, help to strengthen the abdomen and improve suppleness in the muscles of the lower back and the trapezius around the shoulders. This supports the spine and improves flexibility. Twisting and rotating positions help to strengthen back muscles and are also thought to stimulate certain neural pathways that help to relax us and moderate and balance our response to stress.

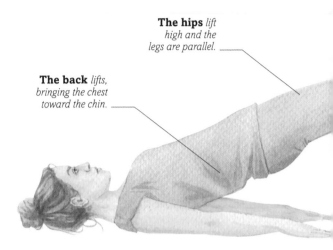

The hips lift high and the legs are parallel.

The back lifts, bringing the chest toward the chin.

BRIDGE POSE

This spine-stabilizing position strengthens muscles in the lower back and glutes, which often hold tension when we are stressed. Lifting the heart above the head also stimulates blood flow, releasing mood-lifting endorphins.

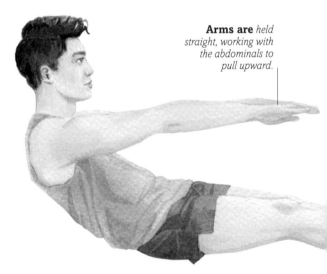

Arms are held straight, working with the abdominals to pull upward.

ROLLING UP

As well as strengthening the core, rolling up involves keeping the shoulders relaxed away from the ears to avoid scrunching the neck. Focusing on this action helps to ease tension held in the shoulders.

KEY BENEFITS

Stretching muscles correctly, ensuring that the shoulders are not lifted and limbs are aligned and fully extended, helps to strengthen the body and correct areas of weakness, in particular in the spine, where stress can lead to pain.

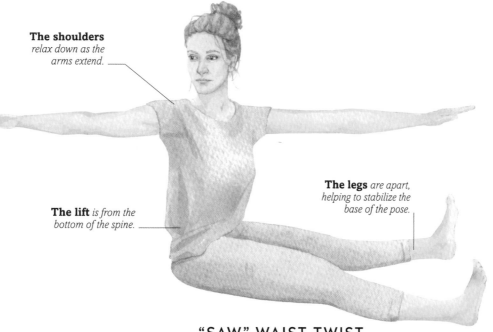

The hips *stay centered as the trunk twists around.*

The ribcage *opens and stretches upward.*

The arm *stretches out fully, lightly touching the floor.*

THREADING THE NEEDLE

Poses that rotate the body are thought to have an impact on neural pathways that are linked to our fight-or-flight response to stress. The action of rotating is thought to help manage these responses to promote a feeling of calm.

The shoulders *relax down as the arms extend.*

The legs *are apart, helping to stabilize the base of the pose.*

The lift *is from the bottom of the spine.*

Feet remain *grounded, legs extended.*

"SAW" WAIST TWIST

This lifting up and twisting position opens up the spine and chest, helping to release tension held in the back and expanding the heart space to help promote deeper and more relaxed and open breathing, which can ease anxiety.

PILATES FOR INSOMNIA AND DIGESTION

A low mood can affect restful sleep, leading to chronic fatigue that can make us feel mentally sluggish and affect processes such as digestion. Pilates exercises can help to promote relaxation and support digestion.

When stress, lifestyle, or a low mood slow us down, the body and mind can feel restless—unable to relax and sleep but lacking motivation to "get up and go." An inability to relax and unwind makes it difficult to achieve restful sleep. Problems with digestion can also be caused by lack of rest and activity, which slow down the processes in the gut.

Pilates poses that open up the body or that fold the body inward can help both to stimulate digestion by stretching the abdominal muscles and also giving them an internal massage, and release stress that can affect our ability to wind down and fall asleep.

QUIETENING AND OPENING POSES

Exercises and positions that bring the head and chest toward the legs can be deeply relaxing, helping to soothe the nerves and shut out external distrations so the focus is on the body and the mind becomes quiet. Stretching out the body fully can be extremely beneficial if you spend a lot of time sitting at a desk and hunching forward. Unfurling the spine and pulling up the chest gives a full stretch to the abdominal muscles, massaging them and stimulating digestion.

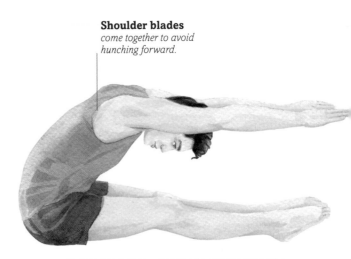

Shoulder blades *come together to avoid hunching forward.*

FORWARD SPINE STRETCH

Forward stretches, as well as stretching out the spine to help release tension, also quiet the mind and allow us to focus our attention inward, promoting calm and relaxation that can support healthy sleep.

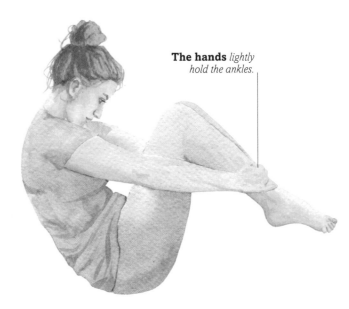

The hands *lightly hold the ankles.*

ROLLING LIKE A BALL

This flowing movement, which involves rolling back in a controlled way, massages the spine, rolling out tension, and stimulates the nervous system, helping to promote relaxation and tackle insomnia.

KEY BENEFITS

Dynamic stretches can stimulate circulation and release stress, helping to unwind and promote restful sleep. Bringing the legs into the body helps to massage the abdominal muscles to stimulate digestion.

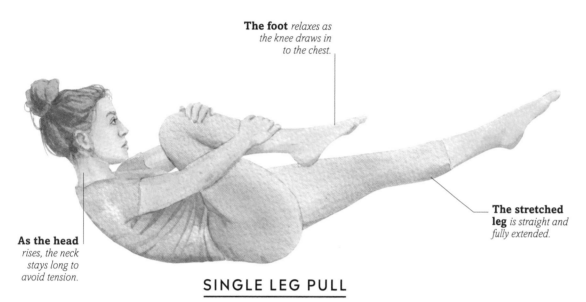

The foot *relaxes as the knee draws in to the chest.*

The stretched leg *is straight and fully extended.*

As the head *rises, the neck stays long to avoid tension.*

SINGLE LEG PULL

Stretching out one leg while pulling in the other helps to both extend the body, stimulating circulation and releasing stress, and fold it inward, giving the abdominal muscles a massage that helps to stimulate digestion.

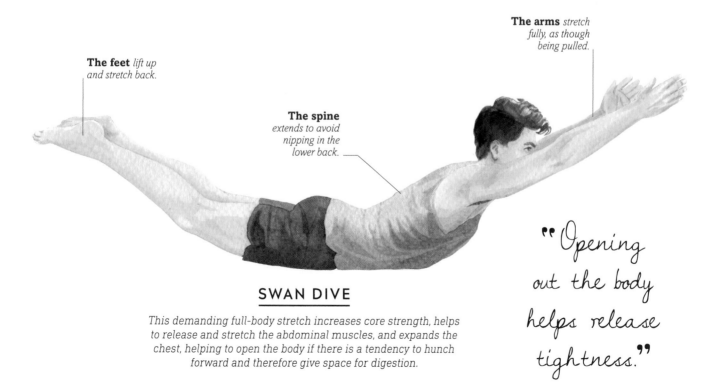

The arms *stretch fully, as though being pulled.*

The feet *lift up and stretch back.*

The spine *extends to avoid nipping in the lower back.*

SWAN DIVE

This demanding full-body stretch increases core strength, helps to release and stretch the abdominal muscles, and expands the chest, helping to open the body if there is a tendency to hunch forward and therefore give space for digestion.

"Opening out the body helps release tightness."

T'AI CHI

Also called t'ai chi chuan, t'ai chi originally developed as a gentle martial art in 13th-century China. It involves slow, flowing, meditative movements that help to improve balance and flexibility and induce relaxation. T'ai chi is a noncompetitive form of exercise and movement that can be done at each person's own pace. Today, it is practiced worldwide as a health-supporting exercise.

WHAT HAPPENS DURING T'AI CHI?

This meditative form of movement is accessible to all ages and abilities. It does not require equipment and can be practiced indoors or outside, where natural settings enhance its meditative focus. It is particularly suited for older age groups who want to raise activity levels gently, and many movements can be adapted for those with a disability. The low-impact exercise involves slow, gentle movements executed without pause, so one action flows seamlessly into the next. Movements are accompanied by focused breathing.

THE EFFECT ON OUR MENTAL HEALTH

T'ai chi has been shown to reduce levels of stress hormones such as cortisol and increase endorphin levels. It also helps to reduce inflammation in the body and support immune and adrenal function, all of which are placed under strain by chronic stress. Regular t'ai chi practice is linked to reduced anxiety, improved mood, and increased energy, balance, and stamina. The focus on posture, movement, and breath stimulates a part of the brain known as the "attentional control network," which helps govern our ability to focus and concentrate. Focusing on the here and now also quiets the mind. As well as relieving symptoms of depression, there is mounting evidence that t'ai chi helps alleviate depressive symptoms linked to conditions such as fibromyalgia, arthritis, multiple sclerosis, heart failure, and mild dementia.

"This meditative form of movement helps to reduce the levels of stress hormones in the body."

MEDITATION
Focused meditative movement helps those who struggle with seated meditation.

NERVE CALMING
The meditative movement calms the body's sympathetic nervous system, which activates the fight-or-flight response.

MIND-BODY AWARENESS
Slow, deliberate movements increase awareness of how the body moves.

BALANCE
An emphasis on being grounded and stable helps to increase balance awareness and enhances well-being.

MUSCLE STRENGTH
Regular practice helps to improve muscle strength in both the upper and lower body.

PRINCIPLES
T'ai chi follows the Chinese philosophy that energy—or chi—flows through channels in the body, and that blockages can lead to reduced mental and physical well-being. The movement is thought to help chi flow freely without hindrance.

MOOD ELEVATION
Increased endorphin levels with t'ai chi are linked to an improved mood and reduction in depressive feelings.

COGNITIVE TOOLS
Focusing on set movements can help increase cognitive function in older people.

BREATHING
Maintaining slow, steady breathing during t'ai chi keeps the mind focused on bodily sensations.

T'AI CHI TECHNIQUES

Chronic stress and anxiety can hamper our ability to concentrate and leave us depleted of energy. T'ai chi involves slow, flowing movements that focus the mind and relax the body.

When tension is held in the body, muscles tend to stiffen and can lose flexibility over time. This, in turn, can lower energy levels, leave the mind feeling sluggish, and affect mood. The continuous, meditative movement that is used in t'ai chi helps to calm the mind and give the muscles a gentle work out. The mind–body action promotes relaxation and helps increase focus and concentration.

The balancing element involved in this flowing practice is especially beneficial for older people. The easily mastered routines suit all levels of ability and help to increase body awareness and can reduce the risk of falls, building confidence and self-esteem and bolstering mood.

CONTINUOUS MOVEMENT

T'ai chi sequences start with the feet firmly planted to give stability and create a strong base from which to move around, building grace and agility with practice. Postures are not static, but rather flow, moving from one pose to the next in a circular fashion seamlessly; the poses opposite represent part of a flowing t'ai chi sequence. Breathing in through the nose and out through the mouth can be used as a conscious accompaniment to the movements. Breathing more deeply into the abdomen, as opposed to shallow chest breathing, brings a relaxing and meditative quality to the practice.

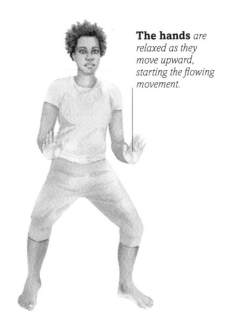

The hands are relaxed as they move upward, starting the flowing movement.

STARTING

A sequence starts with the feet apart, firmly planted to ground and stabilize the body. As the knees gently bend, the hands slowly lift and push outward.

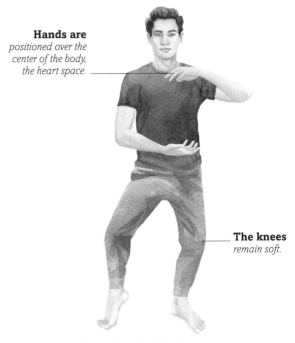

Hands are positioned over the center of the body, the heart space.

The knees remain soft.

HOLD THE BALL

The gaze remains focused ahead, the head straight, and the knees slightly bent as the hands make a ball shape in front of the body, signaling the gathering of vital energy.

KEY BENEFITS

Slow, flowing, meditative movements help to relax the body and mind, promoting a sense of calm while also increasing body awareness.

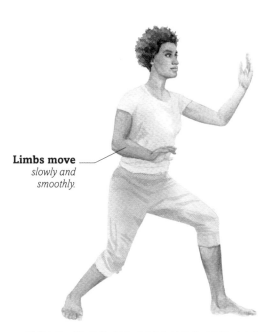

Limbs move slowly and smoothly.

WILD HORSE SHAKES ITS MANE

From Hold the Ball, the body moves around to the side. The knees remain bent while the extended arm "holds the horse's mane" and the other hand moves downward.

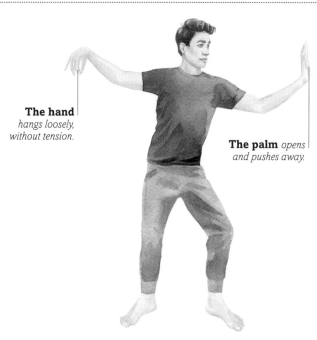

The hand hangs loosely, without tension.

The palm opens and pushes away.

SINGLE WHIP

The arms direct the body, rotating from one side to the other in a flowing action while the weight shifts from one leg to the other. The flow promotes body awareness and good posture.

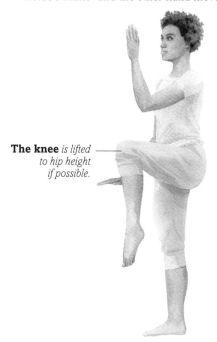

The knee is lifted to hip height if possible.

ROOSTER STANDS ON ONE LEG

This balancing position increases strength and stability. The standing leg remains firmly planted, anchoring the body, as the other knee is raised to the side.

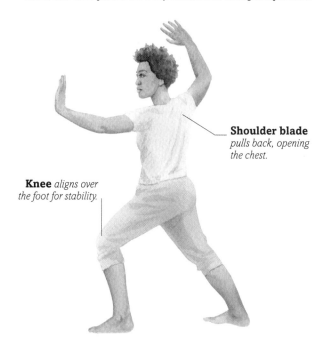

Shoulder blade pulls back, opening the chest.

Knee aligns over the foot for stability.

FAN THROUGH THE BACK

The arms lift and slowly separate, creating a confident, open posture, while the legs crouch low and the weight sinks down, toning muscles and increasing body confidence.

ALEXANDER TECHNIQUE

The Alexander technique focuses on reestablishing the natural connection between the back, neck, and head to increase coordination and self-awareness. It was developed around 1900 by an actor, Frederick Matthias Alexander, who believed that the mind and body work together, constantly influencing each other. Being mindful of the optimal alignment of the head, neck, and spine, he believed, would alleviate pain, breathing disorders, and stress-related conditions.

WHAT HAPPENS DURING THE ALEXANDER TECHNIQUE?

A mixture of physical work and mindfulness, the Alexander technique is usually taught in a series of one-on-one lessons with gentle hands-on guidance and instruction. Its aim is to correct ingrained habits of posture and movement, which lead to muscular tensions that cause aches and pains and that also interfere with our ability to recover from injury and to cope with the stresses and strains of everyday life. In addition to physical adjustments, the technique aims to support emotional well-being to aid calmness. Once the technique is learned, it can be incorporated into everyday life using self-management, so that the benefits are long-lasting.

THE EFFECT ON OUR MENTAL HEALTH

Muscle tension, caused by chronic stress and/or from sitting or standing for long periods in a hunched or tensed posture, causes pain and raises levels of stress hormones in the body. The Alexander technique helps body and mind unwind, promoting relaxation, greater mental clarity, and deeper, slower breathing. Chronic pain also has a profound effect on mental well-being. There is evidence that people who take a course of Alexander technique lessons can experience a dramatic reduction in the use of pain medications. Relieving pain also improves feelings of distress and anxiety and aids restful sleep. For those with body dysmorphia, the Alexander technique can help build greater body confidence.

"The Alexander technique combines physical work with mindfulness."

Correct alignment *of the vertebrae positions the head in line above the perineum and increases height.*

REDUCES PAIN

By identifying and unlocking tense muscle patterns, chronic pain can be relieved, in turn reducing stress.

PROMOTES SLEEP

Releasing tight muscles helps us relax and breathe freely, enhancing the ability to fall asleep and sleep soundly.

A neutral spine *position keeps the lumbar vertebrae curving gently inward.*

CALMS AND GROUNDS

When we hold our bodies correctly, the release of tension has a grounding effect, increasing our ability to be mindful.

BOOSTS CONFIDENCE

Research indicates that good posture can have a measurable impact on self-confidence.

PROMOTES BALANCE

Adjusting poor posture helps body and mind to work in harmony and enables us to respond to stress more effectively.

BRINGS CLARITY

Releasing held-in tension and stress removes distracting pain and improves mental focus and concentration.

POSTURE

Our posture is our body's support system, affecting how we conduct everyday tasks. Correcting bad postural habits can have a profound effect on mental and physical well-being. When we move more efficiently, we enhance our ability to deal with stress, feel more confident, and learn how to relax, which increases mental clarity and stamina.

THERAPEUTIC PRACTICES

INTRODUCTION

THE ROLE OF THERAPIES

We know that our bodies and minds constantly interact. Therapies that take an holistic approach to physical and mental well-being, rather than treating individual complaints, not only address symptoms but also encourage understanding of the root causes of conditions such as depression, anxiety, or phobias. Individually tailored options and suggestions for behavior changes help to address these problems.

HOW THERAPEUTIC PRACTICES HELP

Many complementary approaches have roots in ancient traditional medicine and health philosophies. Often, we turn to these therapies when we feel we need additional support alongside conventional medicine or prefer a gentler, nonmedical approach for less serious conditions.

Complementary therapies place no boundaries between physical, emotional, and mental well-being. Each person is assessed holistically and every aspect of the self is relevant, from posture, lifestyle, and beliefs to energy levels and type of work—the multiple facets of each person's life are believed to play a part in their health.

Embracing complementary therapies provides a way to personalize your path to wellness. The holistic approach draws from a range of appropriate therapeutic options centered around physical therapies, individual or group practices, goal-setting and habit-building practices, and life skills.

Complementary practitioners listen to the person, make a careful diagnosis, and guide individuals on how to take an active part in their own well-being. The consultation process can be a healing experience in itself, ensuring that a person feels heard and that their symptoms are taken seriously. In addition, most therapies, when practiced competently by a qualified practitioner, are generally safe and medicines such as herbs and homeopathy are, for the most part, harmless and nontoxic, with adverse side effects possible but rare.

Practices such as osteopathy, chiropractic, and massage may focus on particular areas of tension, but also treat the body as a whole. And talking therapies or practices such as music therapy, help individuals to explore feelings and patterns of behavior that are detrimental to well-being and, in turn, overall health.

In addition to therapies and practices that are accessed via and carried out by qualified practitioners, therapeutic practices also include simple and accessible

"Taking a therapeutic approach means treating every aspect of the self as relevant in order to heal body, mind, and spirit."

self-care, such as getting out in nature, exploring spirituality, practicing meditation and breathwork, and engaging in mind exercises to keep the brain active, engaged, and agile. All of these support our mental health and well-being and can lead to greater self-fulfillment.

A THERAPEUTIC APPROACH

When mental and emotional health issues become chronic, it can feel as though choices are limited. In fact, most of the therapies in this chapter can be used safely and effectively alongside other natural therapies and more conventional treatment. Massage, counseling, or acupuncture, for example, can be supportive along with conventional antidepressants, while mind exercises and reflexology can support medical therapies that treat cognitive decline. Herbs and meditation or hypnotherapy may for some be the right combination for addressing mild depression or compulsive behavior.

CHOOSING A THERAPY

Exploring natural therapies can help you find one that meets your needs.

Hands-on therapies *such as massage and reflexology are ideal for chronic pain syndromes that can lead to emotional distress.*

Acupuncture and reiki *involve minimal touch, which can suit those with boundary or body issues.*

Group practices, *such as music therapy, time outdoors, counseling, and spiritual practice bring a sense of belonging and connection.*

Approaches such as breathwork, *meditation, Bach flower remedies, time in nature, mind exercises, simple reflexology, and to some extent homeopathy, can be practiced at home to address a wide range of symptoms, including feelings of stress or anxiety, and to improve sleep quality.*

MINDFUL MEDITATION

The practice of mindfulness helps us become aware of our feelings, thoughts, and body sensations. At its most basic level, it is a tool for managing stress, but it is also much more. In a world full of pressure and distractions, where our attention can easily become fragmented, daily meditative practice can bring a sense of relaxation and inner peace, helping us understand ourselves better and grounding us in the present moment.

HOW DOES IT WORK?

Not all types of meditation involve sitting quietly in a crossed leg position. Practices such as t'ai chi (see p.196), for example, focus on meditative movement, combining a relaxed but alert state of mind with slow movements and gentle breathing. Other types of meditation involve visualizations and/or mantras, or extended periods of reflection, while in a relaxed state.

Meditation can also be a component of daily activities—such as mindful chores or an absorbing hobby that allows you to be completely lost in the moment. What links all of these methods is bringing focused awareness to yourself and what you are doing in the here and now.

BENEFITS FOR MENTAL WELLNESS

Mindful meditation can reduce stress, control anxiety, and help us to process and balance our emotions. It also enhances focus and self-awareness and improves sleep quality. In addition, studies show that it can reduce chronic inflammation and bring significant and measurable pain relief, impacting on well-being. For people with mild to moderate depression or anxiety, there is evidence that meditation's benefits rival those of common medications. There is also evidence that it can help manage addictions.

These benefits are largely the result of physiological and neurological changes triggered by the "relaxation response," which lowers stress hormone levels and brings measurable improvements in heart rate, blood pressure, oxygen consumption, and brainwave activity.

"Meditation can be still, or can be a component of daily activities, such as absorbing hobbies."

BRINGS SELF-AWARENESS

A meditation practice helps us assess thoughts and feelings and identify how we respond to stressful situations.

FOCUSES MIND

Meditation helps us stop internal "chatter" when our thoughts dwell on past events or worry about the future, helping to enhance our focus in the present.

GROUNDS

Being focused on the moment releases feelings of restlessness and brings a sense of being centered and calm.

AIDS RELAXATION

Training the mind to switch off, and focusing on one task or thought, helps regulate breathing and promotes relaxation.

UNLOCKS CREATIVITY

Training the mind to avoid distractions can give space for inner creativity and inspiration.

BENEFITS OF PRACTICE

The benefits of meditation are plentiful for mind and body. Setting aside just five minutes a day at first can help you develop the discipline to switch off. With practice, as meditation comes more naturally, the benefits deepen.

MANAGES STRESS

When the mind becomes quiet and less reactive, this is thought to regulate the stress response in the amygdala, the brain's emotional center.

REDUCES PAIN

Meditation is thought to lower stress hormones and help trigger the release of endorphins, our natural painkillers.

ENCOURAGES REFLECTION

Daily reflection helps us explore inner motivations and assess what is important in our lives.

BREATHWORK

We breathe in and out about 20,000 times a day. The process of breathing is so automatic that we take for granted how vital it is to our health and well-being. A combination of factors, including busy, fast-paced lifestyles, stress, and being increasingly sedentary means that most of us breathe in a shallow, inefficient way that reduces oxygen consumption and leaves us feeling sluggish. Breathwork is a way of relearning how to breathe effectively.

HOW DOES IT WORK?

Breathwork is a relaxing component of yoga and meditation and can also be practiced on its own. Often it involves learning how to control, deepen, and slow the rhythm of our breathing. Used on its own it is a simple but effective mental and emotional reset. Deepening the breath increases the supply of oxygen to the whole body via the bloodstream. It can help clear the body of toxins and support the function of eliminatory organs such as the liver and kidneys. Oxygen-rich blood also feeds the nervous system, in particular the brain, which requires three times more oxygen to function than other organs.

BENEFITS FOR MENTAL WELLNESS

The rhythm of our breathing creates electrical activity in the brain that can affect our emotions and enhance memory. Nasal breathing (see below) stimulates the amygdala, the emotional center of the brain, as well as the hippocampus, which processes memory. Slowing and deepening the breath lowers levels of the stress hormones noradrenaline and cortisol, also helping improve focus, process emotions, and calm anxiety.

Yogic breathing techniques, or pranayamas, such as inhaling through the nose and exhaling through the mouth, or alternate nostril breathing (see opposite) have been shown to improve depressive symptoms significantly. They can also be beneficial for those suffering from post-traumatic stress disorder (PTSD).

"Oxygen-rich blood feeds the brain, which needs three times as much oxygen as other organs."

ALTERNATE NOSTRIL BREATHING

This yogic breathing technique helps open and clear energy channels in the body, allowing energy, or "chi," to flow freely. This deeply relaxing practice, which can be done as part of mindful meditation, lowers the breathing rate and reduces stress.

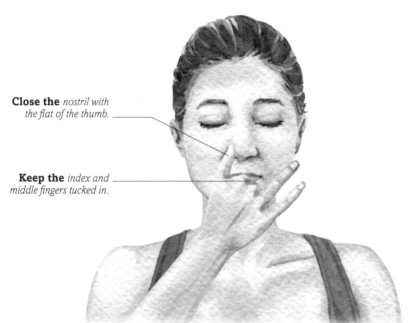

Close the *nostril with the flat of the thumb.*

Keep the *index and middle fingers tucked in.*

1 Sit comfortably upright with eyes closed. Press your right thumb over the right nostril and inhale slowly through your left nostril. At the top of the inhalation, place your ring finger on your left nostril and pause for a moment before the exhalation.

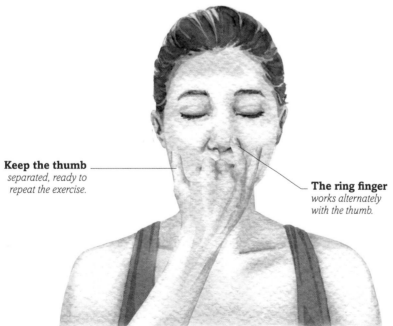

Keep the thumb *separated, ready to repeat the exercise.*

The ring finger *works alternately with the thumb.*

2 Remove your thumb, and, keeping your ring finger over your left nostril, exhale through your right nostril. Start the sequence again by inhaling through your right nostril. Continue in this way for a few minutes.

MIND EXERCISES

Although not strictly a therapy, "brain training" has become a popular way of exercising the brain. The phrase describes a range of activities designed to provide a mental workout, from more traditional puzzles, such as Sudoku and crosswords, to computer games and apps that challenge you to solve tricky problems. There is good evidence that regularly stretching your brain in these ways can improve how well you think, remember, and reason.

HOW DOES IT WORK?

Our mind is like a muscle that needs to be exercised and challenged. The more we learn about the brain's information-processing networks, which are responsible for organizing our thoughts, feelings, and behavior, the more it becomes clear that these are adaptable and responsive to stimulus. Research has shown that with regular challenges the human brain has the ability to learn and grow, changing even as we age. This process is known as neuroplasticity and is enhanced when we strive to keep our brains active.

BENEFITS FOR MENTAL WELLNESS

Apart from exercising your brain, mind exercises can bring a sense of focus and achievement. As an absorbing hobby they can be relaxing, helping to reduce levels of stress and anxiety; regularly practicing a challenging memory game has been shown to reduce symptoms of depression and anxiety in both teenagers and adults. Brain training can also enhance our problem-solving abilities. For elderly people, regular brain training (at least five times a week) does not just boost memory and reasoning skills, it can also improve the ability to carry out everyday tasks such as shopping, cooking, maintaining self-care, and managing personal finances.

"With regular challenges, the brain has the ability to learn and grow as we continue to age."

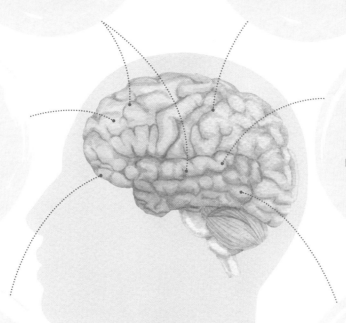

BOOSTS MEMORY

Mind exercises hone memory. Puzzles activate neural circuits in the frontal and temporal lobes, building skills.

LOWERS ANXIETY

Focus stimulates the parietal lobe and creates calm by helping tune out other external stimuli.

ENHANCES EVERYDAY FOCUS

Keeping mentally stimulated encourages neuroplasticity, aiding focus and planning.

PROMOTES RELAXATION

Absorbing the mind with a puzzle is a form of relaxing meditation, stimulating the temporal lobe.

HELPS PROBLEM-SOLVING

Problem-solving mind games increase neural activity in the frontal lobe, honing this skill.

PROCESSING INFORMATION

Evidence suggests that doing brain exercises for six months improves reasoning skills in people over 50.

COGNITIVE TRAINING

Engaging in exercises that involve mental focus helps to keep the mind active and, when done regularly, can have a measurable impact on the brain, keeping neural pathways and connections active and reviving skills that may have declined with age.

TIME IN NATURE

We may not think of spending time in nature as a form of therapy but, increasingly, science shows that getting a daily dose of "green" is vital to mental and emotional well-being. Spending time in natural settings, whether in an urban park or a garden, a forest, walking in the mountains, or meandering by the seaside brings a multitude of benefits and provides an emotional reset in times of stress.

HOW DOES IT HELP US?

Today, many of us are starved of exposure to nature, spending up to 90 percent of our time indoors. However, the human psyche and our whole understanding of the world around us evolved in connection with nature. Our need for that connection hasn't changed just because so many of us spend much of our time indoors or live in cities.

Time in nature can be unstructured and informal or taken as "ecotherapy," a more formal treatment that involves outdoor activities with a therapist. Outdoor activities provide exercise and a chance to socialize, but more than this, science has recently shown that plants and soil in natural environments also release aromatic compounds that work like aromatherapy to encourage relaxation. Mountains, forests, and beaches may also be richer in negative ions, molecules that, once in our bodies, balance levels of serotonin, helping to invigorate and support a positive outlook.

BENEFITS FOR MENTAL WELLNESS

Time in green spaces significantly lowers levels of the stress hormone cortisol while boosting levels of feel-good endorphins. There is ample evidence that city dwellers with access to green spaces have lower rates of mental health distress. Regular contact with nature is restorative, increasing energy, vitality, and focus and reducing negative emotions such as anger, anxiety, and sadness. Time in nature has even been shown to reduce symptoms of ADHD. Moreover, being outside in natural light can be helpful if you experience seasonal affective disorder (SAD). Exposure to sun supports the production of vitamin D, which helps balance moods and can also help increase serotonin levels.

"Spending time in green spaces lowers levels of the stress hormone cortisol and triggers endorphins."

CALMS STRESS RESPONSE

There is evidence that spending just 20 minutes in a natural environment can lower levels of the stress hormone cortisol.

REDUCES NEGATIVE EMOTIONS

Being in a natural environment has been found to reduce activity in the prefrontal cortex, the part of the brain that can dwell on negative thoughts.

IMPROVES MOOD

Spending time in green spaces can quickly distract us from everyday stresses and anxious thoughts, reducing feelings of depression and irritability and lifting mood.

INCREASES SENSE OF CONNECTION

Being in nature helps us to feel more connected with both the natural world around us and with others with whom we share our green spaces.

IS RESTORATIVE AND UPLIFTING

Getting away from computers and screens helps to rest the mind so it can recover from mental fatigue, acting as a restorative, reviving tonic.

THE NATURAL ENVIRONMENT

Getting out into green spaces is increasingly considered key for our mental and physical well-being. Spending just a short time in a natural environment can have measurable effects on our thought processes and stress reactions.

SPIRITUALITY

For centuries, a connection between spirituality and mental well-being has been recognized in Eastern ideologies such as Buddhism, as well as in traditional medicines such as Ayurveda. This is in contrast to the West, where spirituality and religion are not connected to health care. Nevertheless, an holistic approach to health, by its very nature, acknowledges that we are spiritual beings and that attending to this part of our lives can have a profound impact on our overall health and well-being.

HOW DOES SPIRITUALITY HELP US?

There is no single answer as to how prayer and reflection work to enhance healing. Prayer can be a coping mechanism that brings a sense of control, and being part of a spiritual community can bring a sense of social connection, purpose, and belonging. Spiritual practices may also have a physiological effect. Like meditation, they can induce a sense of calm, in turn inhibiting the secretion of stress hormones such as epinephrine and norepinephrine, released by the adrenal glands in response to stress. Chronically high levels of these fight-or-flight chemicals can wreak havoc on the mind as well as the body, disrupting sleep and affecting immunity and digestion.

BENEFITS FOR MENTAL WELLNESS

There is a surprising amount of evidence to suggest that cultivating a spiritual practice can positively impact mental wellness in a number of ways. Something as simple as practicing daily gratitude has been shown to improve life satisfaction and reduce symptoms of depression. There is also evidence that those who pray to a loving and protective God are less prone to worry, fear, self-consciousness, social anxiety, and obsessive compulsive behavior. Young adults who pray daily appear to have fewer depressive symptoms, higher levels of life satisfaction and self-esteem, and more positive outlooks. Anecdotal evidence suggests that religion and spirituality are supportive and grounding to those experiencing crisis, trauma, and grief.

"Practicing daily gratitude can help to reduce symptoms of depression and improve satisfaction."

BRINGS
STILLNESS

Prayer or contemplation lend a sense of stillness, quietening the mind and allowing an inner dialogue to open up.

ALLOWS
REFLECTION

Reflecting on our lives in the context of a spiritual practice can help us feel a sense of support that can reduce stress.

CONNECTS

As well as a connection with a higher being, a spiritual community provides mutual support and avoids isolation.

BENEFITS OF
PRACTICE

For many, a spiritual practice provides an opportunity to take time out from busy lives and enjoy a moment of tranquillity. As well as providing opportunities for quiet meditation that promote a feeling of relaxation and calm, being a member of a spiritual group or community can provide a social support network that is invaluable for well-being.

HELPS LET
GO OF ANGER

Spiritual practice focuses on forgiveness, helping to let go of angry emotions that stress body and mind.

CREATES
POSITIVITY

Prayer fosters positivity by focusing on looking forward with hope and developing a sense of gratitude.

BRINGS
COMFORT

Time spent in prayer helps to face problems and can bring a sense of healing and peace and of being listened to.

HOMEOPATHY

The word homeopathy comes from the Greek words "homoios," meaning "similar," and "pathos," meaning "suffering." It is based on the idea that like cures like, or the "law of similars." This concept was well known to the ancient Greeks and was resurrected in the 18th century by the German physician, Samuel Hahnemann, as part of a less intrusive approach to mental and physical well-being. Considered a gentle but powerful therapy, homeopathy is thought to stimulate the body's own healing processes.

HOW DOES IT WORK?

Minute doses of an active ingredient are repeatedly diluted in a water/alcohol base and shaken vigorously in a process known as succussion. None of the active ingredient remains after this process, but it is thought that the water retains an "energetic imprint," or memory, of the active ingredient, even after it has been diluted in effect millions of times. Repeated dilutions, known as potentisations, are believed to make the imprint stronger, not weaker, which is why in homeopathy higher dilutions are considered more potent. It is suitable for all ages and conditions and can be used alone or as a supportive additional treatment alongside both conventional and alternative therapies.

BENEFITS FOR MENTAL WELLNESS

Tailored homeopathic remedies, chosen to match a person's physical, mental, and emotional makeup, have a track record in treating shock, panic, or fear. Several studies also show benefits for conditions such as insomnia and anxiety. There is evidence that homeopathy can be as effective as certain antidepressants (without the disabling adverse effects) for severe menopausal and postnatal depression, as well as for general mild to moderate depression. There is also evidence that it can be beneficial for chronic pain conditions such as fibromyalgia and chronic fatigue syndrome, both of which can have a profound effect on mental and emotional well-being.

"Homeopathic remedies are chosen based on a person's physical and emotional makeup."

ACONITE

This is a remedy for anxiety, particularly when accompanied by heart palpitations and tension headaches.

PULSATILLA NIGRICANS

Useful if tearful and sad. This remedy can be helpful for those who suffer from mood swings and are reassured by comfort and attention.

ARNICA

For emotional shock and where there is a feeling of fearfulness and/or forgetfulness resulting from trauma.

PHOSPHORIC ACID

Used for loss of appetite with a low mood. This is also helpful for apathy and dulled emotions.

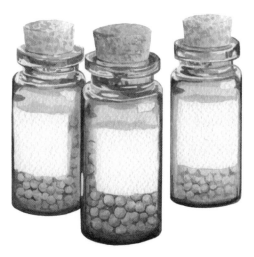

IGNATIA

Supportive for grief and loss, especially for those who tend to suppress their feelings around loss and disappointment.

HOMEOPATHIC REMEDIES

After a consultation, a homeopath will prescribe a remedy based on a range of factors, including an individual's response to events, their emotional landscape, and physical complaints, which may be related to how a person feels.

MATRICARIA RECUTITA

This remedy for irritability also can be supportive when someone is feeling restless and weepy.

ARSENICUM ALBUM

Used as a support for loneliness and when there is a tendency to excessive worry, especially around health.

KALI PHOSPHORICUM

For low mood, nervous exhaustion, and a feeling of being overwhelmed after a stressful period.

BACH FLOWER REMEDIES

Flower essences are a type of "energy medicine," based on the idea that healing energy can be channeled and absorbed by the body to increase vitality in body, mind, and spirit. In the 1930s, Dr. Edward Bach, an English bacteriologist and homeopath, began making the link between his patient's emotional and physical health. He started to experiment with potentized plant essences as an alternative to conventional remedies and found that using the positive energy of a plant could gently return emotional balance.

HOW DOES IT WORK?

Flower essences are traditionally made by infusing plant material in water, usually in the presence of sunlight. The infusion is bottled with brandy or vodka to preserve it, then taken as drops under the tongue. Flower remedies aim to balance the emotions through the use of individually chosen essences that "match" a person's emotional type.

There are hundreds of different types of plant essences, but by far the best-known are the Bach (pronounced "batch") remedies (see groupings, opposite). These safe remedies can be used on their own or in conjunction with other healing practices to provide support through life changes and at times when we feel emotionally stuck.

BENEFITS FOR MENTAL WELLNESS

The most widely used and researched Bach remedy is Rescue Remedy, which is a combination of five flower essences (cherry plum, clematis, impatiens, rock rose, and star of Bethlehem). It is widely regarded as a quick and effective remedy for periods of stress and anxiety. Research shows it can reduce high levels of situation-specific anxiety, such as fear around exams, visiting the dentist, or with job interviews. Practitioners also believe that individually chosen remedies can have long-term benefits. Trials into the use of individual flower remedies for anxiety and stress show they can induce a sense of well-being and improve quality of life.

"Bach flower essences offer support during times of change or when feeling emotionally stuck."

BACH FLOWER REMEDY GROUPS

GROUP	REMEDY	BENEFITS
TO REGAIN SELF-ESTEEM WHEN FEELING DESPONDENT	Star of Bethlehem	*Provides comfort when suffering the effects of shock or grief.*
	Larch	*Rebuilds confidence.*
	Willow	*Offers help in accepting misfortune.*
	Pine	*Is supportive when you experience guilt and feel discontent.*
	Oak	*Provides strength when fatigued from overwork.*
	Elm	*Helps when you feel overwhelmed by responsibilities.*
	Crab apple	*A cleansing essence, this helps with obsessive-compulsive tendencies.*
	Sweet chestnut	*Provides support when events feel beyond emotional endurance.*
TO HELP FACE FEARS	Rock rose	*Offers support when panic makes you feel emotionally frozen.*
	Mimulus	*Helps you express your fears.*
	Cherry plum	*Brings control for those who fear losing control of thoughts and actions.*
	Aspen	*Provides clarity where fears are not understood.*
	Red chestnut	*Helps to stop excessive worry about others.*
FOR SUPPORT WHEN LONELY	Water violet	*Supports in building warm relationships with others.*
	Impatiens	*Builds empathy and helps to avoid feeling impatient with others.*
	Heather	*Provides support when being alone is a struggle.*
TO BALANCE THE NEEDS OF SELF AND OTHERS	Chicory	*Helps to resist being too opinionated.*
	Beech	*Helps to avoid being overly critical.*
	Vervain	*Offers support where being strong-willed leads to exhaustion.*
	Rock water	*Is supportive when someone has high self-expectations.*
	Vine	*Helps to listen and respect the ideas of others.*
FOR SUPPORT WHEN FEELING UNCERTAIN	Cerato	*Gives confidence in own judgement.*
	Scleranthus	*Supports where there is a tendency to be indecisive.*
	Gentian	*Offers support when feeling discouraged.*
	Gorse	*Helps support when feeling hopeless.*
	Hornbeam	*Provides strength when this feels lacking.*
	Wild oat	*Offers insight on which direction to take.*
HELPS GROUND FEELINGS AND AWARENESS IN THE PRESENT	Clematis	*Grounds when feeling unhappy and indifferent.*
	Honeysuckle	*Helps to stop dwelling on past events.*
	Wild rose	*Encourages taking responsibility for your own happiness.*
	Olive	*Revitalizes and helps regain interest in life.*
	White chestnut	*Helps clear the mind.*
	Mustard	*Is uplifting when a low mood descends.*
	Chestnut bud	*Helps to avoid repeating mistakes.*
SUPPORTS WHEN OVERSENSITIVE	Agrimony	*Gives courage to express your emotions rather than avoid confrontation.*
	Centaury	*Offers strength to say "no."*
	Walnut	*Helps to move forward and make important life changes.*
	Holly	*Helps avoid angry thoughts and jealousy.*

ACUPUNCTURE

A key component of traditional Chinese medicine, acupuncture is now practiced worldwide. In Chinese medicine, physical, mental, and emotional health problems are thought to arise when the flow of a person's vital energy, or "chi," becomes blocked. Energy is thought to flow along multiple meridians, or energy channels, throughout the body, each of which is connected to specific organs. Acupuncture aims to identify where blockages are occurring and to stimulate and restore the natural flow of the body's chi.

HOW IT WORKS

Along each of the energy channels of the body there are several powerfully sensitive points, known as acupoints, where the energy flow of a specific meridian can be stimulated. With acupuncture, a therapist inserts fine, sterile needles at specific acupoints along the meridians to stimulate and rebalance the body's energy flow and help promote healing. The needles are extremely fine so generally they cannot be felt. However, if needles are a concern, an acupressure massage, which uses firm pressure to stimulate the acupoints and unblock energy, is an effective alternative.

BENEFITS FOR MENTAL WELLNESS

Acupuncture is of proven benefit in relieving chronic pain, headaches and migraines, and other conditions that can interfere with sleep and/or daily activities, some of which may be linked to depression. It is also deeply relaxing, making it beneficial for stress and symptoms of anxiety, including rapid breathing, palpitations, and digestive upsets. As well as stimulating nerves and muscles, acupuncture also aids the release of anti-inflammatory chemicals into the bloodstream and triggers the release of endorphins, our hormones that offer natural pain relief and lift mood. It has also been shown to calm sympathetic nerve activity, which regulates our heartbeat and fight-or-flight response, and bolster the immune system to promote overall well-being.

"Acupuncture triggers the release of our natural painkillers, endorphins, to relieve pain and relax the mind."

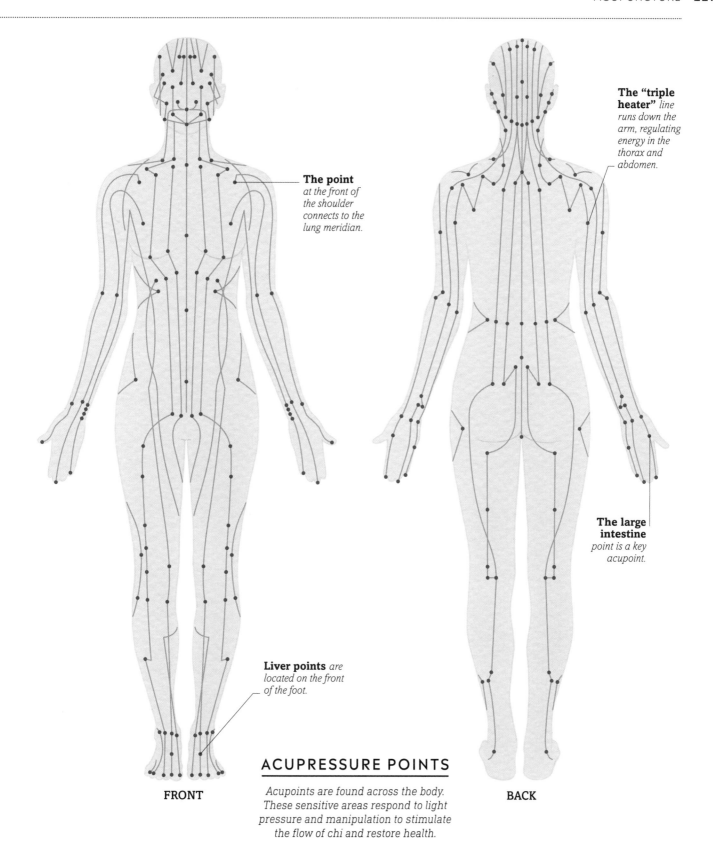

The point *at the front of the shoulder connects to the lung meridian.*

The "triple heater" *line runs down the arm, regulating energy in the thorax and abdomen.*

The large intestine *point is a key acupoint.*

Liver points *are located on the front of the foot.*

FRONT

BACK

ACUPRESSURE POINTS

Acupoints are found across the body. These sensitive areas respond to light pressure and manipulation to stimulate the flow of chi and restore health.

MASSAGE

This healing therapy, which has been practiced throughout history, involves a variety of hands-on techniques that manipulate the soft tissues and muscles in the body. The most widely used form of massage in the West is Swedish massage. Other more specialized techniques include deep tissue massage, trigger point therapy, shiatsu, and Thai massage. Massage can also focus on specific areas, such as the head, hands, and feet.

HOW DOES IT WORK?

Sometimes considered a pamper treatment, we now know that human touch in the form of massage brings with it a sense of connectedness to others and profoundly changes the body and mind. It helps improve circulation and as a result raises body temperature, producing the warm "glow" that many experience after a treatment. Human touch can be deeply relaxing, lowering levels of the stress hormone cortisol. It also triggers the release of the hormone oxytocin—the "love drug"—as well as the two other feel-good hormones, serotonin and dopamine.

BENEFITS FOR MENTAL WELLNESS

Studies into the benefits of massage show it calms the mind, reduces tension, anxiety, and stress and increases body awareness. It also relieves chronic pain, which is linked with higher levels of depression. In addition, massage has been shown to aid mental clarity, lessen fatigue, and increase energy, all of which have a profound effect on mood and outlook. When touch is combined with essential oils in aromatherapy massage, these effects can be even more pronounced. For instance, citrus fragrance used during massage has been shown to raise mood and improve immune system function. Roman chamomile also has a mood-lifting effect, while lavender can relieve anxiety and depression and promote restful sleep.

"A healing therapy, massage calms the mind, reduces tension, and increases energy levels."

Soothe and calm *with light-touch strokes on the head and face (if welcome), which can be deeply relaxing.*

KEY

Effleurage stroke: *long, gliding strokes.*

Petrissage stroke: *short, kneading strokes.*

Release chronic stress *held as tension in the shoulders. After sweeping effleurage to warm the tissues, move on to more vigorous petrissage, to work deep into the knots in the trapezius.*

Bring strokes *up and over the shoulders.*

Make fan-shaped *effleurage strokes up and down the back, avoiding the spine.*

Knead *across the fleshy upper arm to warm and relax tissues here.*

Sweep along *the length of the arm in one long stroke.*

Unlock stress *in the lower back by working deeply down into and across the fleshy gluteal muscles.*

Increase vitality *with sensitive, light-touch stroking of the hands and arms.*

Energize *with a stimulating kneading petrissage on the back and front of the thighs and also across the fleshy calves.*

Release sluggishness *with warming long effleurage strokes along the length of the calf and the thigh to warm up the tissues before deeper petrissage.*

TYPES OF STROKES

Effleurage and petrissage are the two main strokes in Swedish massage. Gliding effleurage works along the back and limbs, while short, kneading petrissage works into fleshy areas.

DE-STRESSING MASSAGE

Chronic stress and everyday anxieties can leave the mind and body tense and unable to let go. Massage can be tailored to soothe and release tight muscles, in turn helping to refocus a racing mind and bring about a state of deep relaxation.

Chronic stress can lead to tight, tense muscles and difficulty in switching off the mind and completely relaxing. This can be the case whether the cause is emotional stress, or a heavy workload, leading to mental stress that impacts on sleep and everyday activity. A full-body massage, using relaxing essential oils if desired, can help to work tension out of the muscles and calm an overwrought mind so that the receiver is able to unwind completely.

RELAXING STROKES

Massaging the whole body using steady, even pressure and following a set pattern of strokes achieves a natural rhythm and flow that soothes and relaxes. When the recipient needs additional help to unwind, emphasis can be placed on particular parts of the body where stress tends to be held, spending a bit longer there. For example, more time may be spent focusing on the back, and giving extra attention to the feet, arms, and head can be especially relaxing.

KEY BENEFITS

Even, steady pressure that is maintained throughout the massage encourages deep relaxation, while a mix of soothing effleurage and tension-releasing petrissage works out areas of knottiness to soothe the mind and body.

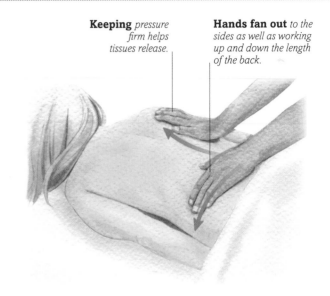

Keeping *pressure firm helps tissues release.*

Hands fan out *to the sides as well as working up and down the length of the back.*

WARMING THE BACK

Long, sweeping effleurage strokes up and across the back at the start of the massage help to spread oil over the skin and warm and loosen the tissues, preparing the back for deeper, tension-releasing petrissage strokes.

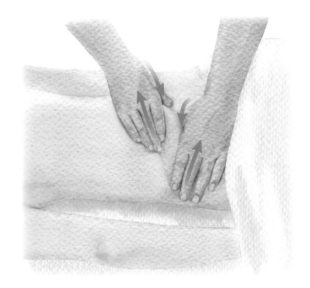

LOWER BACK KNEADING

Once the tissues have been warmed, kneading petrissage strokes across the fleshy lower back and top of the gluteals work deeply into the muscles, releasing held-in tension that may be causing discomfort in the back and legs.

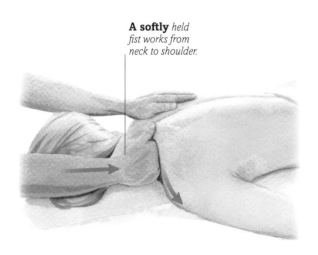

A softly held fist works from neck to shoulder.

UPPER TRAPEZIUS MASSAGE

The trapezius muscle in the shoulders and upper back can hold a great deal of stress. Using sweeping strokes with the back of the hand and knuckles can warm tissues effectively, preparing them for deeper work to release knotty areas.

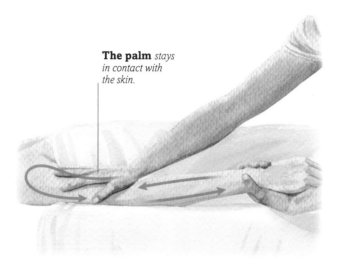

The palm stays in contact with the skin.

GLIDING ALONG THE ARM

Tension in the shoulders can extend into the arms. Using flowing effleurage strokes up and down the arm while supporting the hand can help to ensure that this entire area is relaxed. Working on the arms can be particularly soothing.

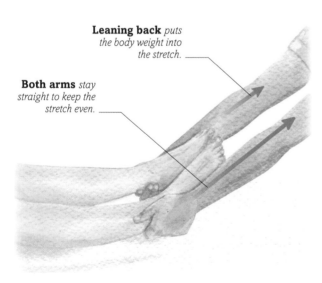

Leaning back puts the body weight into the stretch.

Both arms stay straight to keep the stretch even.

LEG STRETCHES

The large leg muscles can hold considerable tension. When lying on the back, supine, stretching the legs toward the end of a massage can be intensely relaxing, giving the feeling that the body has been soothed from top to bottom.

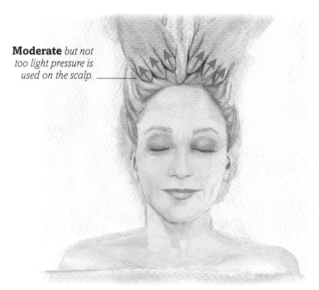

Moderate but not too light pressure is used on the scalp.

SOOTHING HEAD WORK

Working on the head can be profoundly relaxing at the end of a massage. Gentle work around the face can also be soothing if this is welcomed by the receiver. Fingertips glide over the head from the forehead up, easing out tension.

REVITALIZING MASSAGE

The body and mind can feel sluggish and lethargic for a variety of reasons, and tiredness in the body can slow down the mind, and vice versa. Stimulating massage strokes can help to rejuvenate and energize.

As well as causing tension, stress can also lead to feelings of tiredness and an inability to "get up and go." Other physical causes can also deplete energy stores, such as a sluggish digestion, which may be partly due to lifestyle factors, or when recovering from illness. Incorporating stimulating strokes into a full-body massage, using revitalizing and zingy essential oils if desired, can be an excellent way to reenergize body and mind.

STIMULATING MASSAGE TECHNIQUES

Massaging the entire body helps to ensure that all the tissues are warmed and revitalized. Some particularly stimulating and lively techniques can be added into a full-body massage routine, and making sure time is spent on the legs—which can feel sluggish and heavy when tired—and the head helps ensure that the massage is nicely invigorating.

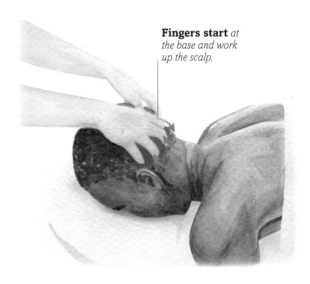

Fingers start *at the base and work up the scalp.*

HEAD CIRCLES

Using fingertips to circle the head before starting work on the back, right at the start of the massage, can be especially invigorating. The fingertips massage into the tissues, not just over the skin, making small, fairly rapid circles.

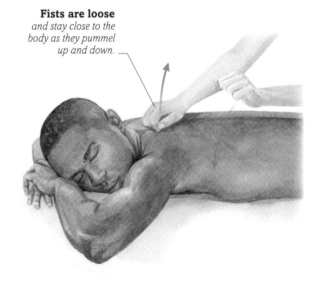

Fists are loose *and stay close to the body as they pummel up and down.*

RHYTHMIC STRIKES

Percussion techniques with a quick, staccato rhythm are a great way to wake up the body and mind. Light fists or the sides of the hands can be used over the back (avoiding the spine) to stimulate blood flow to the whole area.

KEY BENEFITS

As tissues are warmed, circulation to the various parts of the body is stimulated, ensuring that tissues are oxygenated and in turn revitalized, rejuvenating body and mind.

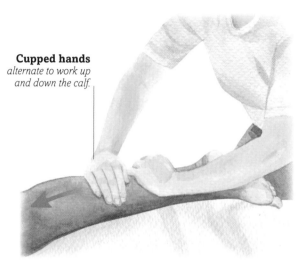

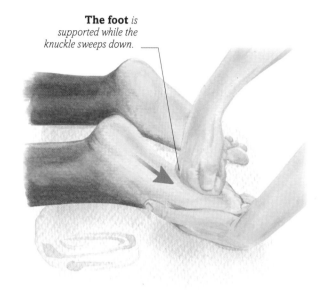

Cupped hands *alternate to work up and down the calf.*

The foot *is supported while the knuckle sweeps down.*

SWEEPING LEG STROKES

Using cupped hands to make sweeping strokes with moderate pressure up the entire leg, starting at the base of the calf, revitalizes and warms tissues and starts to release any tension in the leg muscles that can make them heavy and fatigued.

DEEP-TISSUE WORK ON THE FEET

The feet can feel weary and fatigued when overworked and tired. If the receiver is happy for the feet to be worked on, using deep pressure over the soles can be extremely energizing. Working with the knuckles here stimulates circulation to the area.

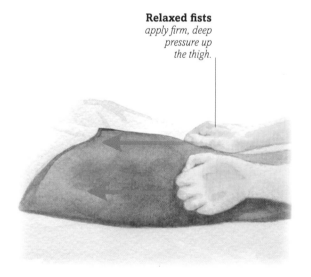

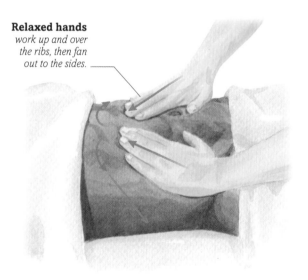

Relaxed fists *apply firm, deep pressure up the thigh.*

Relaxed hands *work up and over the ribs, then fan out to the sides.*

KNEADING THE THIGH

The fists can be used to work deeply into the fleshy thighs once these have been warmed up. Tension in the lower back can radiate down into the hamstrings and quadriceps, making these stiff and heavy-feeling.

STIMULATING STOMACH STROKES

A sluggish digestion can leave the entire body feeling depleted of energy. Gentle, warming effleurage strokes over the abdomen can help to warm the tissues here and stimulate the process of peristalsis, the movement of food through the digestive system.

REIKI

Reiki is a subtle and effective form of healing that seeks to restore the balance of energy in the body. With its roots in ancient Japanese tradition, today reiki is practiced worldwide by private practitioners and in hospitals and clinics. It is used as a way of relieving stress and pain, aiding relaxation, releasing emotional blockages, and promoting natural healing. It can be used alone or in conjunction with other healing therapies. Although it is spiritual in nature, reiki is not affiliated with any particular religion or religious practice.

HOW DOES IT WORK?

Reiki practitioners use a technique called palm, or hands-on, healing, in which the therapist is a conduit, channeling healing energy through their palms to the patient to restore physical and emotional well-being. Although the therapy usually involves the laying on of hands, reiki can be just as effective when the therapist's hands hover just above the body. Research shows that reiki primarily helps to reduce stress, anxiety, and depression. It can also be supportive where there is chronic pain, which can make psychological and emotional symptoms worse.

BENEFITS FOR MENTAL WELLNESS

Widely studied, reiki has been shown to cause beneficial changes in the parasympathetic nervous system—the part of the autonomic nervous system that stimulates processes such as digestion when the body is at rest—and to reduce signs of cellular inflammation. These effects can translate into pain relief, a reduction in anxiety and depression, and improvements in sleep quality, relaxation, and general well-being. For those suffering from "burnout," reiki has been shown to produce a significant relaxation response as well as immediate and long-term improvements in feelings of stress and hopelessness. Combined with guided imagery, whereby mental images evoke sensory responses, reiki has been shown to produce significant reductions in post-traumatic stress disorder (PTSD) symptoms in soldiers.

"Reiki can be a powerful tool for supporting symptoms of stress such as insomnia and anxiety."

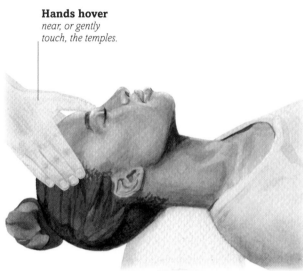

Hands hover
near, or gently touch, the temples.

HEAD

The head is one of the main centers of energy flow in the body. Focusing on this area is thought to enhance consciousness and wisdom.

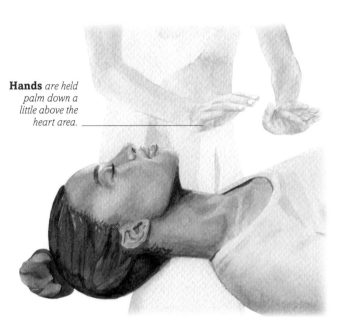

Hands *are held palm down a little above the heart area.*

CHEST

The heart region can be an area where heavy emotions gather. Using healing energy here can help to open up the heart chakra and release held-in emotions.

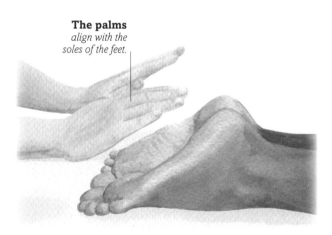

The palms
align with the soles of the feet.

FEET

Often neglected, our feet are full of nerve endings and work hard each day. Giving attention to the feet can be grounding, energizing, and deeply relaxing.

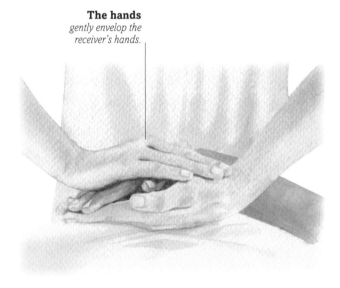

The hands
gently envelop the receiver's hands.

HANDS

Cradling the hand in reiki can be powerfully comforting for the recipient, inducing a feeling of warmth and a sensation of being held.

REFLEXOLOGY

This modern-day treatment has its roots in ancient Chinese principles. A type of massage, reflexology works with the meridians, or energy pathways, that run throughout the body. The practice uses the power of touch—on the feet and hands—to help balance energy and ease physical and emotional symptoms.

HOW DOES IT WORK?

Reflexology uses pressure massage techniques on specific areas of the feet and hands to stimulate healing in the corresponding organs, glands, and structures (see foot map, opposite), working along the body's meridians. In addition to the proven physical and biochemical benefits of massage and touch, practitioners believe that working through the body's meridians has a profound effect on the mind and emotions. This is because in Oriental medical tradition, each meridian has both a corresponding organ and a corresponding emotion. The stomach, for example, is associated with worry and anxiety; the liver with anger and irritability; the kidneys with fear; the lungs with sadness and grief; and the heart with joy and contentment. In this system, healing the physical body also heals the mind.

BENEFITS FOR MENTAL WELLNESS

Reflexology's most immediate benefit is the release of tension and anxiety in both body and mind. Like regular massage, reflexology supports circulation, lowers the heart rate, and helps to reduce levels of the stress hormone cortisol while raising levels of calming hormones such as serotonin, endorphins, and oxytocin. The therapy is a gentle way to relieve tension, improve mood, and encourage relaxation and restful sleep, in turn increasing energy levels and restoring a sense of balance.

"The most immediate benefit of reflexology is the release of tension in body and mind."

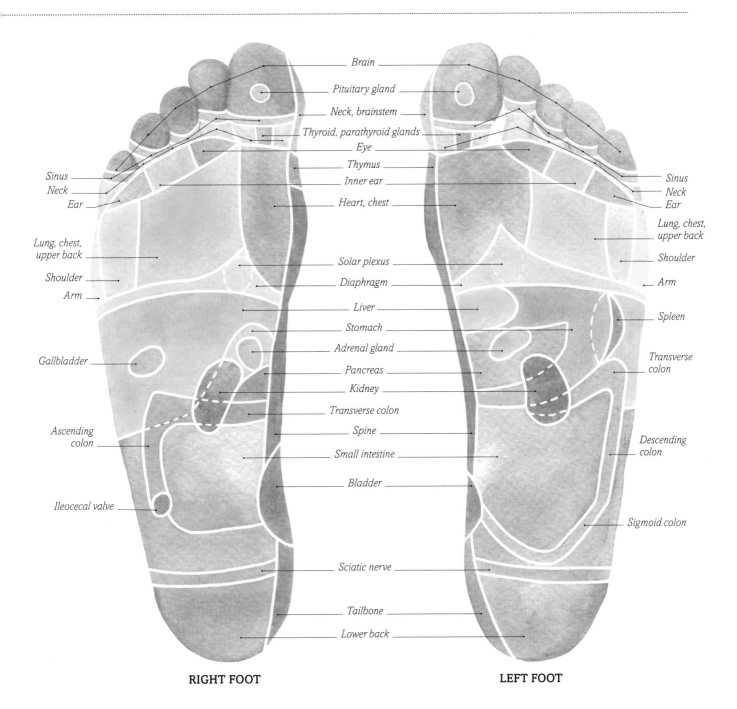

Brain

Pituitary gland

Neck, brainstem

Thyroid, parathyroid glands

Eye

Thymus

Inner ear

Heart, chest

Sinus

Neck

Ear

Sinus

Neck

Ear

Lung, chest, upper back

Shoulder

Arm

Lung, chest, upper back

Shoulder

Arm

Solar plexus

Diaphragm

Liver

Stomach

Adrenal gland

Pancreas

Kidney

Transverse colon

Spine

Small intestine

Bladder

Spleen

Transverse colon

Descending colon

Sigmoid colon

Gallbladder

Ascending colon

Ileocecal valve

Sciatic nerve

Tailbone

Lower back

RIGHT FOOT

LEFT FOOT

REFLEXOLOGY FOOT MAP

The reflexology map, above, divides the foot into areas that link to different parts of the body or specific organs via the body's energy pathways. The right and left foot maps correspond with the respective sides of the body. So the heart zone is larger on the left foot map while the liver area is larger on the right, reflecting their position in the body.

REFLEXOLOGY TECHNIQUES

Over time, the effects of stress in the body build up, affecting our mental well-being and physical health. Reflexology aims to break the harmful patterns of stress in the body and support a return to health.

By working on particular zones that correlate to organs or body systems, reflexology provides a targeted approach to mental health and well-being. Balance can be restored by stimulating areas that are especially susceptible to the effects of stress, causing symptoms such as palpitations and stomach complaints.

Reflexology also helps to increase activity in the brain and is thought to trigger the body's relaxation response, easing tense muscles and calming the mind.

TARGETED PRESSURE

The zones of the feet that correspond to the solar plexus, stomach, and the adrenals may be focused on when dealing with mental health concerns such as anxiety and the pervasive effects of stress. By helping to restore balance in areas such as digestion and promote relaxation, body and mind are energized, anxiety is eased, and the spirits are lifted.

KEY BENEFITS

By targeting the areas of the body that are typically affected by stress and promoting relaxation, these areas can be supported and strengthened.

THUMB-WALKING TECHNIQUE

This technique enables the practitioner to apply steady pressure, bending and unbending the thumb to "walk" over the sole of the foot.

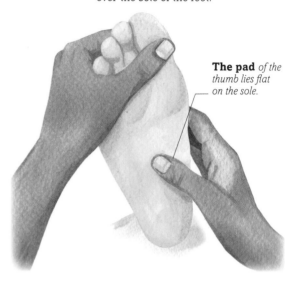

The pad *of the thumb lies flat on the sole.*

1 The upper hand supports and stretches the sole of the foot while the thumb of the opposite hand rests on the sole. The wrist stays low and relaxed, helping the thumb to apply constant pressure.

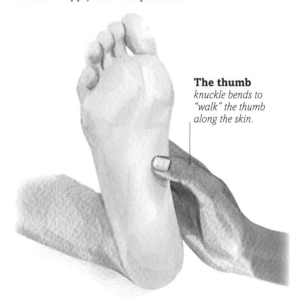

The thumb *knuckle bends to "walk" the thumb along the skin.*

2 The thumb is bent and straightened so that it travels up the foot, keeping pressure steady as it moves. This technique can be done to massage the whole foot or to work on specific areas.

REFLEXOLOGY FOR ANXIETY

Reflexology for anxiety focuses on stimulating and balancing the parts of the body that affect our mood and response to stress. Supporting these areas promotes relaxation and soothes anxiety.

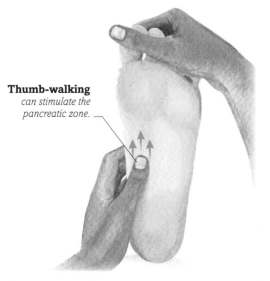

Thumb-walking *can stimulate the pancreatic zone.*

1 The thumb-walking technique can be used over the area corresponding to the pancreas, which regulates blood sugar. Stimulating this area helps balance blood sugars, avoiding mood swings that can trigger anxiety.

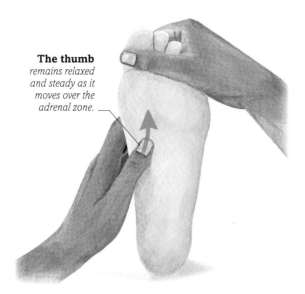

The thumb *remains relaxed and steady as it moves over the adrenal zone.*

2 When the thumb walks over the adrenal area, this supports overworked adrenal glands, in turn helping to regulate levels of the stress hormones cortisol and adrenaline, involved in our fight-or-flight response.

REFLEXOLOGY FOR STRESS

Stress impacts the entire body, affecting nerves and body systems. Reflexology helps to ease stress by supporting areas such as the solar plexus to increase our resilience to stress.

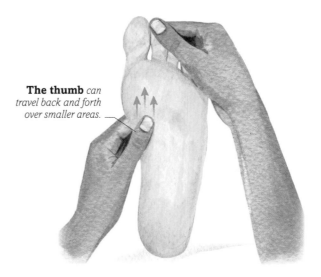

The thumb *can travel back and forth over smaller areas.*

1 Working around the solar plexus as your thumb walks over the foot supports the body's response to stress. The solar plexus, a group of nerves at the top of the stomach, is knotted and tight when we are stressed.

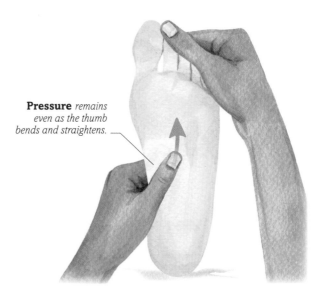

Pressure *remains even as the thumb bends and straightens.*

2 Applying pressure using thumb-walking to the stomach area can help to support and stimulate digestion, where stress can lead to a nervous stomach, or to sluggish digestion.

OSTEOPATHY AND CHIROPRACTIC

These two practices work through the musculoskeletal system and both represent a mind–body approach to health, addressing stresses in the body to improve physical and mental symptoms. Osteopathy uses touch-based manipulation of soft tissue and joints as well as techniques to mobilize the spine to diagnose and treat pain-related conditions. Chiropractic focuses more on spinal manipulation, applying gentle force to the joints and muscles surrounding the spine.

HOW DO THEY WORK?

Both therapies recognize that prolonged muscle tension and contraction can lead to uneven pressure on the spine and skeleton, resulting in physical stress and pain. Relieving this stress by realigning the body has been shown to improve range of movement and reduce symptoms of chronic pain. In addition, it also induces the same relaxation response seen in meditation and yoga, where the heart rate slows, breathing becomes deeper, and there is a release of feel-good hormones such as oxytocin, endorphins, serotonin, and dopamine that can translate into better mental health, physical function, and energy.

BENEFITS FOR MENTAL WELLNESS

Chronic pain syndromes such as fibromyalgia, lower back or neck pain, or migraines are as hard on our minds as they are on our bodies. These chronic conditions are commonly linked with depression, anxiety, fatigue, a more sedentary lifestyle, and insomnia. Apart from the physical benefits of realigning the body and reducing pain, osteopathy and chiropractic have been shown to calm the central nervous system and ease suffering for those experiencing chronic pain, often enabling them to lower their use of painkillers. Studies also indicate that relieving chronic pain helps improve quality of life, reduces fear, and creates a positive outlook that encourages individuals to be more mobile.

" These holistic practices address muscle tension and contraction that result in stress and pain."

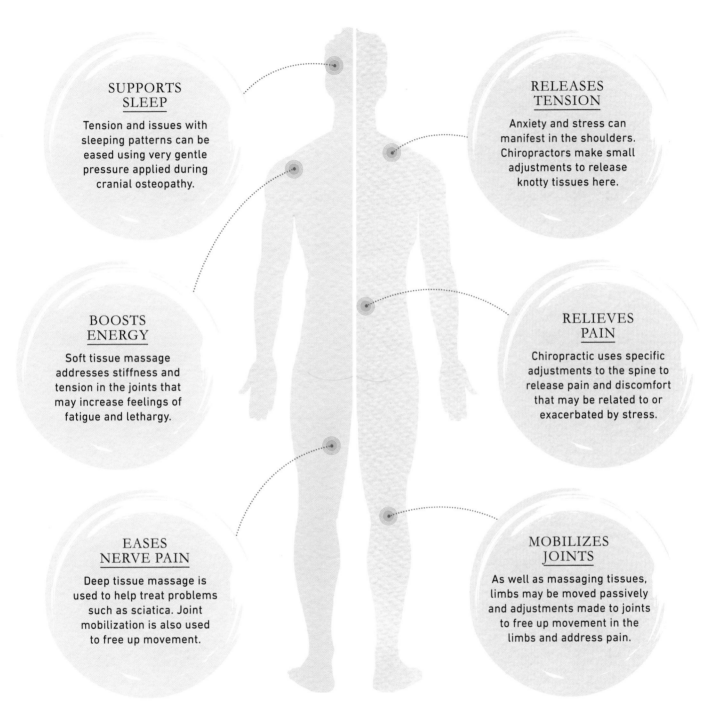

SUPPORTS SLEEP

Tension and issues with sleeping patterns can be eased using very gentle pressure applied during cranial osteopathy.

RELEASES TENSION

Anxiety and stress can manifest in the shoulders. Chiropractors make small adjustments to release knotty tissues here.

BOOSTS ENERGY

Soft tissue massage addresses stiffness and tension in the joints that may increase feelings of fatigue and lethargy.

RELIEVES PAIN

Chiropractic uses specific adjustments to the spine to release pain and discomfort that may be related to or exacerbated by stress.

EASES NERVE PAIN

Deep tissue massage is used to help treat problems such as sciatica. Joint mobilization is also used to free up movement.

MOBILIZES JOINTS

As well as massaging tissues, limbs may be moved passively and adjustments made to joints to free up movement in the limbs and address pain.

OSTEOPATHY VERSUS CHIROPRATIC

Both practices treat the body holistically. Osteopathy focuses on the release of tension in tissues—myofascial release—while chiropractic looks at body mechanics primarily, using small, precise adjustments to address pain, injury, and mobility issues.

KEY

- **Osteopathy:** *primarily soft tissue manipulation.*
- **Chiropractic:** *emphasis on targeted adjustments.*

TALKING THERAPIES

Therapies such as counseling and cognitive behavioral therapy (CBT) provide a variety of ways to identify and resolve difficult feelings. They offer a regular, safe, confidential space for exploring the roots of mental or emotional issues. Talking things through can promote greater self-awareness and clarity of purpose. It can challenge entrenched beliefs or patterns of behavior and offer better alternatives to ways of thinking and behaving that can undermine health, self-esteem, and the ability to develop and sustain meaningful relationships.

HOW DO THEY WORK?

There are different approaches to talking therapies. Cognitive behavioral therapy (CBT) focuses on changing specific behaviors or thought patterns. Counseling and psychotherapy tend to be less directive and involve listening, empathy, encouragement, and challenge, to help healing by reaching a higher level of self-awareness. Mindfulness-based cognitive therapy (MBCT) combines talking with mindfulness techniques such as meditation and breathing exercises or hypnotherapy. In all instances, sessions are carried out with a trained therapist, either one-on-one, in a group, or with others such as a partner or family member, and may be done face-to-face, online, or over the phone.

BENEFITS FOR MENTAL WELLNESS

For those with mild to moderate depression, talking therapies are a well-established and effective form of treatment. There is a good deal of evidence to show that CBT, MBCT, counseling, and psychotherapy can be as effective, and sometimes more effective, than medication, and may be especially helpful and supportive when medication has not worked. Talking cures can take a little longer to work, but because they encourage self-awareness and behavioral change, the results are usually long-lasting. They are also often used as part of a multifaceted approach to serious mental health conditions such as schizophrenia or bipolar disorder. Other evidence shows that talking therapies can effectively help address issues such as anxiety, phobias, addiction, and eating disorders.

"Talking therapies are well-established treatments for mild to moderate depression and anxiety."

COUNSELING AND PSYCHOTHERAPY

COGNITIVE BEHAVIORAL THERAPY

METHOD

Behaviors and emotions are discussed. As trust in the therapist builds, feelings are explored in increasing depth.

METHOD

A goal-oriented therapy, this identifies thought patterns and triggers that affect behavior and well-being and lead to poor choices.

AIMS

By allowing a person to explore problems linked to the past, they develop a greater sense of self-awareness in the present.

AIMS

Exercises and "homework" raise awareness of negative thought patterns and help find ways to alter entrenched responses.

OUTCOME

An in-depth understanding of emotions leads to ownership of issues and positive action to resolve problems and practice greater self-care.

TWO APPROACHES

Both counseling and CBT aim to raise self-awareness. Counseling is less directive, with the therapist encouraging and guiding the person to a point of self-realization; while with CBT, client and therapist work together to actively change behaviors and thought processes.

OUTCOME

Unhelpful thoughts are replaced with positive responses, breaking negative and irrational patterns of behavior and thinking.

MUSIC THERAPY

The healing power of music has been acknowledged for thousands of years. All types of music have the power to relax, to engage the mind, and also to provoke strong emotions. Today, as we learn more about how music affects different areas of the brain, our understanding of the healing power of music, with its ability to reach deep into the mind, has moved from the realm of folklore into neuroscience and legitimate therapeutic practice.

HOW DOES IT WORK?

Listening to, playing, singing, and creating music during music therapy has a physiological effect that can change our perceptions of pain, aid relaxation, and lower blood pressure, respiration, and heart rate. There is evidence that music can trigger the release of feel-good chemicals such as dopamine and opioids and the hormones serotonin and oxytocin, as well as lowering levels of stress hormones. But music is also neurologically unique in the way that it stimulates many parts of the brain at once. This means that even if parts of the brain are damaged, music can still reach other parts.

BENEFITS FOR MENTAL WELLNESS

The overall benefits of music therapy include relaxation, better sleep quality, and improved self-awareness and self-expression. Music therapy is a supportive additional treatment for those suffering with depression and anxiety, and it can also be used as a support with more serious mental health conditions such as psychosis and schizophrenia. The effect that music has on how we interact with the world, on our relationship with language, and on our cognition also makes it beneficial for those with dementia as well as those recovering from stroke or traumatic brain injury.

Studies show multiple benefits, from reducing anxiety, agitation, and depression and supporting clear thinking, speech, and memory to reducing the need for antipsychotic drugs and fewer and shorter stays in hospital.

"Music is thought to trigger the release of feel-good chemicals and hormones."

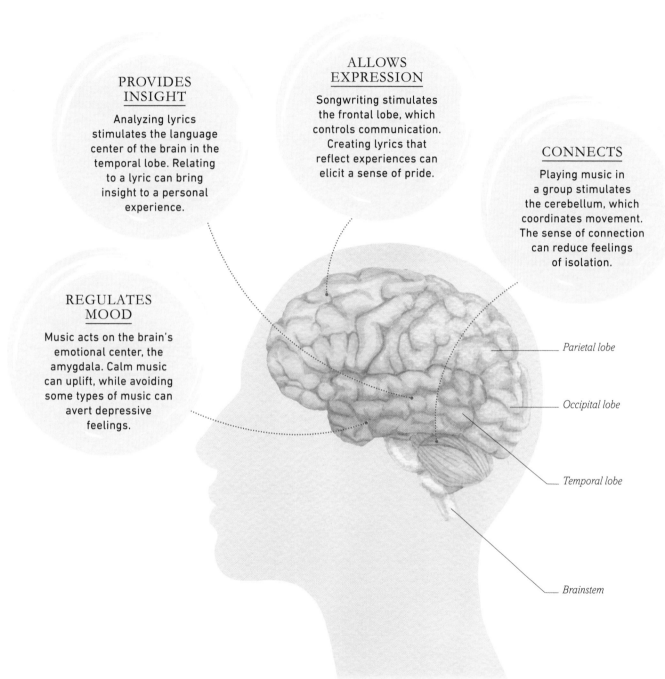

PROVIDES INSIGHT

Analyzing lyrics stimulates the language center of the brain in the temporal lobe. Relating to a lyric can bring insight to a personal experience.

ALLOWS EXPRESSION

Songwriting stimulates the frontal lobe, which controls communication. Creating lyrics that reflect experiences can elicit a sense of pride.

CONNECTS

Playing music in a group stimulates the cerebellum, which coordinates movement. The sense of connection can reduce feelings of isolation.

REGULATES MOOD

Music acts on the brain's emotional center, the amygdala. Calm music can uplift, while avoiding some types of music can avert depressive feelings.

Parietal lobe

Occipital lobe

Temporal lobe

Brainstem

EFFECTS ON THE BRAIN

Using music as a form of therapy has a measurable impact on the brain and well-being. As well as stimulating the parts of the brain involved in language, movement, and emotions, group music therapy can bring a strong sense of connection with others, develop social skills and communication, and build confidence and self-awareness.

HYPNOTHERAPY AND BIOFEEDBACK

Although each is a therapy in its own right, biofeedback and hypnotherapy are very similar and are sometimes used simultaneously. Both therapies provide feedback—and therefore raise awareness—of how our bodies and minds respond to situations. With awareness comes a greater ability to self-regulate our responses and so change behavior patterns. During hypnotherapy, a therapist provides the feedback, while in biofeedback this is provided by a device or computer and then interpreted.

HOW DO THEY WORK?

Both types of therapy involve the use of relaxation techniques to quiet and calm the mind and make it more receptive to changing behavior. The aim of hypnotherapy is to communicate with the subconscious mind to change behavior patterns. During hypnosis a state of deep relaxation is induced, which involves selective focusing—complete focus on one thing—and "receptive attention," the point at which the mind is both alert and receptive to suggestion. In biofeedback, a machine is used to measure changes in pulse, respiratory rate, and/or skin temperature to show when a person is at their most receptive and able to create new patterns of behavior.

BENEFITS FOR MENTAL WELLNESS

As self-regulation techniques, hypnotherapy and biofeedback can be helpful in managing everyday life stressors and sources of anxiety. Both also have a good success rate for treating chronic pain, an important cause of depression and anxiety. Biofeedback can be particularly useful for headaches, especially migraine, and other types of chronic pain that may be linked, or lead, to stress and which cause the sufferer to tense their muscles, in turn leading to more pain due to muscle fatigue. Hypnosis has been shown to improve sleep disorders linked to depression, pain, anxiety, and lifestyle changes. And those suffering from obsessive-compulsive or eating disorders, addiction, or phobias can respond well to hypnotherapy.

"Using relaxation to quiet the mind makes it more receptive to changing set behaviors."

BIOFEEDBACK

HYPNOTHERAPY

METHOD

Equipment is used to measure how the body's processes, such as breathing and heart rate, respond to stimuli.

METHOD

The therapist brings the person to a state of deep relaxation, releasing tension; breathing slows and a trancelike state is reached.

AIMS

The equipment feeds back on the body's responses, raising awareness of them. Methods, such as breathing techniques, are given to help alter responses.

AIMS

Once deeply relaxed, the mind becomes receptive to suggestions to change desctructive patterns of behavior and negative thoughts.

OUTCOME

When faced with a stress trigger, the person uses learned relaxation techniques to control the stress responses.

TWO METHODS

Both biofeedback and hypnotherapy aim to help modify a person's stress response and/or to alter desctructive behavior. The outcome is a raised awareness of responses and the connection between anxiety and tension felt in the mind and its effects on the body.

OUTCOME

Suggestions made in the hypnotic state take root in the subconscious mind, helping to change thought patterns.

CHARTS AND SAFETY GUIDELINES

The information below explains why supplement doses recommended by practitioners for the key mental health vitamins and minerals in the chart, profiled on pages 174–5, can vary from official guidelines. Opposite, general safety advice for medicinal herbs and essential oils is given.

Getting the right amount of vitamins and minerals is key to our mental health, yet knowing what the right amount is can be confusing. If in doubt about which nutrient or amount is best for you, consult a nutritionist and/or doctor to get the correct dosage of vitamins and minerals for your health.

Nutrient Reference Values (NRVs) are the minimum most healthy people need daily from food and supplements to avoid deficiencies. If an NRV cannot be assessed, regulators use Adequate Intake (AI). NRVs are adjusted for gender, age, and pregnancy. Values also vary slightly in different countries. This table gives a general guide for healthy adults.

Tolerable Upper Intake Levels (ULs) are recommended maximum daily intakes generally considered safe. However, nutritionists may advise a higher dose in a supplemental range (SR). For example, if a person has problems absorbing a vitamin or mineral, or has a chronic illness or deficiency that has depleted a nutrient. Also, some conditions respond to short-term supplementation with higher levels to restore balance, followed by a maintenance dose at a lower level.

VITAMINS

NUTRIENT	NUTRIENT REFERENCE VALUE (NRV)	TOLERABLE UPPER INTAKE LEVEL (UL)	SUPPLEMENTAL RANGE (SR)
Vitamin B1 - Thiamine	1.1mg	45mg	15–50mg+
Vitamin B2 – Riboflavin	1.4mg	350mg	300–800mg
Vitamin B3 – Niacin	16mg	40mg	20–80mg
Vitamin B5 – Pantothenic Acid	6mg	ND	20–500mg
Vitamin B6 – Pyridoxine, Pyridoxal-5-phosphate	1.4mg	100mg	10–200mg
Vitamin B7 - Biotin	30mcg	ND	100–1000mcg
Vitamin B12 – Cobalamin	2.5mcg	ND	300–5000mcg
Folic Acid	200mcg	ND	500–5000mcg
Vitamin C – Ascorbic Acid	80mg	2000mg	250–2000mg
Vitamin D3 – Cholecalciferol	200iu	4000iu	5000iu+

KEY

ND = not determined

mg = milligrams

mcg = micrograms

iu = international unit (used for fat-soluble vitamins A, D, and E)

CONVERSIONS

The conversions below can be used for herbal remedies and essential oil blends.

Converting ml to drops for tinctures and oils

1ml = 20 drops

2ml = 40 drops

3ml = 60 drops

4ml = 80 drops

Converting ml to tsp/ tbsp/fl oz for base oils

10ml = 2 tsp

15ml = 1 tbsp

30ml = 2 tbsp

100ml = 3½fl oz

MINERALS

NUTRIENT	NUTRIENT REFERENCE VALUE (NRV)	TOLERABLE UPPER INTAKE LEVEL (UL)	SUPPLEMENTAL RANGE (SR)
Iron	14mg	45mg	15–50mg+
Magnesium*	375mg	350mg	300–800mg
Selenium	55mcg	400mcg	200–800mcg

* Magnesium from food does not count toward the UL. Only magnesium from supplements can have an adverse effect, hence the seeming contradiction between the NRV and UL.

USING HERBS SAFELY

Most herbs can be used safely, but there are times when certain herbs should be avoided. To use herbs safely, follow guidelines and dosage instructions; if in doubt, consult a qualified herbalist and/or doctor. See the cautions provided throughout this book.

CONTRAINDICATIONS
Herbal remedies help to restore balance and, in some cases, can help reduce high doses of medication. However, contraindications exist. If taking over-the-counter or prescribed medicine, especially for heart, liver, or kidney disorders, blood pressure, or for birth control, consult your doctor and/or a qualified medical herbalist before taking herbs. Avoid herbs two weeks prior to surgery. In acute infections, avoid adaptogenic herbs unless advised by a professional herbalist. For acute emotional or psychological conditions, always seek qualified help prior to seeing a herbalist.

DURING PREGNANCY AND WHEN BREASTFEEDING
Medicinal herbs should be avoided if you want to get pregnant (for both parents) and in the first three months of pregnancy, unless advised by a qualified herbal practitioner and agreed by a doctor. When pregnant or breastfeeding, some herbs should not be ingested, as advised in this book.

ALLERGIC REACTIONS
These are rare but can occur. If you have plant allergies, it is advisable to seek professional advice before using herbs.

FOR CHILDREN
The advice in this book is intended, for the most part, for adults, unless indicated. Consult a qualified herbalist before giving herbs to babies and children.

USING ESSENTIAL OILS SAFELY

SOURCE RESPONSIBLY
Sourcing from reputable suppliers will ensure you are using high-quality oils. Be sure to choose oils that are clear about their origins and that reference the botanical name of the plant from which the oil is derived.

PHOTOTOXICITY
Some essential oils, particularly in the citrus family, can cause a skin reaction when exposed to the sun. Cold-pressed oils of bergamot, bitter orange, grapefruit, lemon, and lime can provoke skin reactions, but the steam-distilled versions of these oils, as well as steam-distilled mandarin, sweet orange, petitgrain, and tangerine are not phototoxic. Likewise FCF versions (free from furanocoumarins) of bergamot and lime are not phototoxic. If in doubt, seek advice.

DURING PREGNANCY
In the first trimester, avoid sage, hyssop, and camphor. Cautions are provided in the book. Seek professional advice if in doubt.

WITH EPILEPSY
If you have epilepsy, rosemary, sage, hyssop, and camphor are not recommended since they may trigger seizures. Other oils can indirectly improve epilepsy by removing triggers such as stress. Reactions can vary, so consult a qualified aromatherapist and/or doctor if in doubt.

FOR CHILDREN
Advice in this book is intended, for the most part, for adults. Caution is advised using essential oils on babies and children to avoid irritating their sensitive skin. Gentle oils, such as lavender, Roman chamomile, and mandarin are best, and use well-diluted or diffused.

INDEX

ACKNOWLEDGMENTS

The authors would like to thank: our editor, Claire Cross from DK, whose skill and enthusiasm helped bring this book together; the DK design team, Emma and Tom Forge, who worked so hard to bring the text to life visually; and Neal's Yard Remedies, for continuing to provide a platform through which good information about natural approaches to health can be explored and given legitimacy.

DK would like to thank: Pat Thomas, who guided us throughout, together with all the authors, for their expertise and knowledge.

Proofreading Claire Wedderburn-Maxwell
Indexing Hilary Bird

To access the research and studies supporting the text in this book, visit: **www.dk.com/nyrmw-biblio**